Clinical Judgements

CLAIRE RAYNER

Clinical Judgements

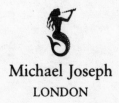

Michael Joseph
LONDON

MICHAEL JOSEPH LTD

Published by the Penguin Group
27 Wrights Lane, London W8 5TZ, England
Viking Penguin Inc., 40 West 23rd Street, New York, New York 10010, USA
Penguin Books Australia Ltd, Ringwood, Victoria, Australia
Penguin Books Canada Ltd, 2801 John Street, Markham, Ontario, Canada L3R 1B4
Penguin Books (NZ) Ltd, 182–190 Wairau Road, Auckland 10, New Zealand

Penguin Books Ltd, Registered Offices: Harmondsworth, Middlesex, England

First published 1989

Made and printed in Great Britain by
Richard Clay Ltd, Bungay, Suffolk

Filmset in Linotron Sabon by
Wilmaset, Birkenhead, Wirral

A CIP catalogue record for this book is available from the British Library.

ISBN 0 7181 3251 3

Library of Congress catalog number 89-83504

For
Basia and Hilary Howells,
two very special doctors.
With love.

Chapter One

Six a.m.

Already the sunlight is so bright it hurts the eyes to look at the big windows in the operating-theatre block and the tall doors that lead to Outpatients, for they glitter ferociously, returning their heat to join the already burning brightness that is spilling over the cracked brown-grassed verges that line the pathways leading to the path lab and pharmacy. The hottest August, the gate porters tell each other as they sit and brew tea in their little cubby-hole and open the *Sun* to the racing pages, the very hottest since records were kept. And they nod companionably at each other as though they can take personal credit for so remarkable a circumstance, and light their cigarettes and build up an even thicker fug as they pore over the day's selections at Doncaster and Kempton Park, and their kettle spews steam all over the grimy windows.

Six-five a.m.

The Accident and Emergency department cat wakes and stretches herself and jumps down from the low wall that curves round from the side entrance to the department as an ambulance comes into the yard. She stares at it, aggrieved at being disturbed so early, and then stalks off to find breakfast, lifting her paws fastidiously as she crosses the asphalt on her way to the kitchen block. Yesterday it had been so hot that one of the ambulance men found his rubber-soled shoe had actually stuck to the ground, an experience that led to a great deal of interested talk in the porters' cubby-hole; and still the heat lingers, adding to the morning's blazing sunshine. How can it be otherwise after so many days of temperatures up in the high eighties and nights that never drop below sixty or so? And the ambulance men jump down and open the back and one of them fetches an agony

1

wagon from the department, complaining loudly at how hot he is already, and that bloody supervisor not letting 'em go into shirtsleeves till after eleven in the morning, he ought to come and try dealing with the sort of rubbish they have to carry about wearing heavy jackets and then he'd know better than to make such bleedin' stupid rules. And the cat stops and stares into the ambulance for a moment as the man comes back with his trolley and then goes on her way, disgusted at humanity in general.

Six-fifteen a.m.

The staff nurse on A and E mutters irritably as the trolley comes in, the stench of the occupant leading the way in great waves, and stares down at the lumpy shape with the same look of disdain the cat had used before stalking away.

'Ye gods, Davy,' she says and makes a grimace at the ambulance man. 'Not another – not at this time of the morning – '

'I told the copper you wouldn't be best pleased, that you'd 'ad a night and three-quarters of it, but all he said was take 'im to St Kitts then. And I 'ad to tell 'im that'd really set the cat among the shite'awks, that would. It's Old East what's on take-in tonight, I says to 'im, and I tell you they've 'ad a really bad time of it. Three BIDs I say and all 'e said was if you don't put a move on this one'll be brung in dead an' all, so what could I do? Sorry and all that, Staff, honest – '

'Not your fault,' says the staff nurse and leads the way to the far cubicle, battering on the staffroom door as she passes. 'I suppose it's what we're here for, though I sometimes wonder . . . What's the story?'

'Picked up over at the dump by Artichoke Hill – where the winos are, you know? Just the other side of the Highway – police was called because one of the yuppies in that new block o' flats at the end of Pennington Street said 'e saw smoke and reckoned it was an 'azard. So the Fire was called out and it wasn't a fire, only the blokes burning their stuff as usual, so the yuppie calls out the police, don't 'e? And they goes and finds this one out for the count and can't rouse 'im. So they reckon 'e's your department and send the rest of 'em on their way.'

2

He grunts as together with the staff nurse they push poles into the calico stretcher and lift the bundle of stinking clothes and blankets on to the couch. 'Not that it'll make no difference, of course. They'll be back tonight. It's them yuppies – it's a campaign they've got to get the 'ole area cleared, so as to make it nice and residential for 'em. I don't see the 'arm it does 'em to let the poor buggers use that patch, been there for years, they 'ave – '

'That's as may be,' the staff nurse says and leans over the man now lying on his back, breathing heavily and with his eyes half open. 'My God, smell him, will you? Uraemia as well as the rest of it – David, get him cleaned up, will you?' The young male student nurse who has come to hover at the entrance to the cubicle looks green and backs away and the staff nurse lifts an eyebrow at him, and he manages a nod and comes into the cubicle as the ambulance man takes his trolley away and the staff nurse follows him.

'I don't know what we can do,' she says. 'I'll get Dr Harker up to see him once we've got him cleaned up and made a few obs, but it's my guess he's a renal. And they're stuffed full and all the medical beds are tied up – '

'Well, 'e'll have to go somewhere,' the ambulance man says cheerfully. 'On account we can't take 'im back where 'e come from, can we? I'll book 'im in then, OK? Anything to 'elp, ducks. We got some info on 'im – 'ad some things in his pockets, surprise, surprise. Prior, 'is name is. William Prior. Forty-five, it says 'ere, got an old driving licence would you believe. Born 1943 – same as me, and looks twice as old. Poor bugger – ' And he nods cheerfully again and goes off leaving the staff nurse to wake Peter Harker, the casualty doctor on call. Not too disagreeable a task, after all, she thinks as she makes for the phone. I've an evening off and broke to the wide. Going for a drink with him could be a worse way to spend the time. And if I wake him now, maybe we can fix a date . . .

Seven-fifteen a.m.

In her flat on the seventeenth floor of Lansbury House on the Tarling Street Estate, Prue Roberts wakes as the baby starts to

3

wail, and lies with her eyes closed as long as she can, praying he'll stop. But he doesn't, of course. He just wails louder and then she hears Danny start, and what can she do? She has to get up. But before she's out of her bedroom door and halfway along the passage to the kids' room she's doing it, retching and heaving, and she knows she can't pretend it's not happening any more. Oh Christ, she thinks as she gets to the bathroom and manages to hang over the lavatory as the baby's shrieks get louder and Danny starts to bawl at the top of his voice and the room goes round and the smell of the honeysuckle lavatory freshener comes up at her in thick cloying waves and makes the retching worse. Oh Christ, I can't manage, not again. They'll have to do something. I'll go up Old East and see 'em, tell 'em they got to do something. The baby's only five months, for Christ's sake, and Danny won't be two till bloody Christmas and how can I be expected to cope, with Gary not back till Christ knows when? All right for some goin' off to bleedin' Saudi Arabia, all right for some. And again she retches and then, slowly, manages to straighten up and stare at herself in the mirror over the washbasin. I look like death warmed up and gone cold again, she tells her reflection drearily. I'll have to go up to Old East and tell 'em – make 'em do something –

Eight a.m.

Kate Sayers closes the door softly behind her and runs down the stairs to the garage, feeling good, her muscles moving smoothly, feeling *good*. And then grins a little to herself, amused at how predictable she is. No matter how tired she is when she goes to bed, if Oliver is randy and takes his time she feels marvellous and no matter how long he manages to keep her going and how much sleep she loses, she feels super next morning. It must have been after three before they fell asleep and here she is, bouncing like a two-year-old. It's always the same. Sex *is* the best remedy, no doubt about it. And she tries to see herself telling the patients that on her ward rounds and grins again as she unlocks the car and throws in her bag. Those poor devils; most of 'em have forgotten what sex is for, let alone trying it for therapy. I should have gone into orthopaedics, not genito-urinary, she tells herself as she starts the engine and pulls the car out into the street. I'm not fair to my patients, feeling like this.

The traffic is building up already; the big BMWs with their sleek drivers shaving with expensive German battery shavers and the cheeky little Renaults with girls with long blonde hair at the wheel clutter up the roads and she shouts insults at them as they get in her way. Oliver finds this behaviour infuriating, pointing out that it's useless since the other drivers can't hear her, inelegant because she looks so silly when she sits there mouthing at people, and maddening to listen to. So she tries not to do it when he's in the car with her, but indulges herself when she's alone. And it does help to get rid of her rage at the halfwits who droop around in the middle of the road with nowhere to go and all day to get there, as she tells them loudly, while she has to get to the hospital early this morning. As on every morning.

But then her sense of wellbeing comes back as the traffic eases and she can get out of the Finchley Road hubbub and into the side streets, heading steadily south. It should be a good day today. Interesting, certainly. And she thinks about Barbara's patient, and wonders how the rest of the ward will cope with him, all the old bladder daddies and the kidney dialysis lot – not used to people as exotic as Kenneth Hynes, that was for sure. And for a moment her lips curve as she visualises Kenneth Hynes walking into the ward dressed as he had been when she had seen him in Barbara's clinic last month. It would be hilarious, and though as a surgeon she shouldn't find amusement in a patient's dilemma, how could anyone fail to find some in Hynes? His own personality made sure you laughed as much as he did. It was his defence against his pain, of course, a veneer.

Le Queux won't laugh, she thinks then and again she smiles but this time a little sourly. If this doesn't turn into a right royal showdown, nothing can ever be done. He's got to see that I'm not his bloody houseman, there to be pushed around. I'm a consultant in my own right and he can get stuffed, however senior he is. If I want to take patients from Barbara Rosen's clinic, take 'em I will. He can't stop me and I won't let him. I hope there is a row, I really do – and she lets her mind create an elaborate scenario, with Keith Le Queux shouting and ranting about Barbara's bloody pansy clinic and truly showing himself up for the pompous ass he is and then retiring defeated, leaving herself the victor.

And then she sighs as she manoeuvres her way through the King's Cross traffic. It won't happen that way, it never does, and she is going to be late this morning after all. And some of the good feeling evaporates, so to get it back she leans forward to switch on the radio, and snaps the buttons till she gets City Broadcasting and hears the trailer for Oliver's morning show, inviting the first callers to stake an early claim to their *Meeting with Merrall*.

'Put London to rights!' cries the announcer excitedly. 'Let everyone know what you think and pit your wits against the sharpest of them all, Oliver Merrall. Eleven o'clock, this spot on the dial, don't be late! The number you need to call is – '

And she grins with pleasure even as she bawls 'Halfwit!' at the black-cab driver in front who has just cut her up. The hell with it. She feels good, she has an interesting day ahead of her, and what more can a woman ask for?

Nine-fifteen a.m.

Audrey settles herself in the seat beside Joe's corner one and glares at the young man in the T-shirt and the earrings who had tried to beat her and failed. If he had any manners she wouldn't have had to push him that way. Sickening it is, the way kids today behave, and she looks at Joe who winks at her, and at once she feels better. He only has to look at her with that droll gaze of his and it always has that effect. Takes all the rage away and the irritation, all of it. And she leans back and tucks her hand into his, trying not to notice how cold it is, even on this hot morning, and murmurs, 'Not bad, eh? We'll be there for half past easy, now. It was only the change at Barking I was worried about.'

'As long as we can take our time walking at the other end,' Joe murmurs as the train speeds up and the boy in the earrings deliberately leans heavily against Audrey's knees with the movement. 'I can't be rushed, love, not on a hot morning – '

'You won't be rushed,' Audrey says firmly and manages to move her foot accidentally as she crosses her legs, so that she kicks the boy in the shins and he can't tell whether she knew she'd done it on purpose or not. 'I'll get a taxi – '

'You won't,' says Joe, looking stern, but still droll like he always does. 'Throw money around like there's no tomorrow? There is, you know – '

'Of course there is,' Audrey says quickly, too quickly, really, and holds his hand tight. 'Never mind, ducks, we'll see when we get there.' And they both sit and stare out of the window, and Audrey is glad when Earrings gets out at Plaistow and she can think quietly without wondering if he's going to kick her or something.

Not that she really wants to think. She and Joe, together thirty-seven years come November, never did have to talk a lot to be comfortable. They could always sit quiet and think together and be very easy that way. People used to talk about it a lot, saying how they was the perfect couple; and so we are, she thinks fiercely suddenly, so we are. But I can't sit quiet and just think no more. Better to talk.

So she talks, all the way, watching the stations go by. West Ham and Bromley-by-Bow, and Bow Road and Mile End and chattering about everything and nothing. The roses in the gardens they go by and the dirt on people's windows – wouldn't you think they'd have more pride even if they do live by the railway? – and how it used to be in the old days of a Monday when there was always lines of washing, everywhere washing, only nowadays why put the washing out? It's all dryers in the launderettes now any old day of the week, not like it was when we was first married and I did all that big wash in a copper on Mondays, do you remember, Joe? Stepney Green and White-chapel and time to change to go to the last station, to Shadwell and Old East, and she would get a taxi for him, no matter what, because however hard he tries he can't fool her. Exhausted he was, dead exhausted – very exhausted, she corrects herself swiftly, really very tired. And she holds his hand hard and lifts the case down from the rack and slowly they move through the hurrying morning crowds at Whitechapel station on their way to Joe's deathbed. He knows it and she knows it and what can anyone say about that?

7

Nine-thirty a.m.

Ted Scribner puts down the phone and stands there staring at it, trying to think what to do. He's been up so long getting everything ready, making sure his bag is properly packed with his special pyjamas and the sponge bag and the soap and the shaving things in their own special container inside, and giving Mrs Carroll next door the food for the cat, and turning off the water and the gas, and now he doesn't know what to do. It's like he's trying to think with cotton wool instead of brains. It wasn't his fault. It wasn't being old or any such bloody rubbish as that. He wasn't old for a start, not seventy yet, not quite, and anyway what was seventy nowadays? His old dad had gone on to be eighty-three and he'd been as sharp as a bloody tack till the day he died and then his mum had always said it had been the booze what had done it. He, Ted, had never been a boozer, not ever, and that was what made it so hard he had to have all this trouble now. Taken good care of himself he had, even after Enid had died, hadn't been like some, letting everything go. And now this.

Four times. Four times he'd been promised this operation, four times he'd had a date and now to stop him again, this close! Another ten minutes and he'd have been out of the house, locking up, walking down the road to get the bus to take him along the Highway, and into the hospital. He'd been really looking forward to it. Not that any man ever wants to be put to the knife and made ill; he'd had enough of being ill in the war when he'd got the frostbite on Salisbury Plain and been on the sick for five months, but when you got a problem like this, what are you supposed to do? Seven times he'd been up to pee last night, seven times. No wonder he got so tired and couldn't think out of his cotton-wool brains. He needed this operation, needed it real bad. He'd be able to hold his water properly afterwards, that Mr Le Queux had promised him faithful, and now this. The bed gone, taken by an emergency, they'd let him know as soon as they could when he could come in. Soon as they could.

And he stands and stares down at the phone and the tears begin to slide down his carefully shaven cheeks, making tracks in the film of talcum powder he'd put on so carefully, so as to look his best when he went up to Old East to have his operation.

8

Nine-forty-five a.m.

They stand in a little huddle, very aware of their shining new uniforms, very uneasy, rustling with anxiety, smelling of it. Alice Abingdon looks all right though, bouncing and full of herself, and some of them look at that round beaming face and ache to share her self-confidence. 'She looks as though she knows it all already,' Clemency says to Suba who looks at her with a scared sort of sideways glance and whispers, 'Yes – ' but doesn't really care whether Alice feels that way or not. She's too scared herself to care tuppence about anyone else and she wishes she was at home, with Mum and Daddy.

Alice looks at Peter Burnett and David Engell, both very neat in their tunics and white trousers and feels her chest get even tighter. She looks awful in her own uniform. They haven't done anything to find one that really fits her, and she can feel it straining across her bottom and flapping at the back and knows she looks silly. Big people don't ever look their best in pink nylon, she tells herself, and smooths her face even more. Never let them think they're getting at you, her mum had said. Keep it all inside and bring it home. *Never* let them know they're getting at you. And Alice stares at the two boys who look back at her and one of them blushes and looks away and for the first time Alice begins to feel it will be all right after all. She *can* do it. And again she puts on her bouncing sort of face.

There is a rustle of chatter at the door and she comes in, Miss Chessman, the senior tutor, and with her Miss Hyte and the tall man with the red hair who always sneers so much, the clinical tutor. Alice can't remember his name at all. All she knows is she doesn't like him much and he doesn't like her.

'Good morning,' Miss Chessman says briskly. 'I dare say you don't feel it is much of a one, but it is, all the same. This is a difficult day for you and we all know it and will make it as easy as we can. Now, do remember once you are on your wards all we told you in your lectures in the Introductory course. No one expects you to know all there is. All we ask of you is to be calm and sensible and to *ask* when you need to. You will be comfortable I am sure, as long as you don't try to go beyond your own abilities too soon. Now, Miss Hyte will tell you your allocations, and then you will collect your timetables from Mr Muncey. Make sure you keep them with you at all times, in case they are required for alteration, and if you have any problems you can always talk to one of us, or to Mr Kellogg, who's off sick today but should be back tomorrow. We'll be around the wards from time to time anyway. Now – '

'Miss Chessman, may I just ask – ' The tall girl with the very short hair – a crew cut really – and the small gold earrings speaks loudly and Suba looks at her and wonders how she can do it, in front of all these people. She has been at the lectures and so forth for three months now and still is frightened to speak, and this one is never frightened, not even this morning. 'Miss Chessman, I wanted to ask you about that business of talking to people – '

'If this is the matter of first names and surnames again, I really don't think – ' Miss Chessman begins.

'But I still don't see why,' the tall girl says loudly. 'Why should the sisters and the staff nurses be allowed to call me by my first name and me have to call them Miss this and that? If they can say Sian to me, why can't I say Jane or whatever to them? Why can't I say Edna to you?'

'I think we've spent quite enough time on this issue, Miss Bevan,' says Miss Chessman frostily and turns to Miss Hyte. 'Now, if you will, please?' and she, after a sharp glance at the now sulky Sian Bevan, begins to read her list.

And one by one, the new nurses make their way to the wards where they will spend the next twelve weeks. Alice Abingdon is sent to Paediatric Outpatients, which comforts her greatly, for children, surely, can't cause her any problems; and Suba Mahmoudi takes a deep breath of happy relief as she is told she is to go to Gynaecology. To be with women patients: wonderful! That should stop Daddy nagging for a little while anyway. She walks through the big double doors into Annie Zunz Ward and, as they sigh closed behind her, feels much better about being one of the new nurses' intake at the Old East.

But Sian Bevan marches into her ward, Genito-Urinary, in a very different frame of mind. This place, she tells herself firmly, needs stirring up, and I'm the one who's going to do it.

10

Ten a.m.

'I rather think I preferred the Elephant House,' murmurs Professor Levy as they make their way through the shining new splendours of the DHSS offices in Whitehall. 'I find dirty paint and the smell of dust much more comforting than this magnificence. How many intensive care beds could I have got for the money they spent here, do you think?'

'My dear Professor, talk that way and they'll never listen to you,' Matthew Herne says anxiously, every inch the hospital administrator trying to soothe an intransigent hospital Dean. 'Not noted for their warm responses to that sort of shroud-waving here, you know, you really mustn't try to – '

'Pooh,' says Professor Levy loudly and likes the sound of it so well he says it again. 'Pooh. It's because no one ever tells these jacks-in-office the truth that they get away with what they do. You can't tell me that they can't see how stupid they're being over this issue? To close us down just because they can sell the land – '

'It isn't just the value of the site, Professor,' Herne says patiently. Too patiently, but he's been through this argument so often and got so little further forward that perhaps he is entitled to show some of his irritation. 'The area's overbedded and that's the truth of it. There's St Kitts, and there's the whole Bart's set-up and Guy's and Thomas's just over the river and – '

'You know as well as I do that that has nothing whatsoever to do with anything,' Professor Levy snaps as the large lift wafts them silently upwards. 'We've all been cheek by jowl for centuries, literally centuries. And we've always had more work to do than we could handle. Do we have empty beds or waiting lists? Do we have short outpatient clinics or massive ones? Are we trawling for patients or sending 'em out half treated to let their poor bloody GPs cope as best they can? You tell me, and try not to insult me with such stuff as overbedding. You tell Le Queux he's overbedded in his renal unit. You tell Gynae they're overbedded – they've got the longest bloody waiting lists of them all and – '

'If they didn't do so many abortions and stopped that very expensive IVF programme they might find it easier to shorten

11

their lists,' Herne says waspishly. 'And it's no use getting angry with me, Professor, because I tell you what the thinking is here. If you don't like the message it's no use shooting the messenger. They say the area's overbedded and – '

'And I say they want to sell our site to put up more million-pound flats for city whizzers. None of whom use the NHS of course, so they don't give a damn for the poor devils who do. The people on our *overbedded* hospital's waiting lists.'

They are still bickering as they reach the big conference room where they are to hear the current views of the mandarins dealing with Old East and St Kitts, and they will go on bickering for some considerable time. They always do and they always will. And the mandarins, as usual, will pay them no attention at all.

Another day at Old East is on its usual creaking way.

Chapter Two

'I think,' Esther Pelham said loudly, 'indeed, I'm *sure* that if I have to put up with yet another round on this ward this morning I shall go bonkers. Not noisily you understand, nothing spectacular. Just quietly bonkers. I shall probably dance naked in the day room. Then everyone will know for sure that Sister in charge of Genito-Urinary is a certifiable lunatic.'

Kate snorted with laughter. 'It can't be that bad. Just Keith Le Queux and me, and I promise I won't take that long.'

'Oh you two are the least of it. And I don't mind you – I mean, you've got a right. It's your unit. But first I had Professor Levy with a bunch of Japanese and Americans doing some sort of study tour and then I had that boring old fart from the Manager's office – you know the one I mean – Puncheon, isn't that his name? Goes around looking like he knows it all and as far as I'm concerned wouldn't know a spigot from a catheter and I could cheerfully shove either one into him. A long way up too. He had a crowd of DHSS characters with him and architects and Gawd knows who else – '

Kate looked up from her pile of notes sharply. 'What did they want? I've heard the rumours. Is there something in them, then?'

Esther made a face. 'Mm – more coffee? Shove your cup over. Not rumours any more. Looks like the real thing. They were talking nineteen to the dozen about the Admin block and one of them said something about was the building listed, being Georgian, and another one said it wasn't, being in such poor condition. And then someone else said something about the Victorian ward blocks as compared with the later ones and then I had to leave 'em to go and sort out Sally Charterhouse, who'd blocked her cannula again. But it sounds bad, doesn't it?'

'I can't see they'll do anything as silly as close us,' Kate said and drank some more coffee. 'There's no way they can, not with the pressure we're under for our beds. Don't worry, Esther – no need to man the barricades just yet. May I have Sally's notes,

13

then? I think I might be able to get her stabilised at home on the League's new dialysis machine. They're more than halfway to another one, they say, bless 'em, so I can put a bit of pressure on, I think, and try to get another patient into the programme – '

'You should be so lucky,' Esther said. 'Mr Le Queux's got his eye on the League's equipment and you know he'll pull rank on you.'

'Damn him,' Kate said, but didn't sound too put out. 'But I suppose I expected as much. Then we'll have to get someone else on to a bit of fund raising and then get another machine. How about talking to some of the relatives who come here? Won't they – '

Esther shook her head. 'They're already busy with the League, and there are all the other funds going too. There's some damned jumble sale or bazaar every other week, it seems to me. What with the new computer the Special Care Baby Unit wants – they've only got one for their seventeen prem baby cots – and the Gynae unit pushing for a laser for the colposcopy clinic and the fund for a breast scanner that Alan Kippen's got going, we're well down the list. Anyway, most of the groups seem to be making posters and banners for a Hands Off Old East campaign. They're really worried – I think I'll go into private, you know. It's getting more and more like a market place here every day.'

'I can just see it,' Kate said, a little abstracted now as she returned to her notes. 'You'd just love poncing around at the Wellington or some such carrying flowers and looking delectable. All for the benefit of fat old Arabs and Greek millionaires.'

'I could do with a nice millionaire,' Esther said. 'Someone to take me away from all this and to hell with Women's Lib. How's Oliver then?'

Kate laughed. 'How you can think of him in the same breath as Greek millionaires, my love, I can't imagine. There isn't exactly big money in radio, you know, and he won't do ads, though they ask him often enough.' She looked a little irritated for a moment. 'I understand what he says about the ethics of it, but I do wonder sometimes – what with Sonia and the children. It'd take a load off his back if he did do the occasional discreet little something.'

'Sonia making trouble again, is she?' Esther pushed her own

paperwork to one side and leaned her elbows on the desk and propped her chin on her fists. 'Do tell.'

'You're a nosy old bag,' Kate said without rancour, but pushed her own notes to one side too. They had ten minutes now to call their own, after all; the patients were eating lunch and the nurses busy tidying the ward for the afternoon, and it would help to clear her head about it all. And who better to talk to than Esther, who'd been her friend for so long? And she looked across at the round cheerful face and untidy curly hair and saw again the student nurse who had stood behind that terrifying old physician whose clinics she had used to take at St Kitts and mouthed the answers to his questions to the worried medical student Kate had then been. And grinned.

'There's nothing really new, I suppose,' she said. 'Sonia rings every other day to change the access arrangements, and she seems always to know the precise times Oliver will be working, and always picks on the days when he can't take them. So then she says he's not interested and when he tries to arrange different days she accuses him of using the children as a weapon between them, when of course she's the one who's doing precisely that. Oliver thinks there's someone at City who's got it in for him who tells her what his diary's like so that she can work out how to make things as difficult as possible for him.'

'The secretary? What's her name – Bridget?' Esther hazarded.

'Bridget? Hardly – she's been with Oliver for years. Thinks the sun shines out of his ears. She'd never – '

'Oh, don't be daft, Kate. Of course she does, and of course that's just why she would. You're very clever, my love, but you can be awfully dumb sometimes. She's got a crush as big as a bloody house on your Oliver – well, I mean, who hasn't? He's very pretty, after all – and if the best way to get rid of you is to make life easy for the repellent Sonia, she will.'

Kate shook her head, dismissing that. 'No, Esther, it's not her. And even if it were it wouldn't make any difference. It's Sonia who's the real problem. She's doing all she can to make life hell for Oliver and doesn't care who gets hurt, especially the children. Her own children, I ask you!'

'Do you get on with them any better?' Esther asked bluntly, and looked at Kate shrewdly, who reddened.

15

'Frankly, not at all,' Kate said after a moment. 'I still find them odious. Barnaby is really the most disgusting creature – spits all the time, at everyone. And Melissa does nothing but whine and grizzle – I get really screwed up because I'm so glad when Sonia ruins the access and Oliver can't have 'em, but that makes him miserable so then I feel awful. I just can't imagine what we're going to do – I have this sort of daydream, you know, that Sonia will just go potty one day and take off to America or somewhere and take them with her, and then Oliver will just have to get used to the fact that he can't have them when he wants to and we'll be able to concentrate on each other.' And she looked at Esther through lowered lids, like a child ashamed of the sin she has been caught committing.

'Better out than in,' Esther said lightly. 'Pretending to like people you don't has to be hell. But even so, if Sonia did do that, would it help? He'd miss them so much, surely? I know you think they're repellent but they're his kids and he loves them.'

'I have to admit they're not nearly as ghastly when he's with them. It's only when I'm around. They must hate me a great deal.' And Kate bent her head and stared down at her hands clasped on the desk in front of her. It seemed a long time since this morning when she had felt so good, driving into the hospital, even longer since last night when Oliver had made her feel so sure, so very sure, that all in their life was wonderful.

She lifted her chin then and looked defiantly at Esther. 'Which is probably reasonable enough, seeing how much I dislike them. They'd be happier without being pulled every which way, surely? I wish she'd take 'em away, I really do. As for Oliver missing them – well' – she tried to speak lightly – 'I could always have a baby, I suppose, take his mind off them with a new family.'

'You want to watch it, my duck,' Esther said, and got to her feet. 'You're getting broody. That'd be a hell of a joker to throw into a game already as messed up as this one. Whenever you talk about Oliver, it sounds more and more like a soap opera than real life. Have a baby yourself? You've got to be potty.'

'Why potty?' Kate collected her own pile of notes and followed her to the office door. 'It's what women are for, would you believe. I seem to remember you thought it a good enough idea a couple of times.'

'I wasn't a shiny new consultant in a shiny new post, was I?' Esther said. 'And let's be brutal, ducks – I wasn't involved with a much-married man who doesn't know how to control a bitch of a wife who's doing all she can to screw up their divorce and their kids equally.'

'No. And you weren't thirty-five and running out of time, either.' Kate followed her out into the corridor. 'It's all very well lecturing me, Esther, but you've *got* your family. How old's Emma? Fourteen? And Davy's a year older. It's easy for you to talk – '

'Point taken,' Esther said and reached out and squeezed Kate's arm. 'Sorry, ducks. Listen, any chance of coming to dinner one night soon? With Oliver or on your own – either way.'

'I'll talk to Oliver,' Kate said. 'He likes coming to you – he says Richard makes him feel so inadequate and boring. It's good for his immortal soul and doesn't do a bad job on his sense of proportion either. What's Richard's latest?'

Esther sighed. 'He's thinking of a sandwich service. Make 'em at home, deliver direct to people's offices. As if it wasn't bad enough he's got the restaurant and that bloody wine bar – I can hardly get into my own fridge for the leftovers. Not that I ought to complain, I suppose. It beats cooking for myself, and the children do well out of it. So do half the school, mind you. They bring the world and his girlfriend home most afternoons. I can tell you, it's a relief to be here at the Old East in among the peepots most of the day. Family life!' And she snorted softly as she led the way out of her office into the ward. 'It's not all it's cracked up to be and don't you forget that before you go getting yourself in the club. Let me know when you can make it. Try Sunday. It's the only day I can count on Richard not having to rush off to an emergency like a collapsed soufflé or a corked bottle of Beaujolais. Now, here's Sally, Miss Sayers, wanting to talk to you about her plans for a holiday with her boyfriend – ' and she slid smoothly into her professional mode as the nurses in the ward straightened up instinctively as Sister appeared at a bedside with the consultant beside her.

*

By the time Kate had finished her round and discussed the various social and emotional problems of her dialysis patients as well as the medical ones, she had got over her irritation with Esther. They were old friends, God knew, but that surely didn't give her the right to be quite so bossy, she had thought as Esther had scolded her about wanting a baby; but now as she left the ward to make her way to the Outpatient department and her discussion with Barbara about her new patient, she had to admit she had been right. It would complicate an already very tangled set of problems quite disastrously if she became pregnant. She knew that perfectly well; but it didn't stop her aching with the desire sometimes. Last night she had wished with all the fervour that was in her that she could somehow persuade Oliver to forget his responsibility, and had been even more abandoned in her caressing and kissing than she usually was, almost as though she were trying to push him so hard and fast that he wouldn't be able to prevent himself; but it hadn't worked. He had timed it perfectly, as always, reaching for his damned condom and putting it into her hand so smoothly that she had it unwrapped and on to him before the idea of deliberately snagging it had come into her mind. But that had been a wicked thought, a selfish and plain wrong thought, and she had been able to banish it completely; till Esther had started her off again –

It was just as well, she told herself now as she reached the courtyard that lay between the high old Victorian ward block which housed the Renal Unit and the rest of the hospital, just as well I'm not a suitable candidate for the Pill. If it was up to me, there's every risk I'd really muck things up, accidentally on purpose. And I'm supposed to be an intelligent, capable woman; and she shook her head at herself in renewed irritation and shoved her hands deep into the pockets of her white coat, and began the long hike across the courtyard to Outpatients.

Around her the sprawl that was Old East glittered still in the blazing late August sunshine and she felt the sweat break out across her forehead and begin to trickle between her breasts. The tar was soft beneath her shoes, filling the air with a faintly antiseptic reek, and she took a deep breath, relishing the smell of it, and all the other scents that joined with it to make up the familiar atmosphere of the place. Exhausted parched grass and sour drains and the dustbins from behind the kitchen block; diesel fumes from the Highway that flanked the hospital grounds and, further away from the south, the smell of Thames water; all mixed up with the heavy pine fluid the cleaners used to scrub the long corridors; and the general carbolicy scent the whole place had, even though it had been decades since anyone had used the stuff. This was the very essence of the hospital, and in many ways, of her life.

She had come here first as an eighteen-year-old medical student from St Kitts, to do a ward attachment during her premed years; a policy of the old Dean, Arnold Duce, who had said every student should know what it was like to mop up sick and empty bedpans as well as how to dissect a cadaver and take blood from a collapsed vein. She had been frightened then, terrified of it all, but she had fallen in love with it in spite of that, and still felt the same now. Seventeen years of her life had been spent in and around this huddle of buildings, one way and another. She had been away for short attachments elsewhere, but always she had been part of Old East, and she stopped now and looked round as though she had never seen it before, remembering what Esther had said about the round made by architects and planners. They couldn't really be meaning to pull the place down, could they? It was unthinkable; and she stared at the big cream-coloured Georgian Admin building, once all the hospital there had been, when the place had been founded at the end of the eighteenth century, but now empty of patients and just a hive of noisy offices filled with a chatter of secretaries and a pomp of administrators; and she grinned at her own elaborate use of language, at the way she was consciously using words to release her impatience with the top-heavy management of the place who made life, it often seemed to her as to the rest of the medical staff, so much more difficult than it need be. Behind her rose the great red-brick blocks of the shabby old Victorian buildings; tall, a little ramshackle now, but still with a certain charm all their own. The high windows with the curtain rails clearly to be seen in the centre, even from this distance, and the clutter of plants and get-well cards on their sills which looked down on the web of glass-covered walkways that bisected the courtyard and which led to the various nineteen-forties and

19

-fifties Nissen huts and pre-fabs, which clustered round the ward blocks like children attached to their mothers' skirts. On all sides there was evidence of growth and spread; here a small hutlike building tucked between two others and clearly of recent origin, there a battered Portakabin brought in to fill a temporary need which had become very permanent; everywhere signs and noticeboards directing bewildered patients to the maze of departments and units that Old East now boasted. Haematology and Histology this way; Maternity and Colposcopy, Gynae, Antenatal and IVF Unit the other; Renal Unit, Outpatients, Cardio-Thoracic, Gastroenterology, Neurology, ENT, Physical Medicine, Rheumatology – the blue-and-white signs were everywhere, bearing mute evidence of the way medicine had spread and burgeoned over this past couple of decades. Even since her own student days it seemed that new specialities had exploded like popcorn until she was almost bewildered by their multiplicity; and if she felt like that, how on earth must the patients feel? For half of them it must seem as though they had newly invented diseases in newly fragmented bodies, and most certainly very newly invented treatments. And by no means all the treatments were less disagreeable than the diseases –

But she had no time, she told herself firmly, as she started to walk again, no time to think of such matters now. There was a time to consider the ethics of her job, but this was not one of them. She had to see a patient with Barbara and she had no right to keep either of them waiting.

'Thank you, Mr Hynes,' Kate said at length. 'Perhaps if you'd just get dressed, and then we can talk again.' And she moved away from the couch and pulled the curtains behind her to leave him in decent privacy, taking with her his beaming smile and murmur of, 'Kim, Miss Sayers, no need to be formal – ' as she went. She looked back through the curtains briefly before closing them, and he sat staring back at her, the blanket held bunched before his bare chest in tightly clasped hands and his eyes wide and dark with enlarged pupils. He had joked with her as she examined him, had made jolly little sallies and giggles, but she had not been deceived. He was sweating with terror, and his hands shook damply. Under the cloud of perfume he was

20

wearing she could smell the tension that was in him, thick and sour in her nostrils. It was a familiar situation, of course, but this patient's fear was not like that of others. He had different apprehensions. And she closed the curtains with a last reassuring nod, and went back to the desk.

She wrote her notes, and Barbara sat and waited, leaning back in her chair and watching her, the smoke from her cigar wreathing itself round her head defiantly. Her colleagues in the Medical Common Room had long ago given up asking her to stop smoking; they could not cope with her sharp grins and her raised brows nor her questions about their own bad habits, because who liked to expose themselves in such a way to a psychiatrist, anyway? Even as cheerful a psychiatrist as Barbara Rosen, with her sleek white hair tied into a cottage loaf sort of bun on the top of her head and her ridiculously red-cheeked face. There were actually some who thought her creepy: no one, they said, ought to be that cheerful and friendly when she had to spend all her working life dealing with such impossible patients. There must be something peculiar about her herself to choose such a field; and they kept their distance.

And it could not be denied that her speciality was not greatly admired by the rest of the consultant staff. She had few allies among them for the work she was doing, few who felt that the many papers she had written for the journals and her two or three books actually brought any renown to Old East's name. How could it be so, when she researched in so esoteric a subject?

'Well?' she said at length, as Kate finished her notes and pushed the folder towards her. 'You are sure you'll do it? No going back?'

'With your endorsement of the patient's determination and your certainty that he can and will cope well post-operatively, I can't refuse,' Kate said. 'I can't pretend I'll feel as comfortable as I might. Mutilating surgery – it goes against the grain, obviously. But looking at him now and listening to him, as well as seeing what your preliminary therapy has done – well, I can operate next week. My lists aren't too long and I can do him at the end – '

'You'll have to learn to change your pronouns, Miss Sayers, after that, won't you?' The curtain had been pulled aside and the patient stood there, smiling anxiously at her. His face was smooth and beautifully made-up with eye shadow that was just enough, and blusher set so expertly that his face seemed to be soft and rounded, even though in fact it was a firm and rather bony one. His lashes were so long and curly that they threatened to touch his upper lids in the middle, but he made sure he kept his chin up and his lids lowered so there was no real risk of that. His hair bounced softly against his shoulders in a profusion of red-gold curls, and the one hand he held casually to his cheek as he stood and gazed limpidly at Kate was long, very white and red-tipped with a perfect manicure. Kate wanted to hide her own rather square-tipped scrubbed hands out of sight as she looked at it.

'Now, which side of the ward will you put me in?' The voice was soft and husky and not a little provocative, and the wide heavily lashed eyes gleamed a little as they fixed their gaze on Kate, who blinked.

'I hadn't thought about that,' she said, 'how very silly of me – ' as Hynes came forward and sat down in the chair that stood on the other side of Barbara Rosen's desk, and crossed one long very silken leg over the other, to show the long kid pumps with the very high stiletto heels more clearly. 'I rather think we should let you have the small side ward. To be on your own might be better for you – '

'No need,' Hynes said, a little more loudly. 'I'm not ashamed. Why should I be ashamed? And anyway, why hide away when all that's happening is that a mistake of nature is being put right? Eh, Dr Rosen? Isn't that something surgeons do all the time? Babies with dislocated hips, and great ugly birthmarks – all that's happening is a cure for an . . . an unfortunate mistake. I am right, aren't I?'

'Yes, Kim,' Barbara said and took another deep drag on her small cigar, letting ash sprinkle itself around her already rather dusty cardigan as she looked sideways at Kate and raised her brows. 'Well, Kate? Is Kim to be fully reassured you can help?'

'Yes,' Kate said after a moment. 'Yes, I'll remove both testes and the penis and make what sort of urethral arrangements seem best as I progress. You realise that I can't fashion you any sort of vagina at this stage – '

22

Kim gave her a radiant smile. 'I fully understand, Miss Sayers. Dr Rosen has explained it all. I can think about that some time in the future. Right now, to know I'm going to get rid of those awful – that ghastly mess down there – well, I can't tell you how happy you've made me. I was so scared, you can't imagine how terrified, that you wouldn't help me, wouldn't operate. You've made me feel – I can't tell you. You're a dear soul, the best friend a girl could ever have. After Dr Rosen, of course – '

And he leaned forwards and took Kate by the shoulders and kissed her on both cheeks, leaving a bright red smudge of lipstick on both of them, and when he leaned back tears were matting his lashes together into spikes above a face which seemed to have collapsed into a crumpled mask of distress. And after a startled moment Kate nodded in some embarrassment and then got up to go, leaving the unlikely pair, psychiatrist and patient, watching her solemnly.

Oh God, she thought as she stood outside the closed door and heard the soft murmur of their voices as they began to talk. Oh God, what have I let myself in for with this one?

Chapter Three

Four of the new intake of nurses managed to get to first lunch, and even though they hadn't been particularly close when they'd been on their Introductory course, still they made for each other like bees for the hive and coalesced into a tight little group as they collected their food from the bored women serving at the hotplate, and went and sat at a small table in the far corner of the great echoing dining hall.

'Oh, my God,' David Engell said, and peered down at his plate, his face creased with distaste. 'This looks even worse than we used to get over at the Annexe. What is it?'

'It said on the board it was a chicken risotto,' Sian said and stared at her own plate with equal gloom. 'Looks more like sick to me. I think I'll change it. I like the look of what you've got better, Suba.'

'You'll get bloody hungry if you try that,' David said, looking over at the long queue that had formed at the hotplate. 'You'll really cop it if you try and cut in on that lot. It'll take ages to get a new one. Anyway it doesn't taste as bad as it looks. Quite nice really.' He had started to eat hungrily, pushing the food into his mouth at great speed. 'Though next time I'll do the same as you, Suba. Looks like it pays to be one of you Muslims.'

Suba went a dull red. 'I'm not Muslim,' she managed. 'I just – I'm a vegetarian, that's all. Lots of Catholics are. It's not religion or anything,' and she began to pick a little miserably at her macaroni cheese.

'Scared of upsetting the dear little animals, are you?' Alice said and laughed. 'I'll bet you've got leather shoes on, all the same.' She had already finished her risotto and was now demolishing custard tart with equal dispatch, eating even faster than David, and her open-mouthed laughter was an unattractive sight in consequence. Suba looked away, redder than ever, hating herself for drawing attention by answering David. She should have said nothing, but how could she have done that? It was so stupid the

24

way everyone always made the same mistake, always thinking all Asians were the same just because they were Asian, and it irritated her to hear it. That was why she had spoken, but oh, how she wished now she hadn't; and she bent her head, wishing too that she hadn't come to lunch at all, but had gone to sit in the garden for her half-hour instead.

'Shut up you,' Sian said unexpectedly. 'Just because you've got no principles, it doesn't mean other people don't. Good for Suba. You eat what you like.' And Suba glanced at her, scared but grateful and not a little surprised. That this odd-looking girl with her almost shaved head and angular face and spiky way of speaking to people should come to her defence was very strange, and for a brief second her spirits rose.

'What's it been like for you lot?' David said. 'I've had a great time and I don't think. I'm on this male medical ward, full of awful old buggers with miserable faces. You never saw anything so dismal. I've done nothing but run around with bottles and bedpans. Oh, yes, and I helped change a wet bed. Big deal.'

'Oh, I've been really busy,' Alice said with great complacency and pushed away her empty plate and began on her coffee. 'Playing with the kids and helping to undress them to be examined and taking them to be examined and taking them to X-ray and all that – no one to nag me at all. They just told me to look after the kids and that's what I'm doing. I dare say it's why I was sent there – they know I can manage on my own well enough.'

The other three looked at her with cold eyes and David made a face at Sian who laughed aloud.

'Yeah,' she said, 'I'll just bet. They sat there in the office and they said to each other, all dead worried, they said which of these wards and departments we have here in this pathetic place is good enough for the towering talents of Alice Abingdon? I mean, we mustn't waste her, must we? She's the best thing that ever happened to Old East – as well as having the biggest arse.'

'Jealousy,' Alice said loudly. 'I know all about you and jealousy, Sian Bevan. You're too stupid to be anything else. It'll be sunrise in the West before I take any notice of something like *you*. Can you smoke in this place?' And she turned her head to peer around the big room. But there were No Smoking signs everywhere and she got up. 'I'll go and find some peace and a better atmosphere some place else,' she said. 'Make sure you keep an eye on the time, you lot, or you won't be back in time to spend your afternoon shifting the bedpans, will you? I'll think of you down in my nice clean clinics — ' And she went pushing her way through the tables with a deliberate swing of her haunches that made Sian laugh aloud.

'I can't think why that ugly bitch is so hateful,' she said. 'I mean, what have we done to her to make her that way? Never got a decent word for anyone.'

'Ask Peter. They've put him on the Psychiatric Unit, you know. He was really scared when they said that. For two pins he'd have cut and run, I swear to you. Thought I was getting the better end of the stick. He should just know. I swear to you I've never seen so much pee in all my life.'

'You'll see more,' Sian said. 'What about you, Suba? Where are you?'

'Gynae,' Suba said almost in a whisper and then, bravely, tried again, more loudly. 'Gynae. It's ever so busy. There were operations all morning. I had to make the beds ready, you know — the operation beds they showed us? And then help lift the patients on when they came back from theatre and make sure they were comfortable. I was with one of the other nurses all the time though. Not on my own. She's ever so nice. She's in her second year, ever so senior, and really nice to me, she was. Wants me to join her group.' It was a long speech for Suba, and she was pleased with herself for managing it. But the morning had been exciting and interesting, not alarming, and telling these familiar faces about it all felt good.

'Group? What group?'

'I'm not sure,' Suba said. 'She said she'd tell me later, because Sister came along and Shirley — that was this second year — she said be quiet till after, so I did. But it was nice of her to be so friendly, wasn't it? I mean, to someone so new — '

'That's the trouble with this place,' Sian said sharply. 'They all think they're doing you some sort of bloody big favour just talking to you, because you're new. As though we're scum because we've only just started! They were new once, for God's sake. It doesn't give them the right to push us around, does it? I called the Sister Esther this morning.' She laughed, pleased with herself. 'It really gets up my nose, all that stuff. Either we're a bloody team the way they said at lectures, or we're not. I may be new but that doesn't mean I'm stupid, does it? Or unimportant.'

'What did she say?' David leaned forwards, agog. 'Did she come on like the Pawn, all ruffles and dignity, or just swipe you?'

'I'm not sure she heard it was me,' Sian admitted. 'There were a lot of people around at the time, and she might have thought it was the staff nurse. All the same, begin as you mean to go on, that's the thing.'

'Is it so important?' Suba was getting braver by the minute.

'Of course it is! It's principle, isn't it? Treating people fairly and equally and so forth – ' Sian began, but David laughed.

'You're getting too political, you are. Joining the Union you'll be, next thing we hear.'

'I already have,' Sian said shortly and got to her feet. 'Did it the first week I was in Introductory, so there. And it wouldn't hurt you to do the same, either. We've got to stick together to get any sort of fair deal – '

'Well, we got the raise, didn't we, without any strike? So what are you on about?'

'It was because the Unions threatened to strike!' Sian said hotly. 'And because the bloody Government saw how mad people were. If it hadn't been for that poncing lot at the Royal College we'd have *had* a strike, and got the raise sooner, and got it bigger. But just you wait, they'll get at us again, you just see. And then you'll be glad there *is* a Union, and you'll be pleased enough to get what we fight for for you.'

David got to his feet. 'Not me, love. I couldn't care less about bloody Unions. I'm here to train, so as to get out as fast as I can and make a decent living. I'll go private, you see if I don't. And bugger the Unions. See you later, then.' He turned to go. 'There's another few gallons of Gawd knows what waiting my care down on Male Med. If you see Peter, be nice to him. He'll probably be foaming at the mouth by this time.'

'Would you join, Suba?' Suba too had got to her feet and she stood uncomfortably trying not to meet Sian's stare. She'd been so nice to her, and it seemed ungrateful not to do what she

27

wanted. But joining the Union – Daddy had been on about that, after he'd seen the nurses on television when the march was on.

'Look at them!' he'd said disgustedly. 'Shrieking and making such exhibitions of themselves, and so messy looking . . . If any girl of mine behaves so I will disown her, and remember that, Suba. Disown her.'

It had been easy to promise Daddy she wouldn't join any Unions because it was the last thing she wanted to do, go marching and shouting. Just to be a nurse, that was the only thing she wanted, to look after people in hospitals, the only thing she'd ever wanted, ever since she'd broken her wrist when she was little and been in hospital herself. So she could easily promise Daddy not to join any marching Union. But it wasn't so easy to say that to this very direct person who was still staring so hard at her.

'I – ' Suba began. 'I'm not sure what I'm going to join. I mean there was that second-year this morning, Shirley, and her group – maybe she meant a Union?' I'm not being honest, she thought miserably. But I've got to say something. 'Let me find out what that's about first and then I'll see – '

'Fair enough,' Sian said after a moment, and to Suba's great relief got to her feet to go. 'As long as you don't go on like the rest of these idiots and ignore things. People like David make me really mad – private work, for God's sake. Nothing but bloody money, that's all his sort care about – well, he'll soon find out. Just you wait and see. He'll find out there's more that matters in this job than money.'

'Oh, yes,' Suba said fervently and went trotting away from the dining room in Sian's wake, glad to be going back to the simplicities of working on the ward. It would all be so much easier, she thought, if she could just be working all the time and never had to talk to anyone, not Daddy or anyone, or think about anything. So very much easier.

Sian was still talking busily to Suba who scurried along obediently behind her as they passed the Admissions office on the ground floor of the main ward block, and Ida Malone, sitting waiting outside, watched them and thought – I used to look like that fair one, once. And she tried to imagine herself in a pink nylon dress with a scrap of a cap on her head, and couldn't. When she'd been that age, she'd been into mini-skirts and thick false eyelashes and dangly earrings; she could never have gone around with a shaven head like this girl; pointed sideboards and a geometric fringe, that was her thing, and she found herself grinning inanely as she stared back down twenty years at the silly giddy girl she'd been. Working in a hairdresser's shop, loaded with money, what had she cared about the future and a career? Not a damn, and she felt the ready tears slide up into her throat again as regret came pouring up.

If she'd had a career it wouldn't have mattered so much, not having a baby. She'd have had something else to do, something to think about. But it was too late now. All these years trying to get pregnant, all these years staying at home to take care of herself because that was what Tony wanted her to do, to have a baby, and then the two miscarriages and – and she reached into her pocket for a handkerchief to blow her now congested nose and thought bitterly about the way these bloody hospitals kept you waiting. It wasn't fair, it just wasn't fair to treat you like you were nothing, just because you had a problem like this. And it wasn't fair she'd had to wait so long to get in to be looked after at all. Five years ago she'd started on this bloody seesaw, trying first of all to find out if she ovulated and then trying to work out the best time to do it, until Tony said he felt like a fucking machine already and went right off his oats. And then all the fiddling around they'd done and still it had got them nowhere, and now at last she was here to be done properly, and what did they do? Kept her waiting in the hall outside their damned Admissions office, like some sort of spare. Oh, she'd tell them, just see what she'd tell them, snotty bitches, when they came to fetch her, she'd have a thing or two to say to them.

The door to the Admissions office opened and a woman put her head out and said peremptorily, 'Next please,' and obediently Ida got up and went in, bobbing her head a little obsequiously as she went.

'Sorry to keep you waiting,' the woman said loudly, clearly not sorry at all. 'Went to lunch late. Some people have no consideration, never come back on time – ' and she shot a venomous glance at the woman at the next desk. 'Let me see — you're Mrs Ida Malone? In for investigation, sub-fertility — '

'Yes,' Ida murmured, very aware of the man sitting in the next cubicle and being talked at by the other admissions clerk, who was studiously ignoring her colleague. 'And I would like to know if — '

'You'll have to ask all your questions when you get to the ward,' the woman said, 'that's not my job,' and pulled a folder over towards her. 'Now, first things first. I'll want your full name and address, and then religion, name of GP and date of birth, next of kin — '

The man in the next cubicle was sent on his way as Ida's clerk muttered over her entries, and his place was taken by another woman, and Ida looked sideways at her, wondering. Was she to come to the same ward? It sounded as though the clerk had said 'Gynae' to her, but her voice had been much lower and harder to hear. Ida hoped so, it would be nice to have someone to go up there with, a sort of friend before she got there, as it were, and she peered at the other woman's face as her own clerk, still muttering, went to look for her outpatient notes to add to her inpatient folder. The other woman caught her eye and Ida tried a small smile, not a grin, that would be too much, just a sort of break in her face to show this other woman she was approachable.

But the other woman just stared at her with round blank eyes and then glanced away and Ida thought — Snotty bitch. Wouldn't have hurt her to look a bit more cheerful, even if she is coming in here. I'm coming in here too and I'm not sitting looking like a lost weekend, whatever I might be feeling like. And she turned back to answer the clerk's next flurry of questions, determined to ignore her companion, even though she now knew she was in fact going to the same ward, for her clerk had spoken more loudly this time. Miserable bitch; well, let her be. Ida didn't care. She could manage nicely on her own, thank you.

'Perhaps you wouldn't mind going up together,' her own clerk said loudly. 'They're too short of nurses to send down to fetch you, and we really haven't the time to go traipsing all over the building. You're both for Annie Zunz, that's on the third floor.

Take the lift at the end of the corridor, turn left when you get out, give this slip to the senior nurse on duty, and tell her I'll send the notes up when I can find a porter or she's ready to send someone down to get them — '

'I'll take them if you like,' Ida said, smiling ingratiatingly, but the clerk pulled the folders towards her possessively and said sharply, 'Confidential documents. They'll go up after. Now then, Mrs Walton, you're on the list for tomorrow it says here, so remind them, will you, that you can't eat anything tonight. They should know, but these nurses — well, it's possible the notes won't get up there in time, so you be sure to tell them. Next please!' And the two women were sent out of the door and on their way to the lift too quickly for anything further to be said.

They were the only people in it, and they stood each side of the shabby cube as it rattled its way upwards and stared in silence at the indicator lights flashing as they reached each floor; until the doors opened and the other woman said to Ida, 'Is this the right floor?' in a husky cracked sort of voice and Ida said eagerly, 'Yes, this is it. Annie Zunz, see the name? It's a funny name, isn't it, for a ward? I wonder where it comes from?'

The other woman said nothing, just lifting a brow slightly and after a moment Ida said as huffily as she dared, 'Well I just thought to ask. Sorry, I'm sure, to — '

Mrs Walton looked at her and then tried to smile. 'Sorry if I was rude. Didn't mean to be. Don't feel too good, to tell the truth, and I was worried about the kids — '

It happened so quickly that Ida felt sick; that rush of icy coldness that filled her when other women spoke of their children. It wasn't fair, it was so wicked of them to do it. Why did they always dig at you that way, reminding you how special they were and how useless you were? Wasn't it bad enough she, Ida, had to be coming into a hospital about it, without having someone have a go at her about what she couldn't help? And what was she doing here anyway, this other woman, if she had kids? She ought to be told, the selfish bitch, ought to be made to see how wrong it was to hurt other people that way —

'Oh, I am sorry,' Ida said. 'You don't look too well, now I come to see — I didn't mean to — '

31

They were out of the lift now and walking in the direction of the signs to Annie Zunz.

'Well, you know how it is. I do nothin' but throw up all the time – not kept anything down for weeks. Call it morning sickness they do, say it's over in three months, but I know different. It was the same last time, sick all day and every day. Right up till she was born, so it was, only a few months I was all right really – What about you? D'you get the same?'

I hate you. I want to kill you. I hate you, Ida thought. You bitch, you lousy bitch – 'No,' she said. 'No, I'm not – I mean, no.'

'Oh,' Mrs Walton said. 'Well, I suppose you're just lucky then.'

'Yes,' Ida said. Oh, God, I wish you were dead. I hope you die, you and your bloody children too. I hate you, I hate you. 'I suppose I am.'

The big double doors that led to the ward whispered open and a nurse came out and, seeing them, held the door invitingly open. 'Can I help you?' she asked and seemed to mean it.

'I'm here for an operation tomorrow,' Mrs Walton said. 'They said to tell you I'm on the list for tomorrow and I'm not to eat tonight, the notes are coming up later – ' Suddenly she put one hand to her mouth and went pushing past the nurse into the ward, shoving Ida to one side too.

'Feel sick,' she mumbled, and the nurse ran after her and set one arm over her shoulders and half led her, half pushed her into the lavatory that led off the left-hand side, leaving Ida standing with her small case clutched in her hand, outside the main doors and not knowing quite what to do. But after a moment she took a deep breath and pushed the doors open and went in, and stood waiting for someone to tell her what to do. The nurse, who came back to find her, having led a now very shaky Mrs Walton into the ward, smiled at her, seeing the bent shoulders and the defeated expression on her face and, feeling sorry for her, led her into the ward too.

'We'll soon get you settled, my dear,' she said, all professional heartiness and classroom assurance. 'No need to look so worried. It's all going to be fine, I do promise you.'

And Ida smiled back at her and thought – Stupid bitch. How

does she know it's all going to be fine? No one does. It can't be. It never has before, has it? So why should it be this time? I wish they were all dead, all the hateful bitches; I wish everyone was dead, me and Tony too.

But all she did was smile politely and follow the nurse to a bed.

Chapter Four

———————∽∾∽———————

They were, Audrey conceded, quite nice, considering. At least they had made an effort to show Joe he was welcome on the ward, and that helped a lot. And, what was more, they were nice to her too. None of the way it used to be with that 'You wait outside Mrs Slater, we'll call you if you're needed Mrs Slater, and keep out of the way we're busy Mrs Slater' stuff that used to make her so mad. Now they treated her properly and she felt the ice inside her melt a little as the round-faced nurse with the rather bushy curly hair bobbed her head at her and grinned and said, 'We'll show your husband to his bed, Mrs Slater, and then see about a nice cuppa for both of you – '

But then as she followed the nurse along the ward the ice came back, colder than ever. Back in the early days of this illness, two years ago when they'd all been so offhand with her and getting anyone to pay any attention had been so hard, no one had known how ill Joe was. Now, having them all being so kind underlined it, and she felt suddenly bitterly alone as she walked along behind them, watching Joe's feet dragging a little on the floor as he walked, because he was so tired. I hate you, she thought with sudden fury. I hate you Joe, doing this to me – and felt sick with the pain of such wickedness. She'd need that cup of tea, she told herself as the curtains rattled around Joe's corner bed, need it real bad when she got it. And she began to unpack the little case she had brought for him. Being busy, that was the thing.

The cup of tea duly arrived, brought by a young man in a white tunic and trousers, and Audrey looked up at him suspiciously and then peered at the label badge pinned on his chest. 'David who?'

'Engell,' the boy said and smiled at her a little shyly. 'I'm the nurse who's going to help get Mr Slater settled.' He sounded pleased with himself, and put the tea down on the bedside table and went round to Joe's other side to help him take off his shoes.

'No need for that,' Audrey said sharply. 'We can manage well enough,' and she pushed past the boy to kneel in front of Joe and began to untie his shoes. 'Ta for the tea and all, but we'll manage fine. Joe likes me to do things for him, don't you, Joe? We'll call you when we're done – '

The boy hesitated and then went away, his expression a little hangdog, and Joe said, 'Hey, you don't have to be so sharp with the boy, Audrey. He meant no harm.'

'Yes, well,' Audrey said, her head down as she took off the shoes and then the socks. 'I can't be doing with them and that's the truth of it – men nurses, I ask you! All nancy boys, I dare say. What sort of a chap does a job like that?'

'The doctors do,' Joe said mildly and then began to cough, and full of compunction Audrey said even more sharply, 'Now just you be quiet, Joe Slater! Let me have those trousers – that's it – ' And she bustled about him, taking his clothes, putting on the nice clean pyjamas she'd ironed so carefully last night and helping him on to the high bed. It wasn't difficult: he'd never been a big man, her Joe; ever since young Mary had been born, she'd outweighed him by a good two stone or more; but he'd always been sturdy. Compact she'd called him in her mind, her Joe. He'd been compact. But not now. Lifting him now he felt like a bird, a bag of bones that moved uneasily inside the tired stretched skin and she felt the traitorous tears fill her eyes as she pulled him into place against the piled-up pillows so that he could lean back and recover from his coughing bout. His face was reddish-blue with the effort but the skin around his mouth looked white and his eyes seemed glazed with the struggle just to breathe; but then, slowly, it eased and he looked a bit better. But only a bit.

She had turned her back on him to fuss over his clothes, folding them neatly to repack them in her little suitcase. There was no room in the ward, the admissions office clerk had told her firmly, to store patients' day clothes. Audrey must take them home and bring them back when he was to be discharged; and she had said a heartfelt thank you to the woman for that, as though her talking about Joe's discharge and saying his clothes would have to be brought back actually meant it would be that way, even though Audrey had known it wouldn't. She'd never bring these clothes back, not again, not ever . . . and she folded and refolded, smoothed and resmoothed, to give the tears a chance to reabsorb inside her eyes and run back down the back of her nose to be swallowed so that she could present him with a calm face when she turned round.

'Now, I'll put your Lucozade here, on your locker, and there's your paper hankies and the magazine Mary sent for you – and here's your soap and flannel and razor and all like that – you make sure those nurses keep it all nice and tidy for you, now. I think that's all you'll be needing.'

'Packet of fags,' Joe said and grinned at her, a wide-mouthed grin that showed his teeth, dull little yellowish teeth that showed no gleam of reflected light at all.

'Well, I suppose you think that's funny!' Audrey said but she managed a smile all the same and he stopped grinning and closed his eyes and said, 'Funny, really. It was the first thing they gave you when you got back out of the fighting. A cigarette they'd give you, and then fill your pockets with 'em while you lay on your stretcher. Funny, when you think of it.'

'Yes,' Audrey said. 'Very funny. I'll go and get you some chocolate now, Joe, from the shop down in the courtyard. Like I said, even if you don't want it yourself, you can always give some to the nurses. They like a bit of chocolate, nurses do – ' And she smoothed the counterpane over his thinness and then bent and kissed his cheek. 'I'll send that there nancy nurse, then, and I'll be back soon. Just you behave now and have a little rest. You must be tired – '

And he nodded on his pillow, not opening his eyes. He was indeed very tired.

The new patient in the corner bed had slept all afternoon, once his wife had gone, and David was disappointed at that. Sister Sheward had said he could take a special interest in him, make observations to discuss with Mr Kellogg, the clinical tutor, when he came round, and he'd cheered up no end at that. After a whole morning doing nothing but the dirty work, it felt like a bit of real nursing. But Mr Slater had gone to sleep, and there wasn't much you could observe about a man asleep.

But things improved once the teas were served. David woke

Mr Slater up for his tea, though he said he didn't want any, thanks all the same, and David was just trying to persuade him to try a bit of bread and butter and jam when Sister arrived at the foot of the bed together with a doctor. David was too busy with Mr Slater, trying to lift him up without spilling the tea on the counterpane to pay much attention at first, but then Sister leaned over and whisked away the tea tray and put it on the bed table – where really it should have been all along – with a sharpish look at David when she did it, he noticed with a little knock of fear against his ribs, and came and stood beside the head of the bed. David stood there too, not knowing what else to do, and looked over to the other side of the bed where the doctor had gone to stand, and this time the knocking feeling against his ribs was quite different.

He was, David decided, the most marvellous-looking man he'd ever seen. Not big – David never felt really safe with big men – but nicely made, very nicely made, sort of solid without being fat. He had close-cut curly hair, a bit white at the edges, and big round glasses which he kept pushing up his nose with a long forefinger as though they were slipping, and behind the glasses his eyes were dark and friendly. Even when he was looking at the patient, David could see that. The eyes were so wide and dark you could see into them even if they weren't looking right at you.

'Hello, Joe,' the doctor said and the patient blinked and peered up at him and then gave a big smile, the biggest he'd given anyone since he'd got on the ward.

'Hello, Dr Carr! Well, it's nice seeing you! I thought I wouldn't, seeing they sent me to this ward. I said to them in Admissions I always go on to Andrew Green Ward, Dr Carr's ward, not Mr Byford's, I said, but they said not this time, so I thought, maybe I won't be looked after by Dr Carr no more – '
He began to cough, after the effort of saying so much, and Dr Carr sat down on the bed and set one hand lightly on Mr Slater's chest.

'Oh, you've got me, all right, Joe. I wouldn't let anyone else look after you! Remember what I showed you, Joe?' he said and David thought – It's a smashing voice. Nice and friendly like his eyes and not a bit stuck up like most of them are. 'Breathe easily

37

and pace yourself. You need to take your time with what you have to say, not run at it like a bull at a gate.'

The old man in the bed, still coughing, tried to do as he was told, but that made him splutter and for a moment there was a bustle of activity as Sister Sheward and Dr Carr together eased him forward with concerted and skilful movements that had the old man upright and breathing more easily, so quickly that David had hardly been aware of how they had done it, and he thought – One day I'll be as quick as that. I'll be the one that'll stand on the other side and help him instead of Sister. I'll be the one he smiles at and says 'Thanks' to like that –

'That's better, Joe,' Dr Carr said as the coughing at last stopped and the two of them eased him gently back so that once again he was leaning against his propped-up pillows. 'Slow and easy, that's the ticket. Now, let me tell you what's to happen. I explained it to your wife – I saw her downstairs before she went home. She'll be back later this evening, I dare say, but I promised her I'd explain it all to you. We'll try the chemo again, Joe – '

The face against the pillow seemed to go yellow with anxiety. 'You said I didn't have to have no more of that, Dr Carr,' he said fretfully. 'After the last time you said it wasn't right to make a man feel so ill – '

'I know I did, Joe,' Dr Carr said and pushed his glasses up his nose yet again. 'I had great hopes it wouldn't be necessary. But the thing is that it did help. Not as much as we'd hoped, I can't deny, but it helped. It stopped the tumour growing and pressing on your windpipe. You remember how that felt, now, don't you? Of course you do. Well, it could happen again, going by last week's X-rays. That's why I've brought you in again. To try again. A short course, and that should give you some consider-able relief to your breathing. Do you see, Joe?'

'It's like drowning, sometimes,' Joe said and his voice was lower now, and he stared up at Dr Carr with unblinking intensity. 'Just like drowning.'

'I know, Joe. It's no fun. That's why I want to try another short course of the chemo. It's worth it, even if it does make you feel a bit off colour for a while.'

'Off colour!' Joe said. 'For a while!' And began to cough again.

'It'll stop the coughing too,' Dr Carr said.

'I'd rather have cough medicine,' Joe said. 'That linctus I had last year — it helped a lot, that did.'

'It won't help now, I'm afraid. Not where there is a pressure, you see. That's what's causing the coughing. Pressure on the windpipe. We'll sort this out, just a short course. Sister here will look after you just like the nurses on the other ward did, if that's what's worrying you. She used to be one of my staff nurses, eh, Sister, before these cardiologists got hold of her — ' And he looked over his shoulder at Sister and smiled and David felt a stab of pain as real as if a knife had slid between his ribs.

'We'll take perfect care of you, Mr Slater,' Sister said in her bright cheerful voice. 'You'll see. We'll take you to have the first injection tomorrow, and it'll be over in no time at all. Don't you worry — '

'It's not the injection I worry over,' Joe said, and then closed his eyes, as though the lids were too heavy to stay up any longer. 'It's not the injection — '

There was a little silence and then Dr Carr said softly, 'That's right, Joe. A little nap'll do you a world of good.' And he got to his feet and walked to the foot of the bed. Sister followed him; and after a moment David did too. No one had told him not to, after all.

'Are you specialling him, Sister?' Dr Carr said as they reached the nurses' station at the end of the ward, and he looked over his shoulder at David who felt his face turn brick red.

'Hmm? Oh,' Sister too turned to look at him. 'No, this is a new student today, first year. He's writing notes on Mr Slater for his clinical tutor. I'd use a more senior nurse if he needed a special, but I don't think he does. And there's his wife, of course. She wants to be here most of the time, I gather, so we can press her into service. Just as well. We're very pushed, you know. I've got three of Mr Byford's cardiac catheterisations in at the present. He's keeping the theatres very busy.'

Dr Carr lifted his brows at which David felt his chest get even tighter, it looked so marvellous. 'Then he's off again? Looking for a suitable transplant candidate? I'd heard a few whispers — '

Sister positively snorted. 'They're no rumours. If he can get a donor he's off again all right. Any one of the three'll do, I gather.

39

I don't like it, I must say. Place overrun with people – but at least they won't be on my ward. I just have to have them for the catheterisations. Then they go to Surgical Cardiology or Intensive Care as the case may be – '

'Will Byford fuss over my having one of his beds? If I leave Slater much longer he'll suffocate, you realise that. This treatment's only palliative, of course, I don't know how often I can do it, but we'll have to hope he'll get toxic and dies comfortably that way before he reaches occlusion. You realise, young man, what this patient's problem is?' And he looked at David directly, who went redder than ever.

'Er, yes, sir. I mean no, sir, I mean I think I do, a bit,' he said and knew his voice sounded silly.

'Well, tell me then.' He sounded friendly enough; it was Sister who was staring at him accusingly as though daring him to make the sort of fool of himself he knew he was going to.

'Er – well, sir, I think he's got cancer.'

'Well done, that boy. Where?'

'Er, trachea, sir?' He did tell the man it was his windpipe, didn't he? David thought feverishly. Didn't he?

'Not quite. He has pressure on the trachea. That's causing the breathing difficulties Mr Slater is most aware of, of course, and the coughing attacks. It's quite a high lesion. No, it's not tracheal. He has bilateral upper lobe carcinoma of the lungs. Used to smoke thirty cigarettes a day. Do you smoke?'

'Er, no sir,' David lied.

'Just as well. You see what happens to people who do. Right, Sister, I'll see Mr Slater in Andrew Green in the morning and send him straight back to you. I'm sorry we're so full we can't take him and very grateful to you for making a space for him. If Mr Byford is worried – '

'He won't be,' Sister said with a certain grim relish. 'What he doesn't know won't hurt him. And we'll see to it that Mr Slater's bed is curtained and we're busy with him when he does his rounds. I'll get Dr Azzopardi to write up the night drugs and the premed, shall I?'

'If you would, Sister. And talk to Mrs Slater will you? She's finding it more difficult to cope than she shows, I rather suspect. Needs a woman's touch, and so forth. Good afternoon Sister.'

And he went, his square back disappearing through the double doors as another doctor came towards them from the corridor. But David didn't pay any attention to the newcomer. How could he, when the other one was so much more interesting?

'Ah, Neville,' Agnew Byford said and stopped in the doorway. 'How are you? I haven't seen you for a long time. Been on holiday, have you?'

'No,' Carr said, and managed a thin-lipped smile. Bastard, he thought, smooth bastard. 'I've been extra busy, in fact. My wards are chock-a-block.'

'Really? Sorry to hear that, indeed I am. Though you can't be much worse off than we are here.' He stopped then and looked over his shoulder at the ward which stretched away behind him. Sister and her attendant acolyte, he noticed, had disappeared from view behind one of the glass partitions which had been put up to break up the vista of the old Florence Nightingale racetrack arrangement, and he frowned. 'Have you been seeing one of my patients, then? I can't recall one with any need for an oncological opinion – '

Carr, cursing silently inside his head at the mischance of the meeting, pushed his glasses up his nose and said cheerfully, 'No, not one of yours, dear boy. One of mine. I've got an urgent chap for palliative chemotherapy and we're bulging at the seams. I found out there was a spare bed here, and put in for it. I'm sure you won't mind. I can't send a dying man out, now can I? Not when there's a bed available here on the medical side – just imagine the sort of fuss there'd be if I did that. Especially if you're doing another of your transplants. Can't damage the publicity for that, can we?'

Agnew's cheeks mottled suddenly. 'Who told you that?'

'Common knowledge, dear boy,' Carr said airily and began to move away. 'X-ray, was it? Or did I hear them discussing it in theatres? Anyway, it's common knowledge. Must hurry. Got a chap waiting in OPD,' and he went, leaving Byford to stump angrily into the ward.

But the anger didn't last. He had much too good a reason to feel pleased with himself and the way things were going for him to be annoyed by a character like Carr. He'd soon get him out of

41

the place; no risk of anything different happening. But anyway it didn't matter. Not now.

'Sister!' he called imperiously. 'Sister Sheward!'

She made him call twice more before she appeared and then came down the ward at a pace so calm that it verged on the impertinent and he wanted to snap at her, but had the wit to hold his tongue. This was not a time to antagonise the woman. But he'd have to talk to the Nursing Admin Office. This was getting intolerable. Thought she had the right to put anything she liked in front of him, and whose ward was it, damn it all? But now it would all be different, and he smiled widely, a happy smile that showed his teeth to very good advantage.

'Ah, Sister, looking after Dr Carr's patient, were you?' he said a little spitefully, momentarily forgetting his good intentions. 'You always had a soft spot for oncology, didn't you? Surprised you came over to me and cardiology – but there it is! Unless your soft spot was more for the consultant, hmm?' And he laughed fatly as Sister stared stonily back at him.

'Your catheterisation patients are all ready to be seen, sir,' she said with a faint and undoubtedly insulting emphasis on the 'sir'. 'They've all been prepped and I've had the forms signed. You can start as soon as you like – '

'Well, they can wait for the moment,' he said in high good humour. 'Just for the moment. Now, Sister, we have some special arrangements to make – yes, special arrangements.' And he actually rubbed his hands together like an eager cook about to set to work on a table full of rich ingredients. 'Who have you in the far corner bay?'

She looked startled. 'Just one non-cardiac patient, sir. A Mr Slater.'

He looked at her sharply and then grinned even more widely. 'Dr Carr's patient, no doubt. I don't recall the name, so I imagine – yes. Well, he'll have to be shifted. And who else is in there?'

'The other three beds are your catheterisations, sir,' she said. 'As I think you know.'

'Well, they'll have to shift down to this end – I know it's easier if they're all in the same section, but needs must when the Devil drives, hmm? And the Devil is surely driving today. I want those four beds tucked in wherever you can get them, to release the whole of that unit at the end.'

'Why?' she said and frowned even more sharply. 'I can't pack the beds more closely than they are – not and leave a whole unit empty. If you need it for a transplant patient, well, I'll have to tell you, sir, I don't have the facilities here. It's got to be the ICU, you know that. I can't just – '

He put up one hand and smiled again, clearly enjoying himself hugely. 'Nothing of the sort, Sister. I wouldn't dream of having my transplant patients anywhere but in my own ICU with nurses I know and feel sure of' – at which Sister glinted with anger – 'and this patient who is coming here is not for surgery. No, not for surgery. Yet.' Again he rubbed his hands gleefully. 'But he is a very important patient indeed. He's coming in for close observation, possibly for catheterisation and if necessary a bypass, though I hope to avoid that. But first of all, I want him here for a few days to do a really exhaustive work-up on him.'

'Well, why does he need a whole four-bedded unit to himself? Why do I have to crush up my beds so that – '

'Because, Sister dear,' Byford said triumphantly, 'because this patient is only Mr Edward Saffron.'

She stared at him and then said, 'Who?'

'Edward Saffron, Sister,' Byford said, and then repeated slowly, breaking up the syllables insultingly, 'Mis-ter-Ed-ward-Saf-fron, the Junior Minister of Health.'

'I know who he is and what he does,' she said tartly. 'I just want to know why he's coming here, and turning my ward upside down. Why don't you take him into the St Andrew's Wing? He's a private patient, surely? And that's what we've got St Andrew's Wing for, isn't it? Private patients . . .'

He raised his eyebrows at her, almost pityingly. 'My dear Sister, how can he be a private patient? He is the Minister of Health. There'd be an uproar if he went into the Private Wing. No, he's got to be here in an NHS ward. On my NHS ward.'

'Oh,' Sister said and then lifted her brow at him. 'And how are my nurses to cope with the extra fuss there's sure to be?' And the emphasis she put on the 'my' was unmistakable. 'I'm short-handed as it is, with a new nurse straight out of Introductory and – '

He waved his hand airily. 'Oh, no need to worry about that. He'll have his own nurses coming in. And he'll need extra telephones – two – and a desk in there. For his secretary, you know. And you'll need a spare corner somewhere for the security people. He's a considerable security risk you see – he was Northern Ireland in the Cabinet before he was Health, or have you forgotten? So the security will be considerable.' He looked almost dreamy-eyed for a moment. 'I'm afraid the publicity will be considerable, Sister,' he said. 'Really considerable – '

Chapter Five

Prue Roberts sat in the corner seat and waited for Jerry to fetch the drinks from the bar. The place was full of smoke already, and noisy too, but the doors to the street were wide open and that helped a little. It was getting cooler, at last; it had been another pig of a day, hot as hell and just as sickening, and as the word came into her mind she felt her gorge rise and she closed her eyes to concentrate on preventing the feeling. And blessedly it settled as Jerry came and set her fruit juice in front of her and then sat down with his own beer.

'When I said have a drink I meant a drink,' he said, sounding aggrieved. 'What's this orange juice kick, for Pete's sake? You're not driving or anything, after all.'

'I like it,' she said shortly, and sipped the stuff. It was warm and sticky but it seemed to help a little and she felt a bit better.

There was a long silence between them as they sat and drank until he could bear it no longer. 'So all right, ducks, tell me what it is,' he said at length when he'd swallowed half his beer and she still hadn't spoken. 'Don't hang about.'

'What do you mean?' She looked at him and then let her eyes slide away.

'Here,' he said, and pulled on her shoulder. 'Look at me. See? Pink and lovely, that's me. Nothing green is there, anywhere? Not even my eyes. They're as pink as the rest of me. So, come on, Prue. After all this time, you can't pretend you said you wanted to have a drink with me just to sit shtoom. Or to cuddle up. You made that bloody clear the last time. So it's got to be you want something.'

She took a sharp little breath in through her nose. 'Well, all right. Money.'

He lifted his brows at that, and pushed his tankard away. 'Who doesn't? I thought you were all right, you and your bloody Gary. Coining it, isn't he, working for the bleedin' A-rabs? Why ask me for money? I offered you the lot once and you didn't want to know. Why ask me now?'

'Because I don't know no one else who'd help me out, that's why,' she said with some desperation and reached for her glass and then pushed it away as another wave of nausea lifted in her at the sight of the bright orange stickiness that clung to the rim of the glass; and he peered at her more closely and said with a sharper note in his voice, 'Hey, what's this? You look like a bloody sheet, you do. You all right? Come on, I'll get you out of here before you show us both up – ' and he tried to lift her to her feet.

She managed to shake her head and then took a deep breath and leaned back. 'I'll be all right,' she said after a moment. 'Just give me a minute – ' and he watched her as she sat with her head back and her eyes closed as around them the pub roared into even noisier life as a group of young people, some in hospital uniforms, came pushing in through the wide-open doors, chattering and shouting at the tops of their voices.

'I'm all right now,' she managed. 'Sorry, Jerry. It's just that – ' She made a face. 'In the bloody club again, aren't I?'

'Christ,' he said after a moment. 'Don't mess about do you, you two? How old's the baby?'

'Five months,' she said drearily. 'I know. It's awful. But what can you do? These things happen.'

'Aren't you on the Pill?'

'Can't take it. We used – you know. Anyway, what's the odds? It's happened. And I've got to get rid of it. I can't have another – I can't – ' and her voice rose a little and he looked back over his shoulder, embarrassed; but the young people at the bar were making such a din that no one had heard.

'Well, tell the quack, then. Or go up to Old East, get them to fix you up – '

'I've been,' she said savagely. 'Been, haven't I? First thing I thought of. And they just sends me off, like some sort of bloody tart or something, they're full up in their wards, they can't take me no more, go to the GP, see what he can do, no good coming to them. So I goes to the GP and my regular one's retired and this new one sends me packing. He doesn't believe in it, he says, it's all wrong he says, and gives me a bloody lecture about it. Some

46

bloody Paki telling me what's right and wrong, what does he know? So I told him to piss off and he could do what he liked with his fucking lectures and – ' A tear appeared in one eye and began to track down her cheek. 'I didn't know what to do. I'm in dead trouble now. I can't go back to the doctor, not after the things I said to him and what if the kids get ill? I got to get a new one and I can't just walk in and say hey, gissa'n abortion, can I? That'll do a lot of good, that will. So now what?'

'There's people,' Jerry said uneasily, watching her. 'I've seen the ads down the underground.'

'Life!' Prue said bitterly. 'I called 'em. They don't do abortions, for Christ's sake. They talk you out of them.' She shut her eyes again, but it didn't stop the tears which kept on streaking her face. 'And then I tried the other ones, but they said I'll need some money. And anyway – ' She opened her eyes and stared at him. 'Anyway, I've cocked up everything. Gary sends me money but I'm always getting in a mess over it and now there's the new welfare rules I can't even go to the Social and – please, Jerry. I didn't know who else to ask.'

He sat in silence for a while and then laughed softly. 'What my old dad used to call a right turn up for the book, 'n't it? You give me the push so you can marry that bugger Gary but when he goes off and leaves you in the club and on your uppers who do you come to? A right turn up – '

She began to get her things together then, her thin blue cardigan and the old white handbag, keeping her head down. 'Sorry I bothered you,' she said in a high voice. 'I'd better get back. Left the kids on their own and they might wake up. The baby's due a feed anyway – I'd better get back.'

'Oh, don't be in such a bloody rush,' he said and pulled on her arm to make her sit down again. 'Who said I wouldn't help? I just said, what a turn up for the book, that's all. Christ, bloody nurses. The row they make! Listen, let's go back to your place, all right? You can see to the kids and I'll pick up a Chinky and we can talk, all right? We'll sort something out – come on – '

David and Peter saw the two seats fall vacant and made for them like a shot as the others went on shouting and chattering at each other at the bar. 'My feet are killing me, I swear to you,' Peter said, almost groaning, and eased himself into the corner seat gingerly as the thin pale girl and the big bearded man who had been there pushed their way out past the crowd to the street. 'Ooh, thank God to sit down! I could cry with it, I really could.'

'Listen, you didn't really pass out, did you?' David slid in beside him and settled himself for a long gossip. 'It's not as though you were on a surgical ward or anything – I mean, what can there be on a psychiatric unit? All those mad people, but no blood or anything. Why faint, for God's sake?'

'You don't want to believe everything that cow says,' Peter said, throwing a malevolent glare at Clemency Strange who was holding court in the middle of the crowd, throwing her long curls around with great abandon and a good deal of eye-flashing to back it up. 'She wasn't there, so how does she know? She only heard about it afterwards – '

'Well, what did happen? If you don't tell me, I'll believe Clemency and you'll never live it down. Peter Burnett fainted on his first day on the wards, did you hear? Peter Burnett fainted – '

'I didn't! I just came over – well, anyone would have. You too. I was with this man, you see, who gets violent, they said, if he's upset, but he was all right; and then when they took him down to X-ray for something they said to go to fetch clean sheets from the linen cupboard to make up the bed, and I suppose I was a bit uptight with having been worrying about whether this bloke'd suddenly go berserk or something, and I dare say that was what did it. Anyway, I went into the linen cupboard and it's not very light in there – just one low bulb, you know how it is – and I almost tripped over something and when I bent down to look there sticking out from under the bottom shelf was this leg, wasn't there? A bloody leg. Brown shoe, striped green and red sock, pin-striped trousers – I tell you, I can still see it just while I'm telling you! And I thought, Christ, that bloody man must've killed someone and no one knows but me and I just turned and ran out of the cupboard and right into this staff nurse and – well it had been hot in the cupboard anyway and what with that and being so taken aback I can't pretend I didn't feel a bit off. So this staff nurse – she's got tits the size of bloody water melons, gorgeous she is, a right cracker – she picks me up and holds me against her and I'm not stupid, am I? So I kept my eyes closed and just stayed there all cuddled up and made the most of my chances. Well, I mean, who wouldn't? Well, maybe you wouldn't, not for a pair of water melons, but I did, believe me! And they all made a lot of a fuss, but it wasn't anything, really – I didn't actually *faint* you see – '

'Peter, for Christ's sake!' David was staring at him aghast. 'The leg – what about the leg?'

Peter laughed. 'Oh, that, that wasn't anything. I mean it was, but it wasn't to worry about. Bloody artificial leg, wasn't it? We've got this manic depressive, lost his leg in the war. Comes in regularly it seems, and won't use the leg in the ward. Just hops around on crutches, so they shove it in the linen cupboard for him. You'd think I'd have realised there wasn't room under the shelf for a whole body, wouldn't you? But I was being stupid. Worth it though.' He grinned reminiscently. 'Those tits – I'm going to like that ward. Got time to talk to each other, people have, you know?'

'You're a randy devil,' David said. 'One of these days it'll catch up with you, just you see if it doesn't.'

'So are you in your own way,' Peter said, and grinned. 'Though the ward they've shoved you on – Male Medical, isn't it? All those old buggers – not much talent there.'

'I wouldn't dream of getting involved with a patient,' David said and ducked his head, but too late; Peter had seen the flush and let out an uproarious laugh.

'Hey, get you! What's happened to you, then? Seen love's young dream, have you?'

'Shut up!' David said furiously and got to his feet. 'That's not funny. We're not all like you, you know, the original three-legged man, nothing in our heads but our bloody pricks.'

'Oh, shut up yourself,' Peter said equably. 'And get in another. And give us a fag – '

'I haven't got any,' David said, as he went off to get the drinks. They'd had spats like this before, but they never really amounted to much. And as the only two men in the intake they had to stick together, after all. 'I've given up. As of today.'

'They're not really going to, are they?' Barbara Darwood, one of the juniors from Outpatients, said, and her eyes were as round as saucers. 'Not all of it, I mean – are they? How will he – you know?'

'How will he what?' Sian said and teetered back on her bar stool. She was having a marvellous time, all of them standing there and staring and listening. 'If you're going to be any good at this job you've got to learn to be honest. Not so mealy-mouthed.'

'Well, how will he pee for a start?' Barbara said and slid her eyes sideways to look at Frances, her friend from Female Geriatrics, and the black girl, Fatima, both of whom were as round-eyed over Sian's revelations as she was, and then giggled, and the others did too.

'Nothing very complicated about that, I imagine,' Sian said, with all the lofty certainty of total ignorance. 'They'll leave the urethra patent, of course. Put in catheters I dare say or something of the sort. Anyway, they're taking the lot, I promise you.'

'It's wicked,' Fatima said suddenly. 'I mean, poor man – how can they do it to him?'

'Because he wants to have it done,' Sian said with exaggerated patience. 'He said to me when I helped him get undressed, he said this was the best day of his life knowing they were going to do it for him.'

'He's mad then,' Fatima said. 'And that makes it even worse, doing things to mad people who don't know any better.'

'He's as sane as you are, ducky. More than most, in fact. I like him a lot. He's funny and nice. It's just he says that he's suffered a terrible mistake of nature all his life. He's known since he was a baby, he said, that he was trapped in the wrong body. All his life. But he's done the best he can and he's been really incredible. He's a designer, you know. Did the training, got all the exams, went to night school, the lot. He works for this firm of dress manufacturers now, and he says they're a good lot, they understand, and let him stay on when he started to change.'

Barbara leaned forwards, a little breathlessly. 'How? I mean, what happened?' she said in a low voice. 'How did he change?'

Sian wriggled into a more comfortable position on her seat, even more pleased with herself as one or two of the others standing at the bar came and joined in, as interested in her information as her existing audience of three.

'Well!' she said, in a low voice. 'He went on hormones, for a start. Mind you, Dr Rosen – she's the psychiatrist in the Gender Identity Clinic – she said he had to pass as a woman for two years before she'd do anything, so before the hormones he had masses of electrolysis – can you imagine? Having all those hairs taken away with electric needles. He had to go twice a week for months. Not that he had a lot of beard, he said, and none on his chest which was just as well. He says that was one of the ways he knew he was supposed to be a woman. Like the size of his hands and feet – quite small really. Anyway, he had all that, and then the hormones, and that made his breasts grow.'

She made a face then and looked down at her own narrow chest. 'He's got better boobs than I bloody have,' she said and a great laugh went up from the listeners, and a few more came and collected around Sian.

'Anyway, that went on a long time, almost two years I think he said, and then they started talking about the surgery. He'd had some plastic surgery already at a private clinic, nearly bank-rupted him that did, he said. They've built up his breasts a bit as well as what the hormones have done. He's a B cup, thirty-eight, would you believe? And now he's going to have this operation – '

'What'll they do exactly?' someone from the back of the group said.

Sian's voice became even more confidential. 'They'll remove his whatsit, and take away the testicles as well. He says they'll save as much as they can of the skin of his – you know – the scrotum so they can use it to help make a false vagina later on. He says it's a technique that Miss Sayers' not used before but it's been done in America – '

Frances drew in a little hissing breath. 'Oh, it's sickening, it really is. They shouldn't do such awful things to people! It's not what we're for, is it? I mean, I never thought they'd do operations like that. I thought it'd be things like appendixes and hernias and things like that – '

'Where have you been all these years?' Sian said scathingly. 'They do those on day patients these days – have it in the morning, home at night, pop back to have the stitches out. All part of saving on the NHS, that is. The things we keep them in for are much bigger. Important things – '

'You can't tell me cutting off a chap's whatsit's a big thing!' Frances said hotly and went red as several people around her hooted with laughter. 'I mean it is, but it isn't what ought to be in hospitals, is it?' And she appealed to Fatima.

'I don't know – don't ask me,' Fatima said and turned away. 'I said it was wicked and I still think so, but don't ask me – '

'Well, I'm going to ask about it,' Frances said. 'I'm going to ask at the next Branch meeting, that's what I'm going to do. Isn't that a good idea, Sian? You said if we joined for you we could talk about all the things that bothered us, and I tell you, this bothers me – '

'Oh, don't be daft,' Sian said, and now she sounded even more scathing. 'The Union's for things like pay and conditions and equality. It's got nothing to do with who has what operations, has it? Anyway, it's none of your business. I only told you because it was interesting, that was all.'

'Well, I'm going to ask someone about it,' Frances said stubbornly. 'Because I think it's awful. I'll ask Mr Kellogg or the Pawn or someone.'

'You do that,' Sian said and jumped down from her stool. 'And a fat lot of good it'll do you. Anyone coming back? It's been a hell of a long day and I'm going to bed – '

Ted Scribner hadn't meant to come in for a drink. He'd never been a drinker, just the occasional nip at Christmas or out with friends. Seen too much of the damage it did with his old dad; and anyway it wasn't good for him the way he was. Years it had been since he could risk a half-pint of an evening. But it was nice to hear a bit of life, have a bit of company, even if you didn't know anybody actually to talk to. And he had sat and nursed his glass of Cola hoping people would think it was something stronger because no one likes to look a fool, and listened and watched.

And now, as the nurses began to drift out and he watched them go, he didn't know what to do or what to think. Here he was, sitting here drowning his misery in Coca-Cola because there wasn't a bed for him at Old East, and what did he find out?

It was wicked, that was what it was, downright wicked. All the years he'd paid into the National Health, all the years he'd spent fighting for his country – and with damp-eyed nostalgia he

52

looked back down the long dusty corridor of his own history to the four years he'd spent on Salisbury Plain as a storekeeper – all that he'd done and been, and now this. If he hadn't heard it with his own ears, he wouldn't have believed it.

But what had he heard? He sat and stared into the depths of his glass and tried to remember. He'd had nothing to drink really, no proper booze, so his head ought to be clear, but it wasn't easy to work it out. There'd been a lot of people laughing and that stupid juke box grinding away and of course the noise of the machine in the corner they were always playing with, which pinged away like some sort of demented clock, so it hadn't been easy. But that girl had had a clear voice and there'd been no mistaking that she was talking about Old East. Well, all of them were. New at it he shouldn't wonder; showing off, they were, new and pleased with themselves, all talking about what they'd done and the patients and all. But that one with the hair like a lavatory brush, the common-looking one, she'd had the loudest voice of all, even when she was being quiet and trying to keep things down. He'd heard it all right.

Someone having a fancy operation the others thought wasn't right to do. Something dirty it was. People only laughed like that when it was dirty, somewhere between belly button and knees, the way his old mum used to say it. And that meant the same as himself really, didn't it? This man, whoever he was, who was having an operation, was in the same ward he, Ted, was supposed to be in. That nurse had said the Genito-Urinary ward, the ward he would be in tonight if it hadn't been for an emergency. Was this man having this peculiar operation – she had said he was to have his whatsit chopped off, hadn't she? He couldn't have imagined that, it was such a crazy thing to imagine, it had to be true – was he having it in the bed he, Ted, should have been in if only he'd left home that bit earlier this morning, and not got that phone call?

He sat and thought a long time, long after the last of them had disappeared out into the street, staring at the sugary rubbish in his glass and thinking hard about what he could do, and then got up to go to the Gents, as usual, still thinking. There had to be something that would sort it out. If this man who was having an operation in his bed was really having what that spiky-haired nurse had said he was, then people ought to be interested. The question was, of course, to decide who were the people who would be interested.

He walked home, still thinking, all the way along the Highway, not bothering to get the bus, only having to stop once in a dark corner for the usual, and by the time he got there and found the cat waiting on the step for him, he knew he was going to do something. He wasn't sure what, but something. They'd pushed Ted Scribner around quite long enough, thank you very much.

Chapter Six

———————∞∞∞———————

'Bean salad,' Esther said gloomily. 'And aubergine purée. He's been on a Turkish kick at the wine bar and it didn't go as well as it should.'

'It's lovely,' Kate said loyally, and reached for another piece of pitta bread. 'Though I didn't know it was specifically Turkish.'

'It isn't,' Richard said. 'But what the hell — what do they know in Gants Hill? That's why I'm going to close it and use the place as the base for the sandwich service. I can sell 'em a lot more tuna mayonnaise than I can aubergine purée, and anyway I'm bored with the wine bar. Got to stay open too late to make money. The sandwiches will go better, faster, and I can shut up in good time to get over to Acton.'

'It wouldn't be so bad if the various places were closer together,' Esther said and refilled glasses all round. 'But the way it is, I ask you! Here's us living in Highgate and me working in Shadwell, and Richard belting around between the far East and the far West just to keep everything going. Spends more time in the car than he does in the kitchens. Mad, if you ask me — '

'Like hell it is,' Richard said and leaned back in his chair and stretched widely so that his shirt parted over his undoubtedly rotund belly, showing it hairy and expansive. 'I get a chance to be on my own with no one nagging me and I can listen to Oliver on the radio and shout back at him when he trots out all that socialist stuff of his — '

'God help me if you ever get a car phone,' Oliver said equably. 'Stay in the car, Richard, do me a favour. I've got enough problems with the rest of my listeners without you mucking in.'

'I've got a car phone,' Richard said. 'But there's no way I'd use it to call in on your show! Not worth the money.'

'Lovely fella, Esther,' Oliver said. 'Where the hell did you find him? No wonder everyone says "love her, hate him" — ' And he grinned at Kate.

'Lying around somewhere scruffy,' Esther said. 'So I just scooped him up out of pity. I've got baklava. Anyone interested?'

'What's that?'

'Greek pastries, dripping in honey, and sweet as all get out. Nice enough, though – '

'I thought it was a Turkish kick? How did the Greeks get in there?' Oliver said and held out his hand for the plate Esther offered him. 'Or can't you tell the difference between 'em, Richard? Still stuck in the Cyprus of the fifties are you?'

'Better than being stuck in the Britain of Wilson and his crew,' Richard retorted. 'That chap you had on Friday, ranting on about the bloody welfare state being eroded – where do you *find* 'em, for God's sake? Time these lazy buggers were made to get up off their arses and work for a living the way the rest of us do. If they spent half the energy working they spend skiving at the Social Security offices they'd be sitting pretty – '

'Like hell they would,' Oliver fired up at once and Kate sighed. It was too easy for Richard to rile him; why couldn't Oliver see that the man was just being outrageous and trailing his coat? He was nothing like as right wing as he always pretended to be when Oliver was around; he couldn't be or Esther wouldn't put up with him. She wasn't a political person at all, but she had a clear view of what she thought was right and what wasn't, and she'd never have stayed with Richard so long if he didn't share most of her opinions about the way the world was run; of that Kate was convinced. But as soon as Oliver was within hearing he was off, castigating everything from the Race Relations industry, as he called it, to the 'halfwits knocking on all the time about nuclear disarmament' and anything else in between he could think of to annoy Oliver. And every time Oliver rose to the bait like a trout to a tickling finger while Richard sat and grinned and pulled at his beard and laughed at him. Bloody man; and she caught Esther's eye, who looked as bored with the two men as she did, and without exchanging a word the two of them got up and began to collect the dishes to take them out to the kitchen.

'I really resent this sometimes,' Esther said as she scraped plates and stacked them into the dishwasher. 'I mean, why shouldn't they clear up after us? But it's the only way to get any peace – '

'I wish Richard wouldn't do it. Oliver's too easy a target, to be honest – '

'That's why he does a good programme,' Esther said. 'If he didn't care, it'd come across. At least he's talking. When you got here I thought he'd brought his own private thunderstorm with him.'

Kate flushed, and bent her head over the wooden salad bowl she was oiling, rubbing hard so that she didn't have to look at Esther. 'Oh, we had a bit of a natter on the way,' she muttered. 'Sorry it showed – '

'This is me, remember?' Esther said and put an arm across Kate's shoulders and hugged her briefly. 'Like, I notice things about you. Always did – so what is it this time?'

'What do you think?' Kate said bitterly. 'It's always the same, isn't it? Those kids of his. I'm trying to make a plan to get away for the last week in October, just the two of us, and he says he can't, it's half-term, maybe the children will come over, and he knows and I know Sonia'll find some way to screw that up. And I said so and then – ' her voice dwindled away. 'And it all went downhill from there.'

'I know,' Esther said and her voice was sympathetic and warm. 'I know. They're buggers, these men, aren't they?'

But of course she doesn't know, Kate thought. She doesn't know at all. It had been one of the worst fights they'd ever had; he'd even parked the car at the side of the road to shout at her, not able to trust himself to go on driving, and then she, to her own fury, had wept and at once of course he'd been all compunction and had apologised desperately and admitted that he was wrong; it was just that whenever the children came into any equation he couldn't get things to work out at all and he didn't mean to hurt her, and then he'd wept too, and that had made her feel appalling, and she had reached for him to kiss him, and that had been like a fuse newly lit to him; and there, in the car at the side of the road they'd made love in the craziest fashion, like a pair of petting teenagers as the headlights of passing cars in the evening dusk threw fitful glares over them and the roaring engines went by making the car shake, and neither of them had cared as they groped at each other and rubbed and hugged and clung; until both had climaxed virtually simultaneously and then collapsed against the windows of the car, rubbing away with their shoulders the steam their excitement had set there, and breathing heavily.

They'd laughed of course after that and tidied themselves and finished the journey to the Pelhams, arriving, amazingly, only twenty minutes late. But though Oliver had grinned at her secretly from time to time there had been no doubt in her mind. He was more than usually distressed by what was happening with Sonia and the children, and that made him remote, unreachable in a way. And she felt a little chill of fear move in her and she thought – It's time I had a baby. And didn't know why the two thoughts should have melded themselves like that because of all reasons to have her own baby, fighting with Oliver was definitely the worst.

By the time they came back into the dining room with coffee, the two men had left behind the argument about the welfare state and its benefits and were on to hospital closures. Richard was well away, pontificating loudly – he'd had rather more of the rough red wine than the rest of them – on the crazy waste of money the NHS represented.

'There's you lot at Shadwell,' he said to Esther. 'And St Kitts up the road and God knows how many more hospitals littered around the place, all within a stone's throw or two of each other. And yes, I know you're all busy, but that's only because you're *there*. It's a law of commerce and it's got to be a law of everything else too. Where something's offered, made available, people turn up to use it. I opened a restaurant in Acton on a shopping parade where there'd never been a restaurant before, and what happened? Within months I've got a regular clientele and plenty of passing trade. What did those people do before? They went without, ate at home or whatever. Well, it's the same with hospitals and doctors. Set enough of 'em up and the customers come. In the old days when people couldn't afford to be ill, because they had to pay doctors and hospitals, they didn't *get* ill. Now, they get ingrowing toenails and right away they've got to have doctors and treatments and bandages and all the rest of it – and a cash handout too if it's going. Money chucked away because the toenail'd get better by itself left alone. Or they'd deal with it themselves the way people used to – '

'Oh shut up, Richard,' Esther said wearily. 'You know that's all a lot of cobblers. Look at the wine bar, for Christ's sake. You opened that where there'd never been one before and what's happened? Even aubergine purée doesn't bring 'em in and suddenly we're making sandwiches till they come out of your ears, and God help us all if that doesn't work because the freezer'll explode with them. You're just complaining because you want me to give up my job. I've been there before, ducky, heard it all. And I'm not leaving Old East and there's an end of it.'

'You'd better not,' Kate said, alarmed. 'Hey, what is all this? I can't do without you in my ward, Esther! Richard, what are you on about now?'

'I'm on about common sense,' Richard said. 'There she is, putting all that effort into that place, and getting flumpence for it, and if she worked with me in the restaurant, I could open another, really make the business take off. We'd be working for ourselves, not for some gobbling welfare system that eats up money and spits out misery. It's all it does, and you know it. How many people live that much better a life because of what you lot do, eh? Kidney dialysis? Big deal – they live another year or two, and that's it. Transplants? Forget it, cost too much to be practical and anyway there aren't enough to go round. It's all so *daft*. Let someone else do it – time you showed a bit of common sense and started to work for your own.' Richard was getting belligerent now as the level dropped in the third bottle of wine, and Esther looked at him and made a face and then threw a comical look at Oliver.

'Ignore the slob,' she said cheerfully. 'He always starts on this when he's had a good supper. Gets ideas about making us into the Fortes or the Mario and Franco of Highgate, I shouldn't wonder. He'll change his mind by tomorrow. If he really had me around all the time, he'd go out of his head – '

Oliver was staring at Richard. 'Do you really think that?' he said suddenly and Richard looked up and blinked at him owlishly.

'Mm? Think what? Mario and Franco – '

'No,' Oliver said even more abruptly. 'That illness is encouraged by the availability of care. Honestly now, I know you send me up and argue just for the sake of it most of the time, but this is a new idea. Do you really think that if hospitals closed and doctors went away people'd be better? Less ill?'

Richard squinted down at his glass. 'Let me think. I suppose I was shouting off my mouth a bit but – well, yes I do. Not all the way, I suppose. I mean people break legs, get cancer and so forth – but half the time you hear about people being ill, having treatment and what for? I've got a girl, a waitress, has to have psychotherapy every other day for God's sake – NHS doing it for her – and why? Because she's hooked on these drugs, what d'you call 'em – tranquillisers. GP's dished 'em out for years, and now she's trying to get off them, gets attacks of panic, all sorts of crazy things, so she sees this chap for an hour at a time, must be costing a bomb. And she wasn't ill in the first place, was she? Just scared, or miserable or sorry for herself or something – '

'You're a hard devil, Richard,' Esther said. She was sitting now holding her coffee cup in both hands and staring over the rim of it at her husband. 'Until you get something wrong yourself of course. If you had an ingrowing toenail, I can just hear the way you'd shriek.'

'But I wouldn't go off to some damned quack over it,' Richard retorted. 'I wouldn't start swallowing happy pills when I got fed up with it, would I? So I wouldn't need a psychotherapist at Christ knows how much an hour, paid for by the taxpayers, thank you very much. It's all a con, you know it is – you told me yourself. Half the work you do there at that bloody Old East of yours is a waste of time. They're either dying and no one can do anything or it's their own bloody fault. Smoked or ate themselves half to death and then – '

'Or drank themselves sick,' Esther said dryly and moved the bottle pointedly. 'And well, yes, you've got a point. A lot of the things we do for people are needed because they were so daft in the first place. Like that chap in the side ward; remember him, Kate? The one who died last week – I warned him that would happen to him if he went on drinking the way he did, and what did he do? Destroyed his liver as well as his kidneys – but all the same, they need to be looked after. You can't say, "It's your bed, lie in it", can you?'

'Why not?' Oliver said, and stared at Esther with a sharp

direct sort of stare that made her uncomfortable. 'When people are the engineers of their own sickness maybe they ought to be left to stew a bit.'

'Ha!' Richard said. 'Some bloody socialist you turn out to be under the skin!' And he laughed. 'My God, my living has not been in vain, I swear. I've talked to the man for half an hour and I've converted him to common sense!'

'Like hell you have,' Oliver said and grinned at him. 'But you've given me a great subject for my big Friday Debate programme next week. Bless you, you old villain. I'll make a good thing out of that.'

'You see?' Richard appealed to Kate. 'You see what sort of bloke you've got here? Talks about principles and then uses them shamelessly as programme fodder to help him earn his fat salary. It's a rotten old world, that it is, that it is.'

'Now just a minute!' Oliver said and leaned forwards over the table and Esther threw up her hands and got to her feet. 'That's it, Kate,' she said. 'Let 'em get on with it. Come upstairs and help me choose what to wear for Danny's school prizegiving. He'll kill me if I don't get it right and as far as he's concerned I'm the worst frump that ever drew breath anyway. And we can talk sense while these two shout at each other – ' And indeed Oliver was already in full flight, defending the importance of bringing real and important issues into his programme and denying vehemently that money played any part at all in his thinking. And Kate looked at him, at the rough untidy greying hair and the sharp-cut lines of his nose and cheeks and sighed. Life would be a lot easier if Oliver weren't quite so intelligent and quite so thoughtful. Thinking too much was beginning to drive both of them apart. And she went upstairs to go through Esther's wardrobe feeling as miserable as she could remember being for a very long time.

Ted worked for a long time over his letter. He'd had to buy a special pad to do it on, for a start; he had some writing paper somewhere around the flat but to tell the truth it was so long since he'd had to write to anyone that he couldn't for the life of him remember where it might be. So, early on Sunday, when he'd walked down to the corner shop to get his *People* just as he had

61

every Sunday for the last thirty-odd years, he'd bought writing paper and a new ballpoint pen and a packet of envelopes. The stamp he'd have to get tomorrow when the post office opened, but never mind; he'd need time to get the thing done properly, and it would give him something to do in the morning. So, he'd made his lunch as usual – a couple of rashers of bacon and an egg as it was Sunday – and then settled down at the kitchen table to do it.

But it was a lot harder than he'd expected. Knowing how to start was the first problem. He had vague memories of the right way to do it: 'in response to yours of the ult – ' or something of the sort, but that didn't seem right. And it had to be clear and properly done. He didn't want people thinking he was just an old fool whingeing on. He had a good case and it mustn't be spoiled by telling it wrong. And sheet after sheet of the new pad was torn up as he struggled on to get it right.

But he managed it at last and read it carefully, several times, and then set it neatly in its envelope and propped it up on the mantelpiece ready to be taken tomorrow to be stamped and posted. And then sat down to watch the telly for the rest of the evening.

But there was nothing on; just a lot of talking on one channel and shouting on the others and he was restless and bored by it, and something more too. He was angry. He'd felt bad enough over losing his bed and his operation, and pretty cheesed off at the pub when he'd heard those nurses talking; but now he felt even worse. It was writing it all down that had done it, that was the thing. The words he'd used went round and round in his head as he sat and stared at the stupid images on the screen; and suddenly he decided he knew what he'd do.

He wouldn't wait till tomorrow and the post office. Why should he? He'd do something about it now, right now, and he got up and went round his flat with his usual methodical neatness, getting it ready to leave, locking windows, dealing with the cat, all of it. And then put on his coat and went out, taking the letter tucked into his pocket, neatly encased in a new blank envelope now. He'd have to see where he could deliver it, that was the thing. Newspapers were in Fleet Street, that much he knew; so he'd just get a bus at the end of the Highway and go up to Fleet Street and see which of the newspaper offices were open. Then he'd walk in as calm as you like and talk to them and show them his letter and hear from them right away what they were going to do. The whole idea was so sensible he couldn't imagine why he hadn't thought of it before. Just writing the letter had seemed all that was needed to start with, but of course he'd been wrong about that. It was making sure he told someone what was in it that mattered. And that was what he was going to do, right now.

Oliver and Kate drove home to Finchley in silence, she huddled into the corner of her seat and he driving with his shoulders held very straight and with elbows held stiffly as he clutched the steering wheel and stared directly ahead all the time, never looking at her. There seemed little to say; by the time they had left the Pelhams Richard had been well tanked up and Esther a little flustered and they had hugged her warmly as they left and asked her if she wanted any help with him, but she had laughed grimly and said she was used to Richard on Sunday nights; not to give it a thought. So they hadn't, and now they sat in a far from companionable silence as the car slid through the dark uncrowded streets, making the lights dance in their eyes as it bumped over the occasional studs and broken asphalt.

Kate stirred when he stopped outside the house, instead of driving straight into the garage, and frowned sharply.

'Aren't you putting the car away?'

'Of course,' he said. 'But I want to nip on to the studio first. Do you mind? I won't be long, but I'd rather pick up some of the things I'll need tomorrow before I go to bed. I'm not too sleepy and – well, I should read it up. I should have thought of it when I left on Friday, but you know how it is on Fridays. Big day, Friday – '

'Yes,' she said, and depression settled over her like a thick old blanket. The last time he'd behaved like this, needing to go off on his own, just to drive about and think his own thoughts, they'd nearly broken up. She remembered it all too painfully, as well as the long weeks of his silence and spurts of anger and then the huge row that had at last ended it and cleared the air with such intense sex they'd both been exhausted. But this time they'd had the row and the air-clearing first; did that mean that after he went off driving around this time he really would decide they couldn't stay together? That had been the problem last time, and clearly it still was. Bloody Sonia, she thought with all the venom she had in her. Bitch Sonia. I wish you were dead, dead. I really wish you were dead. And the sour taste of guilt filled her mouth for feeling so.

'So you don't mind?' he said, peering at her in the dimness, and she could see the troubled glint in his eyes and felt, for a moment, a little better. If he was worried about how she felt, wasn't that a good sign?

'Of course I do,' she said, as heartily as she could, trying to sound natural. 'I want you in bed with me. I need to curl up with someone warm. But I can hang on if I must. Don't be too long.'

He managed a grin then. 'I won't,' he said, 'because I really am going back to the office for some papers. I've got that bloody man from the Environment Office in tomorrow about the Green Belt. Believe me, I need to bone up. I'll be home before – ' He squinted at the dashboard clock which read eleven-ten. 'No later than half past midnight. OK?'

'OK,' she said and stood there on the pavement watching the red rear lights of the car driving away into the distance. She felt awful, even though he'd said that. Because why on earth hadn't he just asked her to come with him? She would have gone, he must know that; and the thought slid into her mind like a worm under a stone.

Is he going to see Sonia?

Chapter Seven

Suba was beginning to enjoy herself. She still got tired quickly and her feet hurt a good deal, as did the muscles down the backs of her legs, but it wasn't so scary any more. Now when she pushed open the big doors to Annie Zunz Ward each morning there was no sick feeling of cold fear; just familiarity. The patients had stopped being terrifying strangers but were people she knew, like Mrs Walton and Mrs Malone, old Mrs Halliwell and Tracy and Dawn.

She liked Tracy and Dawn, a pair of giggling teenagers who seemed not to mind at all that they had to expose their most private parts the way they did when they had their dressings. Why they had needed the operations they had had Suba didn't know, and really didn't want to; all she knew was that twice a day both of them had to lie there on their beds behind the screens, knees bent and flung wide apart while Sister did all sorts of odd things to them. Suba would stand there and carefully not look, though she was supposed to be learning, because she just couldn't, and the girls would giggle and Sister would tease them cheerfully and it was all — well, to Suba it was all very odd.

But still, she was enjoying her work now. Whether bedmaking or bedpanning, helping with feeding the older patients or cleaning up after Sister's dressing rounds, she was Nursing. She always thought of it like that, with a capital letter. She was Nursing. And it was wonderful.

She liked her room in the nurses' home, too. Some of the girls in her set had opted to live out, some of them with their families and one or two of the older ones, who had a bit of money of their own it seemed, to share flats not too far away, but she, together with Sian and Alice Abingdon and Barbara Darwood and one or two others, had a room in the big old house that abutted the Private Patient Wing. A small room, undoubtedly, but it had all she could possibly want; a bed, of course, and a wardrobe and a sort of combined dressing table and desk, and in the corner a small handbasin and mirror. She had arranged all her things neatly and put up a few photographs of the family and her holy pictures too, on the pin-board that was fastened to one wall, and had bought a rubber plant for the window sill so that it all looked cosy. And she had glowed when she had looked round at it all because it was so much nicer than home where she had had to share her bedroom with her two sisters. For the first time in her life she had her own place as well as her own choice of career. Not bad, she told herself with a glint of wickedness, when she thought of how her father had resisted her. Not bad for someone like me. I may be quiet and stupidly shy but I get what I want in the end.

She was even beginning to make friends. She had had some of a sort at school of course, girls she knew in her class, but they'd never been *real* friends; they'd always chattered and giggled about boys and that had always embarrassed her so much she had been aloof, so to be making so close a friend now was lovely. She liked Shirley Farmer a lot; she was a second year here on the Gynae ward, very senior to just a new first year, but still she was friendly and helpful to Suba and that was unusual, as Suba well knew from what the rest of her set said when they gossiped over meals. Most of the other nurses treated the new people as though they were dirt; it took a long time before a new intake was allowed to feel they really had a right to be at Old East. But Shirley wasn't like that and Suba knew she was lucky to be working with her. A tall thin girl with a rather heavy face, she cared a lot about what she did, pernickety and careful to the point of being rather slow at her work. There were times when Sister would complain at her for taking so long over a job, but as Shirley said to Suba, 'You only make mistakes in a hurry.' So Suba would help her whenever she could, so that Sister would leave Shirley alone. And that helped their friendship too.

They talked about a lot of things, but mostly about Shirley's group. 'You'd like it, Suba, really you would,' Shirley had told her earnestly as together they sorted out the linen cupboard, which had somehow got into a terrible tangle of sheets and pillow cases. 'A lot of the people are Catholics like you, you see – '

Suba would slide away from that. She'd promised Daddy she

wouldn't join anything, not even a group where other Catholics belonged. He went on about it a lot. 'We're entitled to be here, Suba,' he had said. 'We're legal immigrants and never let anyone ever say otherwise. But it doesn't do to have your name on lists anywhere. To be members of groups and parties and so forth – that gets people into trouble. Remember what happened to your Uncle Sanjiv and his family – '

'But they weren't here legally – ' Suba had murmured but he'd run over that, refusing to listen to her.

'They were caught and sent away because he joined the Labour Party. I told him he was a fool to get his name down anywhere but he wasn't one to be told, ever. What could I do if he wouldn't listen to me? But you listen to me. No joining anything. No names on computers, you understand me?'

She had tried to explain this to Shirley who had stared at her with blank eyes and then shaken her head impatiently.

'This isn't a political party!' she said. 'Of course it isn't! We're just people who know it's wrong to do what they do here and want to stop it. You don't have to put your name down anyway, if you don't want. Just come to some meetings and you'll hear what it's all about. And then you can do what's the right thing to do and everything'll be fine. You won't have joined anything but you can still help with the important work.'

'But you belong, Shirley, and you can do it, can't you?' Suba had ventured. 'So you don't want me as well.' But Shirley had just snorted at that.

'I'm not on duty all the time, am I? Nor are you – and sometimes one of us is on and one is off and then what happens? It's necessary to be ever vigilant.' And then she had said that again, carefully quoting: 'Ever vigilant.'

So Suba had agreed at last because she wanted to be Shirley's friend so much and Daddy need never know. She needed her, that was the nub of it; to be alone in so very big a place as Old East was not nice and though some of the others were pleasant enough – Sian was all right, sometimes, for example – no one had ever been as kind and as interested in Suba as Shirley was. So Suba went to the meeting of her group.

It had been rather awful. A small hall, behind the church in Hooper Street, a scruffy grubby place, dull and dirty. But there had been a lot of people there, at least a dozen, and someone had made tea and handed round biscuits which had made it seem a bit less miserable. But then they'd shown the film and Suba had sat there with the crumbs of the biscuit sickly sweet in her mouth and the smell of the overstrong tea in her nostrils and watched and felt sick.

It wasn't that she didn't know about such things; of course she did. The nuns at the convent had told her it happened and what a sin it was, and she knew that for all that, there were people who did it. But to see it, in colour, even on a small screen and a rather jumpy scratchy film, was different. They showed her the baby growing in the womb, and then showed, with cartoon-like pictures, how these wicked people introduced their instruments and destroyed the baby, tearing it apart, pulling off its head and arms and legs; and the taste of biscuit in her mouth had gone sour and she had been afraid she would be sick. Her mother had warned her right from the start when she had said she wanted to be a nurse that she had a delicate stomach and was sick easily, and she had had to work hard to overcome that in the wards. Now she could deal with bedpans and people being ill and manage to keep her own insides under control even though she had to look away sometimes, but this film nearly finished her, it was so awful.

Because after they showed the diagram pictures they showed close-ups of the real thing, the pieces of dead baby on a gauze swab. Well, the voice in the film said it was a dead baby though it was hard to be sure; all she could see were great red blobs and lumps but that was enough for her stomach. And she closed her eyes and waited till the wave of sick feeling went away, trying not to hear the deep voice on the film dwelling in such detail on what the instruments did and how the baby suffered this terrible pain and anguish –

After that she tried not to listen so much when Shirley talked about it, but it wasn't easy, because Shirley was obsessed with it. She went on and on whenever they were together and doing anything without people able to overhear them, about the awful way women behaved and how they had sex without caring and then destroyed the babies they carried, just like *that*; and Suba would nod and agree, for of course she was right. Hadn't she been told that all along by the nuns? But all the same she wished Shirley wouldn't go on about it quite so much.

And then there was the matter of Mrs Walton. That really had made things difficult with Shirley.

It had been a busy week, one of the busiest, Sister had said, this summer, and Mrs Walton's operation had been cancelled twice because emergencies had come in and they just couldn't take her to theatre. She'd been ever so upset about it, Mrs Walton; she'd cried and then she'd shouted at Sister when she tried to tell her she'd have to go home for a while and come back later when they had a bed and she'd refused to go and they'd had to send for the medical social worker as well as the consultant, and Suba had heard what it was all about because she was making up the bed next to Mrs Walton's while they were all talking behind the screens and she explained it all to Shirley afterwards.

'She's got three children, quite small ones, and they had to go to a foster mother so she could come in here, and she didn't want to upset them taking them home and then having to send them away again. So that's why she won't go until she's had her operation. And then the consultant said – what's her name? – she said – '

'Miss Buckland,' Shirley said and seemed to sneer a little. 'She's Miss Fay Buckland. Always on the telly she is, on about Women's Lib. She's public enemy number one, the group says, the way she is. Does abortions all the time. She's *awful*.'

'Well, she was very nice to Mrs Walton. Said she understood and of course she wouldn't have to go until the operation was done. And then she said it was going to be a difficult matter because of the dates – '

Shirley lifted her head sharply at that. 'Is she another one of them then?' and she sounded positively eager. 'I'm supposed to count up all the abortions they do here to tell the group.'

'But she's not – I mean Miss Buckland's allowed to, isn't she?' Suba said. She didn't like abortions any more than Shirley did, knew they were wrong, but it wasn't as though they weren't legal. It was one thing, Suba thought, to make a fuss if people did things against the law, but what was the point of making a fuss if it was allowed?

'How can it be allowed if it's wrong?' Shirley said hotly. 'It

69

doesn't matter what the law says. It's what's right and what's wrong that matters – '

Suba had stared at her over the bed, holding in both hands, tightly, the pillow she had been fitting with a clean cover. 'But it *is* different, Shirley. I mean, I know what you mean about not wanting abortions and when that man at the group said about trying to get the law changed, well, I can see that. But what's the point of reporting Miss Buckland if what she's doing is legal? I can't see that it makes any difference – '

'It does,' Shirley said darkly. 'You see if it doesn't.' And she had finished the bed rather huffily, not saying another word to Suba, and that had made her miserable.

And then Sister had called Suba next morning and told her she could go to the theatre with Mrs Walton. Shirley was off duty so there was no one Suba could talk to, and she had stood and stared at Sister blankly when she told her that and didn't know what to say or do.

Sister looked at her. Suba quite liked Sister, a cheerful open sort of person, with a broad Welsh accent that sounded friendly and familiar, a bit like some of the family, really, the ones who still had an accent from living in India, so she wasn't scared when Sister looked at her so directly. She just stood and stared back.

Sister Morgan sighed a little and leaned back against her desk and folded her arms.

'All right,' she said. 'Out with it. You're a Catholic and you don't want to look after her, I suppose? Why do I keep on getting you people on this ward?'

Suba went scarlet. 'I – well – it's just – I'm not sure that – '

'Why you girls come into nursing in the first place beats me sometimes,' Sister said. 'Why not train in one of your own convent hospitals, for pity's sake, and then you'd never have any problems? As it is – this is the big real world and you can't do just what you fancy you'll do, you know.'

Suba could feel her face red and hot. 'I'm sorry, Sister,' she said miserably. 'It's not my fault. It was just that – ' she almost said Shirley's name and then adroitly changed the words just in time ' – that someone told me Mrs Walton's having an abortion and – well, I don't know what I ought to do. It's legal, isn't

70

it?' And she stared at Sister wretchedly. 'It's not as though it was against the law or something, is it?'

'For heaven's sake, girl, of course not. And especially for this woman!' Sister had straightened up and stood there with her hands on her hips staring down at Suba who was very aware suddenly of being only five foot three. 'Have you read the notes?'

'Oh, no, Sister!'

'Then you should!' Sister said crisply. 'And I'd see you did so now if it wasn't that Miss Buckland's taken them. Now just you listen to me, young woman. This lady has three children under the age of six. She is a one-parent family – her husband left her when the last one was born. So now she is not only pregnant – and that is her own affair so don't look so shocked at me – but she has a severe cervical lesion. We thought it was just CIN 3 but now it looks as though it could be invasive. She doesn't want this baby, and couldn't cope if she had it. And its father's left her too. Just as her husband did. And now she needs surgery to make sure it doesn't metastasise. You know about the risk of metastases?'

Suba stared back and said nothing and Sister took a sharp little breath in through her nose and closed her eyes for a moment.

'Spread, Nurse Mahmoudi, spread. She has a lesion in her cervix which is cancerous, it's gone beyond treating with just a laser or cone biopsy. And though if she wanted the baby we might be willing to risk holding on till she delivers early with a Caesar and then do the hysterectomy, she is adamant she can't cope and wants treatment now. And so Miss Buckland has agreed to do the operation today. Do you understand?'

'I – I'm not sure, Sister,' Suba said, still miserably. She thought she did, but it would have helped to have Shirley here to explain it more simply.

'She has cancer, girl! If she has a hysterectomy today there's no risk to her future health from secondary spread. Her scan is clear. She'll lose the baby of course, but since she doesn't want it, that doesn't really come into the matter, does it? Now, if you want to refuse to take a patient to the theatre because she is to have a hysterectomy, that is a very different matter from objecting on conscience grounds to helping with an abortion, as I see it – '

'I suppose it is,' Suba said and straightened a little. 'If she might die if she doesn't have the hysterectomy – '

'Well, her life isn't precisely in the balance at the moment,' Sister said dryly. 'But the time could well come. In fact it definitely would. Right now, I haven't time for all this chat. I'll send someone else to theatre with her – you go and – '

'No, Sister!' Suba said breathlessly. 'I'll take her. I'd like to, really. I mean, it'll be interesting – '

'So I should think!' Sister said, and nodded at her approvingly. 'That's better! I must say I hoped you'd see sense, and I'm glad I was right. I promise you I won't try to send you to deal with any other abortions, the social ones, but this one is different, and I'm delighted you've the sense to see it. Now, collect the resuscitation tray and help me get her on to the trolley. We'll give her her premed in ten minutes and then she can go down. You stay with her till she's in theatre, right? And – let me see.' She looked at her watch. 'If you didn't mind taking a short lunch break you can stay to watch. You'd find it most interesting.'

Amazingly it was. Suba had been so afraid she would make a fool of herself when she first got to the theatre, being sick or, worse still, passing out, but she didn't. They had made her take off her cap and tie her hair up in a sort of white helmet and then she had had to put on a gown and mask over her uniform because she was to go into theatre with her patient, but that had been rather fun. She had caught a glimpse of herself reflected in the glass door of an instrument cupboard and she had felt herself blush with pleasure behind the mask. She looked very dramatic and sort of real, like a character from *Angels* on the telly, and she liked that.

And Mrs Walton had been so nice, very sleepy and woozy, but awake enough to be worried and to want to hold hard on to Suba's hand, and she had felt really useful as she stood there beside her while the anaesthetist chattered to her and gave her an injection and then, as Mrs Walton's grip on her had eased, slid the big tube with the metal end into her mouth and then attached her to the anaesthetic machine. After that the anaesthetist made Suba help him while he set up the drip, putting the needle into a vein in the back of Mrs Walton's hand, and she had liked the way he had muttered, 'Good girl,' at her when she obeyed all his instructions and it all went up as it should, smoothly and easily and without any problems.

Inside, the theatre had seemed quite mad to Suba for a moment or two, for there were so many people, all shrouded in gowns and masks, and such a powerful mixture of smells and sounds that her head swam. The reek of anaesthetic and disinfectant, the pinging of the anaesthetic machine and the monitors, the clatter of instruments and the loud chatter of the nurses and the surgeons had made it all seem like a scene in a particularly frenetic film; but there had been no time for her to worry, because they made her help them lift Mrs Walton into place on the high narrow table and then there was the bustle of putting towels on her and fussing over her; and Suba stood and watched, wide-eyed over her mask, too enthralled to think about what was happening to Mrs Walton or how she felt herself or anything but the drama and excitement that was all around her.

Even when they started on the operation, and Miss Buckland, unrecognisable behind her mask, had made a long incision right across Mrs Walton's belly, just above where the hair had grown before it had been shaved off, she didn't feel bad. Miss Buckland was talking to the man beside her, who was helping her, saying what she was doing, and listening to her Suba remembered her anatomy lectures. Skin and then subcutaneous fat and then fascia and then muscle and then peritoneum – 'And we needn't worry about *that*,' Miss Buckland said firmly, 'because that's the uterus, well up as you can see – well developed fundus, isn't it? I'd estimate at least twenty-six weeks, hmm, Edwards?' And she had chatted on as her knife and scissors moved in the gap that had been made in the green shrouded shape that was Mrs Walton while the retractors held by the man addressed as Edwards held the space clear for her. And still Suba felt all right, and was deeply proud of herself for that fact.

But then it all seemed to happen rather suddenly. One moment Miss Buckland was head down over the gap in Mrs Walton and the next there was the large rounded piece of tissue on a dish, and the man Edwards was slicing into it and Suba watched him almost transfixed with horror as she realised what it was. That was the uterus, and inside it was the baby. Was he going to do what they had shown her on that film and pull the little thing apart, head first and then arms and legs? Was it dead or alive inside there?

And she heard a sort of buzzing in her ears and her body felt very cold and the red object into which Edwards was cutting seemed to recede to a long way away. Someone murmured in her ear, 'Hold on, my girl – let your head droop and flex your legs – come on, tighten your leg muscles – ' as someone else said loudly, 'I think it might be worth talking to Mr Bulpitt about this, what do you say, Edwards?'

And then she really did faint, and knew she was doing it and was desperately ashamed of herself and yet grateful at the same time. Blackness was a lot pleasanter than anything else right now.

Chapter Eight

Laurence Bulpitt reached Male Medical just in time to see the last piece of furniture being trundled in and he stood in the door and stared down the ward towards the far end where there was a remarkable amount of activity, and frowned.

'Sister!' he called, but no one responded, though one or two patients looked at him vaguely and then returned to their books and newspapers, or turned over to go to sleep again. And he frowned even more deeply and went marching up the ward, not waiting for the usual courtesy of an escorting member of the nursing staff.

He found Sister in the last bay, a plastic apron wrapped round her and irritability in every movement she made as, with sharp gestures, she directed the men heaving the furniture around, and Bulpitt stopped at the sight and stared.

'Sister, what in the name of all that's holy is going on here? Where are the beds?'

She turned a flustered face towards him. 'Oh, Mr Bulpitt! Don't tell me it's time for your — I'm sorry, it's just that everything's in such a tangle here I hardly know — if you'll just give me a moment, sir. No, Brovery, not there! I gather the wretched man wants it beside the bed, though how the nurses are supposed to get round it, I can't imagine. Still, that's not my problem. Right, yes, that's it. Now make sure the engineers get the phones in, will you? Mr Byford said he'll have him here at three o'clock, and it has to be all ready then.' She snorted softly. 'A press conference! I ask you! Well, Mr Bulpitt — what can I do for you?' and she came towards him, pulling at the apron and readjusting her cap a little.

'I wanted to talk to you about a patient,' he said, staring over her shoulder. 'But that can wait a moment — what's happening here?'

'It's no secret, I don't suppose,' Sister said crossly. 'Mr Byford has a very important patient coming in. Edward Saffron — '

Bulpitt made a little grimace, pulling down the corners of his mouth expressively.

'Has he indeed! He's a jammy bugger, that one – '

Sister grinned suddenly and let her shoulders relax. 'Not for me to say, sir,' she said. 'But I can tell you it's causing mayhem here. I've had to rearrange the whole ward, and make all sorts of awkward arrangements so that the wretched man can have a section all to himself. I've lost three beds, do you see? That means I've had to put an extra one in the side ward, which isn't equipped for it, and heaven help me if we have a patient needing specialling. I just won't have the space or the nurses to give special care, will I? He has to have a battery of phones here too, it seems – why he can't use those new mobile things I don't know, but I gather they don't pick up calls properly here, what with all our other equipment and so forth – I've had some wretched man from the Ministry here for hours fiddling about and driving me potty. Anyway we're nearly there. At least he's having private nurses – and I wouldn't have thought *he* needed specialling, but I'm grateful all the same. Now, Mr Bulpitt, what can we do for you? I don't think you've any problems with me at the moment, have you?'

Bulpitt smiled down at her. He liked Sister Sheward. Everyone did, for she was a lively forthright sort of lady, and undoubtedly efficient; a rare combination. 'Not yet, Sister, but I've got a beauty for you. If you can spare me one small bed – '

'Mr Bulpitt, are you mad?' She almost squealed it. 'Come and look for yourself, please!' And she turned in a little flurry of nylon uniform and led him down the ward, past the serried rows of beds and their humps of patients towards the far end and her nurses' station. 'Do you see? Not an empty bed anywhere and all of them set too close together anyway, because I've had to fit in the overflow from Mr High and Mighty Saffron's section. And – '

'There's an empty one,' Bulpitt said hopefully and pointed at a corner bed but she shook her head.

'Joe Slater, patient of Neville's – Dr Carr's. Bilateral Ca. lungs – he's down having chemo at the moment on Andrew Green Radiotherapy ward. He'll be back soon. Doing not too badly actually, though I thought he was terminal when he came in. You can't have that one, I hope – not for a while anyway.' And she looked at the bed with its covers neatly rolled, waiting for the return of its occupant, and her face looked bleak for a moment.

'Well, what about the side ward? I won't need it for that long and it's very interesting, Sister. You'll like it – '

She sighed heavily. 'Considering I'm supposed to be a medical ward, you know, it's all wrong I get this sort of pressure. You can't tell me that this is a purely medical case you're trying to put on me, Mr Bulpitt.'

'Well, it is and it isn't.' They'd reached the nurses' station now and she sat down at her desk and he perched on it beside her, his rump pushing her notes to one side. But she didn't mind, for he was a cheerful pleasant man and she liked him well enough; his patients all adored him and from Sister Sheward's point of view that was a strong recommendation. 'The thing is I've got the chance to do something rather special, and I'm determined to do it – but I can't do it down on my own Neurology ward because at this time of the year we're jammed with the summer people.'

'Ah,' she said and nodded. She'd been a staff nurse on that ward long ago, in her early days at Old East, and knew of its tradition of taking in severely handicapped patients in order to give their relatives a summer break. 'Still doing it then, are they? I'd have thought they'd have axed that long ago. Not very cost-effective, is it?'

'They don't seem to have noticed in the office yet,' Bulpitt said and lifted his brows at her. 'Heaven help the poor devils when they do. But that's the problem, you see. We've got half a ward full of these Alzheimer's and so forth and I don't think I can add to their nursing burdens with this case. But it's a nice one, Sister. You'll be fascinated. You'd kick yourself if you missed the opportunity to be involved, truly you would.'

'A little less coaxing, sir, dear, and a few more facts,' she said tartly and he laughed.

'More matter with less art? Right. Let me explain – but it has to be – well, it's a matter not to be talked about yet. You'll soon see why . . . Have you heard of the work they've done in Birmingham on Parkinson's? It's a follow-on to some done in America and Mexico, of all places – '

She squinted up at him. 'That rings a bell. Cell implants? That piece in the *Lancet*?'

'Attagirl. Now I know why everyone loves you, Sister. You know what's going on and say it clearly. Not brain transplants – that drives me potty, as though we were doing Frankenstein stuff – but yes, cell implants. The thing is, Fay Buckland's got some tissue for me. She's had to do a hysterectomy on a woman with a twenty-six-week foetus – cervical carcinoma – and she called me because it was still in – well, in good condition when she operated. The tissue's there and if I use it in the next few hours it would make a considerable impact. I've got a patient I've been considering. And he's willing – my God, is he willing! Almost begging me for it. Well, at least his wife is – and it really seems the time is now. I've got the patient, I've got the foetal tissue and all I need is the bed. And of course the nursing. Can you help me out?'

She sat and stared up at him, thinking hard. It was gratifying that so many of the senior men at Old East thought so highly of her; she liked being the one they all came to when they could for special things, but dammit, with bloody Byford's peerage-in-the-making coming in to the far bay and one of Neville's terminal lungs, could she justifiably fill yet another bed with a case that didn't belong in her ward? What would Byford say if she did it again? He'd been nasty enough when he'd discovered she had a patient of Neville's on the ward; and her face hardened as she thought that. Damn the man! If he could use her ward for his political cases, then she could damn well use it for her own ends too. And being the sort of Sister they all wanted to take their difficult cases to was an agreeable position to be in –

'Where is he now, then?' she asked with an air of resignation. 'Because I'll need an hour or two to get one of these chaps here transferred to your neuro ward. An easy one, who won't put any pressure on your nurses. A fair exchange, hmm? If they'll take one of my sad old gents, then I'll take your Parkinson's, though he'll have to stay in Intensive Care for long enough to be safe here without being specialled. I don't have the nurses for that – '

'I could kiss you, Sister,' he said jubilantly, and slid off the desk to his feet. 'I'll set it all up right now! What time are you off? I want to make sure you're here when I get this chap to you – '

'I'm on till eight,' she said and watched him go; it might have been nicer if he actually had kissed her, come to think of it, instead of just saying he felt like it. And she laughed at her own silliness and went back down the ward to harry the maintenance men on their way. Her Very Important Patient was due at any moment, and she was determined that her ward would do her proud in every way. You never knew who might turn up when a chap like that was hanging around the place.

Oliver stood with the rest of them at the Casualty entrance of Old East, the heavy Uher slung on his hip, and hoped with all the fervour he had in him that she wouldn't happen to come past. Not that he didn't want to see her at every possible opportunity, of course, but this was different. The last thing he wanted was any of these other people thinking he had a special 'in' to the place. Bad enough he actually had it; it would be no good thing if everyone knew it.

If only he'd realised what he was letting himself in for when he'd agreed to help old Radlett out; but how could he have done? There was the man tearing his hair with frustration when Oliver came out of the studio after finishing his programme and of course he'd asked him what was wrong; anyone would. And the old man had seized on him and that had been that.

'I know you're a big name star around the station and all that, Merrall,' he'd said in that rattling staccato speech of his. 'But you're still a bloody journalist and I need a journalist so bad I could kill for one. Who'd be a fucking news editor on a station like this, with two daft girls and a lad straight from university for a staff? But there it is – I'm arse over tip in big stories, and now this. That man Saffron is being admitted to hospital this afternoon and swears he's an NHS patient, but we've had a tip-off he's getting such fancy treatment he might as well be in the bloody Wellington or whatever. Everyone's doorstepping, of course, but we could clobber the lot of them and get a piece into the six o'clock if we could get someone there with a Uher. And even if you can't get an interview, you can do a report of some sort, get some of the doctors, a nurse or two; perhaps see if anyone's got any views on Health Ministers who abuse NHS services – you know the sort of thing – '

79

'Hey, I've got work of my own to do, Radlett!' he'd protested, but he knew the old bastard had won. As soon as he'd come out with that line about Oliver being a star on the station he'd known he was defeated. It was the worst thing anyone could call him; Radlett knew it made him squirm, and that was why he'd said it. If only he could be like that chap on the Beeb who was no bigger a pull than he was – his own ratings were far higher, dammit – but who had no shame at all about exploiting it, it wouldn't be so bad. He, Oliver, had never opened a supermarket or taken part in a TV panel game, for Christ's sake. That bloke had; yet it was Oliver who when accused of being a star immediately capitulated and agreed to stand in for one of Radlett's half-baked journalists who were scattered around London on other stories.

I must have been mad, he told himself gloomily now, to let myself be so easily manipulated, and he stood at the back of the crowd praying that Kate would not appear. If he'd realised in time that it was Old East that was the hospital in question he would have pulled out, no matter what Radlett said or how many times he taunted him with so-called stardom; but there it was, he'd got the Uher on his shoulder and his brief ready when the newscar driver had told him where they were going, so what could he do? Not a damn thing –

There was a little wave of movement through the crowd of journalists then, like a wind blowing over a cornfield, and he followed as they turned as one body and headed for a long black car that had just pulled into the yard.

'Mr Saffron,' someone was yelling as the car door opened. 'Mr Saffron, can you tell us why you are here, please sir – ' And then other voices took up the cry and there was a whirr and click of cameras as the driver got out of the car.

But it wasn't Saffron and they retreated, irritated, as a tall figure in a dark suit came out of the door of the Accident and Emergency department so fast it was as though he'd been shot from a gun.

'You people, move away – move away at once – you are trespassing!' he shouted and waved his arms about officiously. 'You have no right to be here at all, no right – go away at once.'

The journalists turned on him, again moving as a single entity as though he hadn't spoken. 'Mr Byford, sir,' one of them called, the thin chap from the *Dispatch* who seemed to know everyone in sight and who had appointed himself the presspack's spokesman. 'Mr Byford, is Mr Saffron to have – '

'I won't have my patient tormented like this!' Byford said loudly and his face was red with the effort of speech. 'Now go away at once,' and at once the journalists crowded closer as the *Dispatch* man rained questions at him, and the black car behind him remained stubbornly closed.

'Mr Byford, is Mr Saffron suffering from heart disease?' Clearly the *Dispatch* man knew all about Byford and his speciality, Oliver thought, and switched on his Uher. He might as well get what there was, even if it was too blurred and noisy for transmission. 'Is he to have one of your operations, sir, the ones you're famous for, the catheter clearance of the coronary arteries? Has he had a heart attack, sir? Is he at risk of severe illness? Is – '

'No comment,' roared Byford and tried to push past them to the car, but the *Dispatch* man stopped him by simply standing in his way.

'It'd be a lot better, sir, if you agreed to a press conference, you know,' he said. 'We're here now and we can't go till we've got the story, can we?'

Someone had emerged from the far side of the car and now was pushing his way through the crowd and as soon as the *Dispatch* man saw him he pounced.

'Mr Welsh! Good to see you – we need a press man here – look, can we have a statement? We've got some of the story so you might as well – '

The thin man, in an overcoat that looked ridiculous in this warm August weather, leaned over to speak in Byford's ear and then stood up and nodded frostily at the journalists.

'Press conference in the Boardroom in half an hour,' he said shortly. 'And after that we'll consider the possibility of one or two of you coming up to the ward to see for yourselves the arrangements. As long as you go now and let Mr Saffron be admitted quietly without all this fuss. Hardly right when he's a – when a man isn't at the top of his form, is it? No – so the Boardroom, first floor Admin building, half an hour. Mr Byford

81

has agreed to be there.' And he looked enquiringly at Byford who, after a moment or two, nodded. 'Is that reasonable, gentlemen?'

Clearly it was, for the pack moved off, with some hesitation on the part of the *Dispatch* man who led the way, and Oliver followed after a moment, though not before he noted the way the photographers had drifted only a short way away and were ready with their lenses trained on the car door to get a picture of Saffron as he emerged.

Well, that was reasonable enough, he told himself as he followed the rest of them towards the Admin building. The great greedy maw of the presses have to be fed with their bloody pictures, never mind the words; thank God I'm a radio man. It's got a little dignity left to it, though not much. And he walked with his head down, praying he wouldn't meet Kate.

He didn't, and he settled himself in the Boardroom near the front, accepting the courtesy the newspapermen usually offered to the recording people, and set up his microphone and organised in his mind the questions he'd have to ask if no one else did; and waited, trying not to think of what had happened the other night. At least being here and being busy helped to push it away. But not for long.

Why had he done it? Did he have to let Sonia drive him so mad? Did he have to dance so willingly to her bloody piping and upset Kate so much? And his eyes got hot as he thought of Kate and her patience with him. He'd behaved abominably to her, he knew that. She loved him in a way Sonia never had, without any of that profit-and-loss accounting that had been Sonia's trade-mark on every transaction in her life, from childhood on: if I do this for you, what's in it for me? She had used the same yardstick for their lovemaking even, when they'd been married, trading kisses and caresses against cash and status. He knew it now even if at the time he'd been too besotted to realise it. And yet, knowing it, he had still let her do it, still let her make her hateful bargains, chaffer like some damned beggar in a market place — and a soft sound escaped his throat as he thought of how it had been the other night.

He had picked up the papers he had told Kate he was going to fetch from the studios — that had been true enough at least — and

82

was on his way back to the car when he'd been stopped by some old man with a tale to tell, and he'd tried to listen to him but been so desperate to get away to make sure he spoke to Sonia that night that he'd been short with him and had just seized the envelope the old man had pushed into his hand and then legged it for the car, leaving him disconsolate on the kerb. He felt bad about that as he remembered; it had always been his way to be polite and kind to the fans, even though they irritated him so much. They had a right to approach him, after all; didn't he come into their living rooms, their bedrooms, their bloody lavatories even, at the turn of a switch? He had no right to be rude to them. Yet he had brushed off that old man just so that he could go and see Sonia to beg her again to let him have his children on a regular basis; and as he had put the car into gear and pulled away he'd looked back through his rear-view mirror and seen the old man staring after him and felt like a shit. But it hadn't lasted. He had gone to Sonia and –

But that was not to be thought of; and he thrust his hands deep into his pockets now as he tried to push away the memory of what had happened, and how once again she had checked him and fiddled her bloody bookkeeping to make sure all the profit was on her side; the bitch, the hateful screwing – and he pushed his hands down even deeper to stop the words coming into his mind.

And then pulled out the right hand, and looked down at the crumpled paper in it. It had been in his pocket and he'd forgotten it and he had a sudden sharp memory of the old man standing on the dark kerb and staring after his car as he pulled away, and felt again the rush of guilt. He'd given him no further thought, and here was his letter. It had been in his pocket like this for almost a week.

And he made a face at himself and smoothed out the envelope and then slit it open and took out the carefully written letter inside.

Chapter Nine

Kate came clattering down the stairs from the second floor of the Admin building, rather pleased with herself. She knew they'd taken off more tax than they should have done as soon as she'd got her payslip last month and, generally speaking, trying to persuade those people in Finance they'd made a mistake was like trying to walk over a ploughed field in high-heeled shoes, but this time they'd admitted their mistake at once and promised to rectify it, so she felt rather good. It was absurd; even completing a tricky case smoothly didn't give her as much satisfaction as showing an administrator he was wrong. And she grinned at herself as she went past the big open doors of the Boardroom and glanced in as she went by. It was full of people, and she wondered briefly who they were and what they were doing and then went on down to the ground floor and out of the building, forgetting them as soon as she had seen them. She had other things to think about.

The ward when she got there was hectically busy and Esther could do no more than give her a distracted 'Good morning' as she hurried past her in the corridor. Le Queux had a theatre list this morning and the patients were positively whizzing in and out of the theatre and into their beds from Intensive Care as he made the usual whirlwind exhibition of himself. Keith Le Queux, some of his colleagues sometimes commented sourly, drew his surgical inspiration from the nineteenth century; he valued his work in inverse ratio to the amount of time he spent on it. The faster the operation, as far as he was concerned, the less important the outcome. But then, as Le Queux was fond of saying, 'They would say that, wouldn't they?', because Le Queux enjoyed a singularly large and successful private practice, which few of his detractors could match for income.

Kate was glad he was operating. That would mean she wouldn't have to see him and she made a small face at herself as the thought came into her mind. It shouldn't be so. They were supposed to be colleagues, albeit with herself very much as the junior partner, and that meant they should be on good terms, especially since they shared a speciality. But that just wasn't possible for Kate. The man patronised her, that was the trouble. He would smile at her and be exceedingly polite but Kate knew, none better, when she was being categorised and dismissed as a 'little woman' and it made her exceedingly angry. Not least because there was nothing she could get hold of, no accusation she could level against him, no way in which she could find a lever with which to shift his maddening behaviour to a more reasonable mode. She just had to let him get away with it, and try not to grind her teeth too obviously. So, it was much easier when she didn't see him.

Her round was a smooth and easy one this morning and she was happy to do it with the junior staff nurse on duty, so leaving Esther to cope with the Le Queux burdens, and she went from patient to patient, talking, checking wounds and dressings, reading charts and path lab results and reassuring the ones she could and comforting those she couldn't. This was in many ways the best part of her work, she thought, the direct contact with patients. Operating was dramatic of course, full of the pleasure of technical skill, the exercise of intellect and judgement, the source of considerable adrenalin highs, but dealing with people who were far less predictable than the behaviour of blood gasses or the routes of nerves and arteries deep inside bellies – ah, there was the real excitement, even if it wasn't the heady operating-theatre brand. And she ended her round and sent the staff nurse away feeling relaxed and pleased with herself. All these years of work and struggle to become a consultant; there had been many times she had wondered if the time and the effort and the sheer concentrated bloodiness of it all was worth while. This was one of the occasions when she had no doubt at all.

'I'll see Kim Hynes on my own, Staff,' she said now as she passed over the list of charts and took Kim's from the stack. 'I'll need to talk for some time and I don't want to hold you up. How has she been?'

'He's been all right,' the staff nurse said, a little pointedly, and slid a glance at her from beneath lowered lids, and some of Kate's pleasure in her morning's work slid away. Oh, damn it all, why had she agreed to take on so complicated a patient? He belonged with Barbara Rosen, not with her. If only he could be nursed on her psychiatric ward after surgery, how much easier it would have been. And then she bit her lip, annoyed with herself for thinking of Hynes as 'he'. Barbara had been rather strong on that.

'You must regard her as much as a woman as she does herself, Kate,' she had said. 'Unless you do, you're going to have major problems in dealing with her.'

And she had tried, very hard, but it wasn't easy. So she had no right to be annoyed with the staff nurse's unspoken but clearly intended criticism. And she watched the girl march away down the corridor back to the nurses' station with a small sigh, and then turned and went into Kim's section of the ward.

It was one of the basic four-bedded units, pleasant enough though cluttered with the equipment surrounding the two beds nearest the window, where both patients were in dialysis. Esther hated having to put any other patients in there, but it was hard enough to make full use of the units available with dialysis machines without deliberately leaving spare beds unused. If the unit could afford all the machines it needed it would be different, as Kate well knew, but as it was, she had to accept that sometimes patients had to be mixed up in a fashion that was far from medically ideal, and that included mixing patients of different genders as well as different therapy needs.

But Kim seemed happy enough. She was sitting up on the bed, wearing a kimono in very soft pale green trimmed with what appeared to be white fur but which was, on closer inspection, clearly synthetic, and looking at it Kate thought how cheap it looked and knew it had cost a lot of money. Clearly Kim didn't stint herself of the frillier things in life. Her slippers, which lay negligently on the floor at the side of the bed, were pale green satin and very high heeled with the same furry trim, and her bedside locker was laden with bottles of make-up and perfume and hairspray. She was sitting with one foot carefully poised on the bar at the end of the bed, painting her toenails a rich scarlet, and looked as perfectly turned out as if she were on her way to a ball. Her mass of tinted red-gold hair was curled and waved and beautifully arranged inside its shell of lacquer and her face had the porcelain perfection of a *Vogue* advertisement in full colour.

'Good morning, Kim,' Kate said, and stood there looking down on her, and at once Kim looked up and flashed a wide smile.

'Oh, Miss Sayers, I've been so looking forward to seeing you! I thought you'd never come — have you come to tell me when we meet in the theatres?' And the smile widened even more.

'There are things to talk about,' Kate said. 'Would you prefer to come down to the treatment room? A little quieter there — ' and she looked briefly at the other patients by the window.

'Oh, that's all right!' Kim trilled and flashed her wide smile at the other women. 'We've no secrets here, have we, girls? They understand — this is Mrs Antrobus, Miss Sayers, and this is Jenny and this is — '

'I know,' Kate said and nodded at the others. 'This is my ward, after all.' And Kim bit her lip and made a little *moue* of embarrassment.

'Ooh, I am silly! Do forgive me — it's just — well, you know how it is in hospitals. Like ships they tell me. You get ever so close to the people you share with, ever so quickly. We're close, aren't we, girls? So you can say anything you like to me in here, truly you can.'

The other women said nothing, staring from their pillows with dull eyes at Kim in her exotic green kimono and Kate thought — She's working so hard at all this, at being one of the girls. It's so sad, to work so hard and for such a purpose — and looked at Kim.

'I'm sure you're on excellent terms with your — er — room-mates,' she said in a low voice. 'And you're right — it does happen in hospitals that way. But all the same I think I'd rather speak to you in the treatment room. So, if you don't mind — '

'Of course. At once.' Kim was all complaisance. 'Anything you say, Miss Sayers.' She touched her big toenail with one equally perfectly painted fingernail. 'I think that's dry enough — I'll just slip into my slippers then — just give me a mo' — ' And she slid to the floor in a little flurry of fur and pale green chiffon, and began to scrabble for her slippers with her long, somewhat bony feet, and then stood ready for Kate, both hands folded lightly in front of her. And Kate looked up at her, for Kim was considerably taller than she was herself, and managed to smile again. Clearly it wasn't easy to be so debonair and relaxed. The air of desperation that wrapped round Kim was almost as tangible as the green chiffon. Kate could smell it, and she returned the limpid gaze from those heavily lashed lids as directly as she could and felt again the sinking doubts about having agreed to operate. Could it really be right, really be what this terrified anxious patient most needed?

The treatment room, blank and antiseptic, helped soothe her, and she led Kim there and waited, her head bent carefully over the notes as Kim arranged herself on the couch.

'I want to have another look at you,' she said lightly then, and set the notes down on the desk in the corner. 'Just to check, you know — ' And at once Kim lay back on the couch and untied the ribbons that fastened her kimono and pulled up the matching nightdress to reveal the body beneath.

It was worse this time. In the psychiatric outpatient clinic Kate had seen Kim as she usually saw her patients; naked under a sheet, just another human body on display for her wisdom and trained hands. That, she knew, was how the patients regarded their posture. It wasn't nudity, it was supplication; and that usually helped her to be as detached as she needed to be. She could actually believe she was as wise and as trained as she wished she was. That detachment had helped the first time, but now, to see those obviously male thighs and belly with their heavy dusting of dark hair right up to the umbilicus, and the penis, flaccid and wrinkled against the purplish scrotal skin, surmounted by fatty humps of breasts with small pallid nipples, all framed in pale green chiffon trimmed with white fake fur, was deeply shocking. And she took a long slow breath in through her nostrils in an effort to control her face, fearing her distaste would show.

But Kim knew, and it seemed to please her. 'It's awful, isn't it?' she said in that trained soft voice that carried a hint of giggles in it. 'It looks grotesque — it *is* grotesque. I'm a freak, aren't I? A freak of nature. But it's going to be put right, isn't it? I've told all the people in the ward what's happening, you know. It's not a bad thing you're doing, you see, it's a wonderful thing and everyone ought to understand that. I was talking to one of the nurses and tried to explain to her, but she just laughed and went away, poor thing. But you understand, I know you do − ' and she ended on a little breathy hiccup. 'You're going to take it all away and make me normal, the way I was born to be.'

'You're quite sure?' Kate said. 'You're here now but you've time to change your mind − you're quite sure?'

'I've never been so sure of anything in my life,' Kim said, and the tremolo in the voice this time sounded genuine and not a trained elaboration put on specially to convince her. 'It's what I've longed for, so long I've longed for it − ' And again that breathy little hiccup that was half a giggle. 'You can't put it in words, really. You can only feel it. And it hurts dreadfully − '

'Do you get erections?' Kate said baldly, hating to have to do it but knowing she had to, and Kim stared up at her and said nothing.

'Well,' Kate said. 'Do you? And won't you − you understand that any possibility of real sexual function will be destroyed for ever by the operation? I can't − I can try to fashion you a sort of vaginal gap eventually. If you really want me to. It won't be easy but − well, I can do it. But I can't give you any sexual response. That simply won't be there. And if you lose what you already have − ' She carefully didn't look at the genitals, staring hard at the belly instead. 'If you lose this, then you may never have any sexual pleasure ever again.'

There was a little silence and then Kim said, 'I thought you understood. The way Dr Rosen does. I thought you understood.'

'Understood?' Kate said carefully.

'Sexual pleasure isn't a great rod sticking up in front of you like some sort of − some sort of − oh, it's horrible! I can't say how horrible it is to have it. That isn't sexual pleasure! Pleasure is silk against your skin and the softness of it, and walking along with your hair bouncing on your neck and − ' Tears filled the wide dark eyes. 'I thought you knew.'

'How can I?' Kate said, trying not to sound brusque. 'I'm not you. I don't have − ' and she made an awkward little gesture that took in the bare belly and the genitals and the green chiffon. 'I'm trying to understand. I have to because I can't mutilate you if I don't really understand, can I? I said I would operate and I

meant it. But I have to be sure. I'm not going back on my word –
if you're certain, then with Dr Rosen's backing, I'll do as you
want. But *I* have to be sure. And that's what I'm trying now to
be.'

'Well, I'm sure,' Kim said flatly and pulled down the nightdress a little, though the genitals remained exposed. 'Have you –
I mean, are you going to examine me or not?'

'Yes,' Kate said, 'of course,' and began to make a cursory
check of the lungs and the belly, using her stethoscope as much
to hide herself from her patient as to hear the lungs sucking and
blowing and the heart beating, and her hands on the belly to put
a wall between them as much as to check for any doubtful areas.

'Well, you're fit for surgery,' she said and pulled the nightdress
down to cover the body at last, grateful to be released. 'In
excellent health.'

'I know.' Kim sounded smug and sat up and ran her fingers
through her red-gold curls to restore them to their perfect
tumbled arrangement. 'I've taken good care of myself. I watch
every mouthful I eat, believe me, every mouthful, and exercise
regularly.' Again the little giggle tripped out. 'I tried going to a
dance class but the prejudice – my dear, these dancers, they're an
odd lot, and they infect all the other girls with their ghastly little
– well, anyway I've stopped that now. I do my exercises with
Lizzie on the TV every morning. Religious I am about it, and it's
paid off, hasn't it?' She was on her feet now, and patted her belly
complacently. 'Flat as a pancake, isn't it? You have to be careful
though – don't want muscles where girls don't have them – '

'Why?' Kate said, baldly, knowing she was being too crude
but needing to be so. 'Most women who worry about their
figures and about make-up and – ' She made a small gesture that
took in the hairstyle and the painted nails and the long artificial
lashes. 'They do it to attract men. Ultimately to get sexual
pleasure – '

Kim looked down at her and then slowly smiled and shook her
head. 'I dare say you're a wonderful surgeon, Miss Sayers, but
you don't really know about being a woman, do you? I know
you are one, but you aren't really. I mean, spending all your
pretty young years studying and being a surgeon. It's obvious
you don't feel like a woman. Short hair and no make-up – not

that you don't look very nice, of course you do. But you keep your nails short and square – I couldn't help noticing because I always thought that surgeons had to have special hands with long fingers. And yours are quite ordinary really, aren't they? Short square nails and all that – and well, you're not what I'd call a feminine woman. Too modern really, I suppose. But I know what a real woman is, and I don't care what the Libbers say about being old fashioned. I like it that way. Soft and gentle and, well, tender, that's what it's about. That's what makes a woman feel so wonderful. When I'm properly dressed and made up I feel – oh, marvellous. It's a much better feeling than that – ' And she gave a sharp little grimace and looked down at her own crotch. 'That's just like – oh, having a blocked-up nose and then sneezing, no more than that. But pleasure – ah, that goes on and on when you're properly dressed and made up and – it's such a *peaceful* feeling. I can't imagine why you don't have it all the time. Born right as you were, why spoil it for yourself? But there, it takes all sorts – '

Kate had listened with her mouth half open, wanting to interrupt, hugely offended at one level but fascinated at another. But she did not interrupt and even when Kim had stopped speaking she said nothing, just standing and looking at her, and after a long pause Kim lifted her brows and made a little face that both apologised and explained, and invited Kate to share the joke and excluded her from it, all at the same time. And Kate nodded at last and said, 'Well, thank you, Kim. I've got your name on the list for tomorrow. I think I'll leave it there. That will mean no solids after midnight tonight and no fluids after six a.m. Dr Hilliard will come and see you tonight – he's my anaesthetist and you'll find him very sympathetic. You understand that post-operatively you'll have some considerable discomfort – catheters and so forth – '

Kim was smiling brilliantly. 'Oh, yes, Miss Sayers. It'll all be wonderful, I know that. Thank you, Miss Sayers. See you in the theatres!' And she turned and went in a clickety-click of high-heeled slippers and a froth of chiffon and white fur. And after a while Kate bent and picked up a scrap of the fur that had drifted off the hem of the kimono and then followed her patient out of the treatment room.

*

Oliver had sat in the Boardroom for some time after the rest of them had gone. He'd got his recording, for what it was worth, and he still had plenty of time to get it back to the studio, edited and topped and tailed ready for the six o'clock bulletin. Now he needed time to think. He could think here as well as anywhere else, and as the last of his fellow journalists went thundering away down the stairs, he opened out the letter again and smoothed it on his knee and reread it.

And after that got to his feet and went down to the yard. He'd find a black cab, that was the best thing to do, and send the tape back to Radlett at the studio and let him do the spade work on it. He'd have to do something about this letter now he was here at Old East. He couldn't just let it go, tell himself – as he'd been trying to do – that it was just a lot of rubbish, a paranoid old chap making things up. There was truth in that letter; he'd dealt with enough stuff from the punters to know a true bill when he found one, and this was a true bill. He was certain of that and equally certain he had to deal with it, even though it seemed possible that it was Kate's own department that was involved. It might cause her some embarrassment, of course. But he shook his head at that thought; it was much more likely to be the man she worked with and loathed so much – Le Queux, wasn't it? Oliver seemed to remember that was the name. No need to fear Kate was directly involved in this matter. Of course she wouldn't be. She'd never let it happen. But if her department was, then she would be able to help him. And by seeking her help, he'd be helping her too, and that would be no bad thing, Oliver told himself, as he reached the yard and went in search of his black cab. No bad thing at all.

Chapter Ten

'Is it true, then, Ida?' Tracy said and winked at Dawn. The day room was blue with cigarette smoke, most of it coming from the two girls, and Ida flapped her hand in front of her face ostentatiously as she came in and made for the corner chair she liked best. You got a good view from there not only of the TV screen but of the long walkway down the ward to the nurses' station. You could watch your programmes and still not miss what was going on.

'Is what true?' she said and sat down carefully in the chair and pulled her dressing gown neatly over her knees. It was disgusting the way some of them sat around, showing everything, no shame at all. Stupid cows.

Tracy giggled. 'Everything,' she said. 'You know everything 't's goin' on. What about that Mrs Walton? What about her? Did they take it all away then and her as far on as she was?'

'You ought to watch your tongue, miss,' Ida said reprovingly. 'At your age I'd have been ashamed to be so knowing.'

'I bet you wouldn't,' Dawn said. 'I bet you was always one what knew everything. What about what that Paki nurse said about the Prime Minister being in Old East then? Is that true?'

'Not the Prime Minister,' Ida said witheringly. 'The Minister of Health. Yes, he's here − ' She hadn't meant to talk to these stupid creatures, with their giggles and their whispers and the lewd way they whistled when the young doctors came into the ward, but there wasn't anyone else in the day room to talk to, except for Mrs Dawes, and she was asleep in her armchair, so what could she do? 'He's got some sort of heart trouble, so he's in the men's ward for hearts and it's so full the nurses don't know how to get in between the beds, but he's got a section all to himself where they've taken the beds out so as to get his phones in. And he's got a couple of men there to watch him all the time in case someone comes to blow him up. And I think it's disgraceful putting all of us to a risk like that − '

'We ain't at no risk, are we?' Tracy looked alarmed. 'How can we be at risk?'

'Because the men's ward for hearts is down under this one, isn't it? And if they blow up the Minister of Health then we get blown up as well, like they were all blown up at that hotel in Brighton, the Prime Minister and all of them that time.'

'You said they had two men watching him so he won't get blown up,' Tracy said. 'So what are you going on about?'

'Ah,' Ida said darkly, 'but suppose they don't see? They had men watching that hotel an' all but they blew that up all the same, didn't they?'

'Who did?'

'Terrorists,' Ida said and waved one hand to take in all the lurking terrorists in Old East. 'They're everywhere.'

'Well, if they're under here and blow us up, maybe we'll just fall down to the men's ward, eh, Trace?' Dawn said and giggled. 'Land on a nice soft bed. Might be a bit of talent down there, you never know. They've got male nurses down there, I'll bet you. I wish we had 'em here.'

'Oh, yes, can't you just see 'em here? Doing the dressings and the stitches and all for everyone, shoving in the catheters and paddling around – '

'Make a nice change,' Dawn said. 'Better than these nurses we got. It's just bread and bread sandwiches when they do you. No fun at all.' And again she gave that coarse laugh that Ida found so nasty.

'What about you then, Ida?' Tracy said after a while, and nudged Dawn as she stared at the woman in the corner chair, her eyes bright with malice. 'Found out, have they, what they're goin' to do?'

'None of your business,' Ida said shortly and stared at the TV screen, on which a group of Australians were jabbering at great length about nothing much at all. That was one of the good things about these soap operas; it never mattered whether you watched them regularly or not, you could always get into them. 'Just you mind your own, and shut up.'

'Why should I?' Tracy said, suddenly pugnacious. 'You're interested enough when we talk about our business, aren't you?

You ask all the questions and get it all out of us. But when it's us asking you, it's all Madam Muck and touch-me-not.'

'It's my personal tragedy,' Ida said, still staring at the TV screen. 'That's what Dr Buckland said. My personal tragedy. I'm not going to make an exhibition of it to you two, the way you go on – ' And now she did look at them, staring hard, her chin up and her mouth tightly closed, and after a moment Tracy looked away and said, 'Oh, come on, Dawn. It's like a fucking morgue in here. Let's go and see what's goin' on down the other end – ' And she got to her feet and pulled her shortie dressing gown up a little higher to show even more leg and went out and Ida watched them go and considered shouting something after them. But didn't. Got to have more pride, that was the thing. Hang on to your pride.

Not that it was easy. She looked across the day room to where Mrs Dawes snored in her armchair, her head thrown back so that her jaw dropped revoltingly, and then back at the screen. It would help a lot to talk about her personal tragedy to someone. It really would. She'd tried to talk to the nurses, but they were always too busy, one way or another, though nice enough. Even the Paki one was nice and did her best. Not her fault she was a Paki, really. And she stared consideringly down the long walk-way towards the nurses' station, trying to see if she was around. Maybe she could talk to her? Not the other one, her friend, who always looked so sulky and stared at everyone so hard, not her. She was creepy, that one. The Paki one, though, talked – well – nicely, not rough like some of the others, but quietly and nicely. Talking to her might be nice. But she was going somewhere. She could see that from here; Sister was telling her something while she was talking on the phone at the same time and she was sending her somewhere. So there was only the Australians on the TV, after all. And Ida sniffed a little dolorously and settled down to watch them more carefully.

Suba felt agreeably important as she went down to Accident and Emergency. To be sent to fetch a very ill patient like this was something that didn't often happen to first years. It had been a hectic morning, really hectic, what with so many people being off sick and the ward stuffed so full of patients, and Sister in a rotten mood as a result, but she'd managed better than she expected. And then Sister had told her when they'd got the dressing round finished at last that she'd done well, so she was glowing with that anyway. Now, to be sent on a job that really a second or third year should go on was extra good. Wait till she told Daddy. It would help him – wouldn't it? – to get used to what she was doing a bit quicker. It was getting very difficult, the way he nagged on the phone about it every time she called home. You'd think she was doing something really awful like being a film star or something, the way he nagged.

A and E was obviously even more hectic than her own ward. She hovered in the doorway for a moment, staring round, all her confidence draining away through her feet, and felt that hateful feeling in her belly come back; it was awful to get so scared when all she was doing was the work she so much wanted to, ever since she had been so very young, and she drew a deep breath and walked in, pretending she had every right to be there. Which of course she had, though it didn't feel that way.

She managed to stop one of the second years she knew by sight from the dining room and whispered, 'I've been sent down from Annie Zunz to collect a patient – can you tell me where – '

'Oh, lumme, don't ask me, ducks,' the second year said and rubbed her face with one hand, leaving a streak of bright yellow skin lotion there. Her hands were covered in it and it smelled powerful and Suba managed not to wrinkle her nose in disgust. 'I only work here, don't I? It's been like Paddy's market all morning. Look, try Sister – it's all right – she won't bite. Not hard anyway.' And she hurried away, leaving Suba to weave her way through the crowded waiting benches to the cubicle at the far side where Sister was standing talking with one of the doctors. He was tall and burly and very black and wore his stethoscope hanging round his neck sideways instead of the usual collar fashion. Suba thought that he looked very dashing and thinking about that gave her the courage to walk right up to them.

'Of course he has to be admitted, Sister,' the black doctor was saying. Suba liked his voice too; very deep and rich and with the sort of accent you only ever heard on the BBC news. 'It's undoubtedly strangulating. We might be able to get it down without surgery but there are no guarantees. I can't think what the problem is. If a strangulated inguinal isn't a surgical emergency, what is?'

'It's Mr Goodman Lemon's take-in day, that's the trouble,' Sister said with an air of distraction. 'If you can just hold him till tomorrow, when it's Alan Kippen, I doubt we'll have any problems But Lemon'll raise the roof if I just admit him. He made it very clear to me that he'll insist on blood tests, and if they're positive – well, let's just say he said I should arrange for them to be done before I send up any doubtful patients. I told him that has to be someone else's responsibility. I can't do it, not off my own bat. But he was adamant. So there it is. If I admit one of them for surgery through this department I have to let him know personally and once I do there'll be all hell let loose, which is rough on the patient. Do me a favour, Mr Monsarrat, and hold him for twenty-four hours on outpatient observation. If you still want him in tomorrow then I can take him – '

'I want him in *now*, Sister,' the doctor said. 'I'm not being responsible for sending home a man with a lump like that in his groin that I can't reduce. I'm sorry about the fuss Mr Lemon might make but there it is. The man's a – ' For the first time he seemed to be aware of Suba standing near to them and his voice dropped. 'I wonder what Lemon'd do if he were working in Cameroon or Zaïre where I was? The incidence there is much higher – and it's both sexes, everyone, anyone. None of this nonsense there. Well, anyway, Sister, I'll arrange the admission and the wretched test. You send him up. And I'll tell him – ' And he went into the cubicle alongside with a swish of the curtain, leaving Sister standing staring anxiously after him.

'Please, Sister,' Suba ventured. 'I've come for the patient for Annie Zunz. Sister said that I was to – '

'Hmm? Oh, yes – ' Sister looked as though she hadn't heard a word Suba had said, but that was misleading, because she turned then and took her to the corner cubicle. 'In here. Her name's Roberts – Prue Roberts,' she said. 'As soon as I can find one, I'll send one of the porters. Thank Sister Morgan for sending you, will you? I haven't a single nurse to spare – ' And she went away, her heels thudding on the terrazzo floor, leaving Suba to look down at her patient, asleep, or so it seemed, on the cubicle couch.

Her first thought was that she had never seen anyone quite so pale. The woman's face looked more than white; it seemed deeply bleached as though even inside the darkest places of her body she was pallid. Her eyes were partly closed with a line of the white showing beneath each puckered lid, and she was breathing rapidly and shallowly. Suba stared down at her and then at the bag of blood which dangled beside her, dripping quickly into the connection to the tube which snaked down to the back of her hand. The cubicle couch was tipped so that the woman's head was lower than her heels and that had the effect of crumpling her face as the pull of gravity dragged her cheeks up to the level of her lower lids. Clearly she was very dehydrated for her skin looked pouched and saggy, even though she was quite young. How young Suba couldn't be sure but there was no question in her mind that the woman was far from as old as she appeared at first glance.

A nurse put her head through the curtains and said, 'You all right? Keep an eye on that drip – make sure it doesn't slow down. She needs all the blood she can get, as fast as possible. Check her pulse every five minutes too, will you? We'll get you on your way to the ward as soon as we can. Sister said to hold on – she'll send a porter in a minute, but the only one on duty's holding down a drunk over the other side. Call me if you need me – ' And the nurse disappeared before Suba could say anything.

And the thick frightened feeling inside her got thicker and spread further as she looked again at the pale woman on the couch and the dripping blood bag. All round her she could hear the roar and clatter of the busy department: voices shouting as well as talking, the rattle of trolley wheels and instruments and the occasional hiss of oxygen cylinders. And yet she had never felt so alone in all her life. There was just herself and this pale woman for whom she was responsible. It was dreadful.

Tentatively she reached for the woman's wrist to find her pulse, and then the fear grew even more for she couldn't find it at all, and in a sudden panic she scrabbled at her, trying to find it, and the woman's arm flopped to the side of the couch and Suba wanted to scream. Was she dead? Had she been standing here watching a woman die and done nothing about it? Not that she could do anything to stop people dying; how could she, a first year with only a handful of lectures behind her and a few classroom demonstrations to back up her few days of work on Annie Zunz Ward? There'd been no dying patients in the classroom to save, so how could she have learned how to do it? And she felt tears begin to choke her as once again she reached for the dangling wrist to try desperately to find that pulse before running to fetch Sister. And this time she felt it, thin and swift beneath her middle fingertip and relief swept over her so lavishly that she felt dizzy with it and could have hugged the silent figure on the couch. She held on to the pulse for a long time before managing to take her watch from her breast pocket to start counting, and even then counted for far longer than she usually did: a full minute. She bit her lip anxiously because it was so fast. A hundred and eighty, whispering away against her fingertip at such a rate and so feebly that it was hard to count individual beats.

But at least she was alive and it was possible for Suba to stand there and let the fear ebb away a little, and as she waited for the porter, her eyes on the dripping blood and her right-hand middle finger still held over the woman's pulse, as though holding it there like that would prevent it from stopping its headlong rush of beating, she could hear other things around her.

Mostly the voices coming from the adjoining cubicle separated from her and her patient by just a curtain. There was the nice voice of Mr Monsarrat and another voice, higher and more fluting and as she listened she thought – He sounds like someone I've heard before, and puzzled about it for a moment, and then even managed to smile a little as she realised who it was. He sounded like Larry Grayson, the comedian who always made her laugh a lot – though Daddy didn't like him much – even though he didn't have the same sort of accent at all. It was more the way he made his voice swoop and seemed to put some of his words into big capital letters with fat exclamation marks after them.

'Well, *honestly* Doctor, what would you have done?' he was saying. 'There I was minding my own affairs – well, you know what I mean, I'm *sure* – and there's this huge extra one! Well, I'll swear to you that's what I thought! Who wouldn't? And I said to my friend, will you just *look* at this, and well, he was in *stitches*, rotten devil. But then he could see it was serious and there you are, and here I am! Came here at once, of course. And I won't pretend I'm not stirred up about it because I am. Here I am with a new shop opening in a matter of days, so help me, and more work to do than you could shake a stick at, and an extra bollock! What *am* I to do? Is it serious? Do tell me – I can take it, you know! Even if it really is an extra bollock, which I doubt a good deal – '

'You have a right inguinal hernia, Mr Slattery,' Monsarrat's voice rumbled reassuringly and Suba lifted her chin, suddenly pleased with herself because she understood what he was talking about. A loop of intestine sliding down into –

'That means that a loop of intestine has slipped into the gap down which your right testicle came from your belly, originally. They develop inside the belly about here, do you see, and then at or around birth migrate down into the scrotal pouch, here. But the gap that is left behind in some men is rather larger than it might be and if a loop of intestine slips in, that's a hernia. Generally the hernia can be reduced – that is, the loop can be gently pushed back into the place it should be – '

'Ooh, *don't* I know it!' Slattery's voice came a little breathily. 'Been dealing with that for *years* – but it's never been that bad. I mean, no *pain* or anything, just a little bulge sometimes to be pushed back. But nothing like this! *Dreadful*, this is. And this does hurt – and getting worse – ' His voice sounded less cheerful than it had, Suba thought. I dare say he is hurting a bit now –

'I'm sure,' Monsarrat said. 'Yes, I'm sure it is. I suspect we'll have to reduce this surgically to make sure the loop of gut doesn't get so pinched that it's permanently damaged. Don't want that to happen. So we'll take you to the ward and keep an eye on you and if necessary sort out with the surgeons what's to be done – '

'Ooh, me under the knife!' Slattery said and managed a fluting little laugh, but it was not very convincing to Suba on the other side of the partition. He's scared, she thought. Well, of course he is. I'd be scared if I had to have an operation. And she looked down at her own patient and wondered if she would need an operation. At least she wouldn't be scared. So deeply asleep – unconscious – as she was she couldn't be feeling anything.

'You'll feel a lot better when it's all sorted out, Mr Slattery,' Monsarrat said. 'Now, just a few things to see to first. I need some blood for tests – '

'Tests?' Now the patient's voice sounded rather different. Sharper, and even more apprehensive, and Suba lifted her chin and wanted to say – It's all right. I used to be scared of injections, but you get used to it. They made us practise on each other and you do get used to it – but the man's voice came again, sharper than ever.

'Just what tests are you planning to do, Doctor?'

'Oh, blood tests you know,' Mr Monsarrat said and Suba could imagine his face, shining black and expressionless, for his voice had seemed like that too.

'Yes, but what *for*? Don't I have to sign a form or something to give permission?'

'Not usually for blood tests, Mr Slattery. Only for surgical procedures.'

There was a little silence and then Slattery said more loudly, so that it almost seemed to Suba he was in her own cubicle with her, 'Well, I think that's all wrong, frankly. I mean I think patients ought to *know* what tests are being done. And *why*. Will you tell me?'

'Ah – haemoglobin in case you need transfusion,' the doctor said. 'To see if you're anaemic, you see. And blood group so that we can match blood if necessary. Why? Are you a what-is-it – one of those who refuse blood transfusions?'

'Me, Jehovah's Witness? Not me! I ask you, Doctor, do I *look* the type? Hardly! No, I don't mind blood transfusions. I just don't want any other tests. Not unless I know what they are and why they're being done. I've the right to say that, haven't I?'

'Er – well, I'm not sure.' Mr Monsarrat for the first time sounded a little flustered. 'We don't usually discuss the details of tests with patients. It's rarely necessary.'

'I think it is.' The jokiness had gone out of Mr Slattery's voice entirely now. He sounded very determined. 'I've heard of this sort of situation with one or two of my friends, to tell you the truth, Doctor, and I've made up my mind to it that I won't be bullied the way some of them have been. If I need an operation, well and good, I'm prepared to have one. I'll give all the necessary signatures for that and no messing about. But blood tests are something else.'

'Why, Mr Slattery?' Mr Monsarrat said softly.

'Oh, come on, Doctor! You weren't born yesterday! You must *know* the fuss some people make about − about some people!'

'You're homosexual, Mr Slattery?'

'Is the Pope a Catholic?' Slattery said. 'Come *on*, Doctor, I'm hardly one of your all-time male hunks, am I? Everyone else I meet spots me the moment I open my mouth and I don't give a damn. I am what I am and if they don't like it they can get stuffed. But I'm not about to be bullied, and that's the end of it. So no blood tests I haven't agreed to. All right?'

'Why not? Have you reason to suppose that − '

'Oh, of course not! It isn't that I think I've got it! Me and my friend − together seventeen years, we are, and fight like cats, but straight with each other, no matter what. I've no reason to fear. But I'm taking no chances. I've got to get a new mortgage on my shop and all sorts of money deals have to be set up − I'm taking *no* chances. So no test for this bloody AIDS, no matter what. Just get this extra bollock out of my way and let me get back to work, eh Doctor? Sounds reasonable enough, doesn't it?'

'I think so,' Mr Monsarrat said after a long moment. 'But I'm not the surgeon. Just the houseman admitting. Well, let's get you into the ward, anyway. Who knows? It mayn't come to surgery after all. Let's just see how things go, shall we?'

And then the curtains of Suba's cubicle parted and the porter was there with the trolley at last, so she had to go. But she wondered about Mr Slattery all the way back to Annie Zunz.

Chapter Eleven

'I cannot of course be held responsible for any aspect of Mr Herne's department and its work,' Professor Levy said smoothly. 'I'm just the Dean of the Medical School. My concern is with such matters as medical education and the provision of the doctors who will look after us all tomorrow. And as a physician, of course, I'm concerned about the welfare of my patients. But I have nothing to do with such things as closure of beds. These major decisions are, I'm afraid, out of my hands.'

The big office showed every scratch of its yellowing paintwork, every film of dust on the shabby old furniture, as the sunshine picked out each and every detail with vivid cruelty, and he was glad of that. He didn't keep his office looking like a sort of academic slum deliberately, of course he didn't, but it helped when people coming to talk about money could see for themselves that there was certainly none wasted here. He could see from the way the people ranged in the half-dozen chairs in front of him had looked around when they came in that his message had reached them, for they looked alert but not hostile, and in a way pleased with themselves, as though they were thinking – Poor bugger – he's no better off than we are.

They were the usual sort of mixed group demonstrations seemed to attract, a couple of blue-jeaned long-scarved students from the Poly up the road, a bunch of minor businessmen in well-brushed old shoes and seventies-styled suits, a gaggle of housewives in over-tight coats, and of course the woman sitting in the middle who was now leaning forward and looking at him very directly.

'Out of your hands? But you're not just going to sit there and do nothing about it – ' A tall fair woman she was, this spokesman for the group, raddled in a sexually interesting way, Professor Levy thought, looking at the way her long bony legs curled round each other as she sat on the edge of her chair as tense as the classic coiled spring, gazing at him with a fierce blue-eyed glare. 'If you don't take an interest, then who the hell's going to – ?'

'I didn't say I took no interest.' Professor Levy was still as sleek as a cream pot. The whole meeting was working out exactly as he wanted it to. 'Far from it. I just said that I can't comment on Mr Herne's threats to involve the police if you bring your picket line into the clinical areas of the hospital. However, there are certain sections of the premises that are under my jurisdiction. Mr Herne would be hard put to it to turn you out of the medical school area, you know. Hadn't you thought of that?'

'I don't know the geography of this place as well as I might,' the fair woman said brusquely. 'I've been in and out of the wards, me and my kids, and the rest of the family, too, come to that, but – '

'The Medical School, Mrs Blundell, is the building that runs along the other side of the courtyard from the Accident and Emergency department. It has its own alleyway leading out to Cornwall Street, you may have noticed, and anything happening in and around that area comes into my bailiwick. If you set your picket lines there, and indeed actually marched from the front to the back of the Medical School, you'd not only be seen by passers-by and – ah – be accessible to TV cameras and suchlike, you'd be clearly visible to the people in the wards. The main ward blocks look down on the other side of the courtyard, do you see?' He smiled then and inclined his head towards his window through which the main ward block could be clearly seen over the way. 'I'm sure the patients would be comforted to know how concerned you were for them. They could see you actually fighting for their hospital and I'm sure that would encourage them immensely.'

He leaned forwards then. 'Even those who don't actually live on the patch like all of you, but who are patients in the hospital all the same, would be able to see you from there, you know. The male medical ward – the one with the cardiac beds in it – it used to be called Cloudesely, do you remember? When your father was a patient in there – '

She grinned suddenly, and that made her whole face light up. 'I didn't think you'd remember.'

'I remember all my patients,' he said. 'He was a very brave man.'

'Yes,' she said and then grinned again. 'Wicked old bugger. Drove the nurses there potty, he did, before he died. Old bugger – '

'Yes,' Professor Levy said and then added with a casual air, 'He was at the far end of the ward, wasn't he? In the corner where the double windows are?'

She shook her head. 'Imagine you remembering him so well! But, no. He was at the end near the nurses' station. It was the only place in the ward they could be sure to keep an eye on him and stop him getting out of bed and wandering about.'

'Ah – I'd forgotten that. I just thought he might have had the same bed as the one the Minister now has – '

'The Minister,' she said slowly and then sat up very straight. 'He's in the Male Medical ward, at the end there? Where you can look out over the yard?'

'Yes,' Professor Levy said. 'Yes, I believe he is.'

'I knew he was here at Old East. Saw it in the news. But I didn't realise – ' Now a look of seraphic delight spread over her face. 'So if we set out pickets there by the Medical School, he'll see 'em?'

'He'd be hard put to it not to,' Professor Levy murmured. 'And if he doesn't happen to notice, well I dare say someone will draw his attention to you. I'd make sure the placards were large and clear, if I were you.'

'Mr Herne'll be right pissed off!' someone said from the back of the group. They had been happy to leave it all to their fierce spokesman so far but as they at last understood what was being suggested, they relaxed and felt better able to join in. And now several of them laughed.

'I dare say,' Professor Levy said. 'But as I said before, I'm really not responsible for any aspect of Mr Herne's department and its work. Or its feelings.' And this time he laughed too.

Oliver was starting to get irritable. He'd been shoved from office to office, room to room and was getting nowhere. It was enough to force a man to be devious, and he hated being that. It had never been his journalistic style to snoop and pick up information illicitly. He'd always preferred to march straight in and announce himself, his job and his employers: 'Merrall of City Radio,' he'd said to them all, and what had it done for him? A freezing of the faces was all he'd got, a scuttling away to consult unseen seniors, a suggestion that he go to see Mr X here, or Mr Y there. But never any information.

So it would have to be subterfuge, like it or not. He couldn't just go up to the ward to ask, of course. He'd considered that, seeing the signs that said 'Urology', and had almost gone marching up there directly. But then he'd remembered that Esther was the sister in charge, and had quailed, because where Esther was, Kate could be. Even though he knew she was operating this afternoon, there was always the risk she'd come up between cases and see him there and though he could not for the life of him have explained why the thought of that was so dreadful, it was. He'd have to get his information elsewhere.

He was making his way back from the Admin block where he had found so little help, on his way to the main courtyard to see if he'd get anywhere chatting up the gate porter – the sort of person who in his experience was often pregnant with information and willing to part with it – when he passed the Admissions office. And, on an impulse, went in, slinging his Uher in its case well back on his hip, so that it would be less visible to the people in there. Not that most people realised what it meant to be carrying that sort of tape recorder; but still, it paid to be cautious.

The woman behind the desk peered up at him myopically and he smiled at her in the most winning way he could, and put on the Scottish accent he used on such occasions to make sure he disguised his all too recognisable voice.

'Ah, I'm sorry to bother you, but I'm wondering if you could give me some information? For my old uncle, you know. He's very distressed, you understand, and as he's so old I said I'd come along and make enquiries for him.' And he gave her the most charming smile in his repertoire.

She seemed unimpressed. 'We can't give no details about inpatients,' she said stolidly. 'Got to ask on the ward. Sister'll tell you.'

'Ah, but that's the point of it,' he said, still with the charming

106

smile well to the fore. 'He's not in yet. He was supposed to be, was all ready to leave the house and that but he got a phone call, from this office, I think, telling him the bed wasn't available. Needed for an emergency – '

'It happens,' the woman said. 'We are very busy here at Old East,' and she looked at him reprovingly as though she personally were responsible for all the patients' care, and was having her time wasted frivolously.

'Well, I just wantd to check, do you see. Poor old Nunk – so upset he was, didn't take it all in properly. Can't remember, he says, whether you told him another date or not. Would it be asking too much for you to look it up for me, so I can tell him? He's Ted Scribner, 17 Juniper Street. He was to have some sort of operation on his – you know – his waterworks.'

'Bladder Daddy,' the woman said loudly and stared at him for another moment or two, and then at last, reached for the keys of the VDU on her desk.

'That's very kind of you,' he said fervently as she began to tap on the keys. 'Scribner, it is. S.C.R.I.B.N.E.R. – '

'It'd help more if you had his number,' she said and sniffed unappetisingly. 'But if he's here I'll find him – here we are. Under the care of Mr Le Queux, yes – due for admission for prostatectomy March 16th – then May 25th – and then – ' She stared hard at her screen, her lips moving slowly. 'Yes, cancelled five times, he's been – '

'Five times!' Oliver's accent slid away from him as he stared at her. 'He didn't tell me that, for God's sake – '

She looked at him sharply. 'Who did you say you were?'

Just in time he reinserted Ayrshire into his voice. 'Nephew – poor old Nunky! He only told me the last time was cancelled. Never said that – dear me, poor old chap. No wonder he's so miserable – '

'Well, it happens a lot.' She hit a last key on the board and the dancing blue letters on the VDU vanished with a dispirited blip. 'I've got people here in these records who've been sent for and then told not to come over ten times. Into double figures they are.' She shook her head with melancholy pride. 'Double figures. So five times – well, it happens.'

'Can you give me any idea how long he'll have to wait for the next offer of a bed?'

She pursed her lips in genuine disapproval. 'It'd be more'n my job's worth to say a word on that. We can't make no promises and so we've been told over and over, Mr Herne himself came down special and told us, no promises, no matter what. There's such a shortage of beds, you see. They keep doing these cuts and then where are you? Just as busy as ever only worse off. There's seventeen beds shut up over on Women's Surgical you know, already. Got no nurses, they say. And now Mr Herne sends round this memo saying there's likely to be more closures yet. So it'd be more'n my job's worth – '

'Yes, of course,' Oliver said. 'I can see that. Um – you've no way of knowing what sort of emergency it was that lost poor old Nunk his bed?'

She turned the corners of her lips downwards. 'How can I say? They're coming in all the time to Urology. Kidney failures and all like that. Not for me to say, more'n my – '

'Yes,' Oliver said savagely, suddenly pushed beyond patience. 'More'n your job's worth. I quite understand – you ought to get the record sometime, you know. It's a funny song. Or supposed to be.' And he left her staring after him with her mouth partly open, and slammed the door behind him.

So now what? Go to Admin again and insist on seeing this chap Herne? He'd managed to be as slippery as a streak of slime all afternoon so far; no reason to suppose he'd be any more accessible now. Go and get Scribner's side of the story in more detail then? An old voice on tape complaining about how he'd suffered – that would be powerful – then come back here and play it to the man Herne. Surely he'd get a response then? Clearly the old man hadn't been just another crank. There was a story here, and it was worth getting at.

And suddenly he brightened as the excitement of getting going on the research for a story at last lifted in him. It had been so long since he'd done this sort of investigation, that was the trouble. He'd been a star front man for too long. His original journalist's fire had dimmed, settled to a dismal low glow, so that he'd forgotten just how tough you had to be, how determined, and how adroit at getting under people's guards so that they parted with the information you needed out of sheer exhaustion.

Get hold of Ted Scribner then, that was the thing to do, and use a recording of his voice to get to the faceless ones. And at the same time, talk to Radlett, see if he couldn't set up a full investigation into what was happening here under an umbrella title that would look and sound good on the ads for the station. 'The NHS: are we at the crossroads?' would be Radlett's suggestion, of course. It always was, whatever the subject. Oliver would have to think of something a little sharper than that. *The Unkindest Cuts of All*, perhaps? Or something very plain and gutsy – *Ted's Operation*. Simple, very direct – that might work –

He was whistling softly between his teeth as he left Old East and headed towards the Highway and Juniper Street. It was amazing how being busy took your mind off your personal problems. Thank God for work.

Audrey, standing in the window beside Joe's bed and watching the traffic in the courtyard below, tried very hard to concentrate on what she was looking at. Three nurses hurrying across with their silken black legs flashing in the sunshine, obviously off duty and hurrying to change. So young and so happy looking; it must be wonderful to feel like them, to be so sure of everything, so comfortable with their own healthy bodies, and she moved her aching shoulders stiffly and stretched her neck and heard the crackle of rheumatism there and slid her eyes away to the people coming in and out of the A and E department. People on crutches and with bandages, and in wheelchairs; at least she wasn't like them. She ought to be grateful for that, shouldn't she? Sound in wind and limb, just a bit stiff now and again. Ought to be grateful.

She turned back from the window and sat down again beside Joe. Grateful for what? she asked herself as she looked at his parchment-yellow face and the line of white crusting around his lips. She'd have to do something about that when he woke up; couldn't let him get sore lips and a foul tongue again like last time. Oh, Joe, don't do this to me! The words lifted inside her head with all the insistence of a silly popular song, and repeated themselves over and over again, unstoppable and uncontrollable. Joe, don't do this to me, Joe, don't do this to me, Joe, don't do this to me – and abruptly she got up and went padding away down the ward to the nurses' station.

'He's asleep,' she said baldly. 'I can't just sit and watch him. Anything I can do?'

Sister Sheward looked up at her from the notes she'd been writing and gazed at her blankly. 'Hmm? Oh, Mrs Slater. Yes – well, that's very kind of you, but I'm not that – '

'There must be something,' Audrey said and Sister looked at her again and saw the desperation there and put down her pen and smiled.

'Yes, of course, Mrs Slater. There is, I'm sure there is. We're so busy, you see, I can't always stop to think – but let me see – ' She looked over Audrey's shoulder down the ward and then brightened. 'I could use Genevieve to help the nurses with the beds at the far end,' she said, 'if you'd take over her tea trolley.'

'Lovely,' Audrey said gruffly, and managed a small smile in return. A good old sort, Sister Sheward. You didn't have to explain everything to her. 'Just lead me to it. I'll get it done in no time. Anyone not supposed to have any?'

'The list's on the trolley,' Sister Sheward said gratefully. 'If only everyone were as sensible as you! If ever you want a job on my staff, just say the word – '

'I might need it sooner than – oh, well,' Audrey said and moved away towards the trolley, but Sister pulled her back.

'Would it help to talk about it?' she asked quietly and Audrey stared at her with her eyes blank with misery and shrugged.

'What difference does talking make? He's not going to respond, is he? He did last time – a bit anyway. This time he just gets yellower and yellower and his breathing . . . it's awful. How on earth am I going to manage him at home like that? The doctor's already said he can't stay here after he's had his chemo, and it's not working. So what's there to talk about? It's all a lot of – '

'The way you feel, perhaps?'

'You sound like those people on the telly, on the news, when there's been a disaster. There's someone just been blown up or found out their kids have been killed and someone shoves a microphone at them and says, "How do you *feel*?" How do you expect me to feel?'

'Angry,' Sister Sheward said after a moment. 'Resentful. Guilty. Frightened. People do, when someone they love is dying.'

'Angry – ' Audrey said. And swallowed. 'How can a person be angry? There's nothing you can be angry about. Not really – it's the other things – I mean, being frightened. Yes. I'm frightened all the time.'

'Of course you are. And angry.'

Audrey shrugged and began to fiddle with the cups on the trolley as Genevieve, the West Indian orderly, went over to help the bedmaking nurses, in response to a little jerk of Sister's head. Thank God for Genevieve, Sister thought; quick to pick up what's going on and with the wit to act on it. Thank God for Genevieve. 'No sense in that,' Audrey said. 'Being angry – '

'A lot of people get most angry with the person who's dying,' Sister Sheward said carefully, and tried not to look at her watch to see how much time she had left to get the notes finished before the afternoon shift arrived to take over. She'd never get away on time tonight, that was for sure, and David with tickets for the Barbican too. But she didn't move from the trolley, and watched Audrey as she set out the cups and began to pour in the milk.

'Not me,' Audrey said in a muffled voice. 'I couldn't be angry with my Joe. He's – it's not his fault if he's like this. How could I be angry with him?'

'Well, some people are. I just thought I'd mention it,' Sister said. 'In case it happened to you and you felt bad about it. Don't. As I said, it happens to a lot of people. Now, I'll let you get on, and thanks for your help. They're dying for a cuppa, these chaps of mine – '

And Audrey got on, pouring tea industriously, checking each bed number off against the list on her trolley for permission to give out the thick brew, and concentrated entirely on her work.

Until she got to the end of the ward, where some of the beds had been taken out. No one had told her not to go into that section of the ward, and she hesitated for a moment. She knew who was there, of course. Everyone in the ward did and had watched with eyes that missed nothing the busy traffic of secretaries and very obvious plainclothes detectives and messengers with heavy files that went in an unceasing stream to and from the end section. The Minister of Health, she thought now, and looked back over her shoulder to where her Joe lay, barely breathing in his sleep, and tried to see him at home, in their little house with the tiny rooms, tried to see herself coping, tried to see Joe getting the care he ought to have –

And with a sharp little movement, she seized her trolley and pushed it, cups rattling loudly, into the end section where usually four patients lay but where at present there was only one.

Chapter Twelve

'Well, I say it's a matter for the Ethics Committee,' Goodman Lemon said, 'and I can't help it if they aren't supposed to meet for another fortnight. I want a decision as soon as possible. They'll have to be told to meet now. As a senior member of the consultant medical staff, I'm entitled to demand that, and so I do.'

'And will it make the slightest difference what they say, Lemon? Even if that were possible, which it isn't,' Professor Levy said wearily. 'It's clear to me you've made up your mind about this, and nothing I say will have any effect. So why should the Ethics Committee affect you?'

Goodman Lemon stared at him and then got to his feet and went over to the window to stare down into the courtyard. 'Look at them!' he said. 'A lot of rabble – you ought to get the police on to them; Herne ought to. It's all the same these days – no one's got any respect for the decencies.'

'They have just complaints,' Levy said. 'And I'd rather people made their feelings clear and tried to take an interest in what happens to them and to their hospital than just lie supine under events. As I say, people should listen to others – '

'Listen to creatures like those?' Lemon snapped and turned back from the window. 'Listen to people like this disgusting man Slattery who has the brass neck to come here begging our help and then refuses to accept our perfectly reasonable caveats? It's you damned do-gooders and your ridiculous ideas that led to this. You did all you could to ruin this country and left us with all these disgusting problems!' He stood there with every inch of his thin body seeming to vibrate with the intensity of what he was saying but looking really rather ridiculous. His sparse grey hair was carefully trained over a bald head, and his scrawny neck peered out of his collar at an awkward poking angle so that he looked sadly like a tortoise, an impression considerably increased by the heavy lining of his face. 'If it hadn't been for all the freedom these creatures were given in the first place we wouldn't have to deal with this dreadful disease now.'

'As for being a do-gooder, perhaps that's a better label than the reverse,' Levy murmured. 'And I have to say I take exception to the suggestion that I and – what was it? – these people like me to whom you refer so vaguely, have had anything to do with the appearance of the human immunedeficiency virus in this country. But let that pass. The crux of the matter is this man has a sub-acute strangulation of an inguinal hernia. He is not coming to us like some sort of humble supplicant for relief, but because he has a right to do so, as does every citizen coming to an NHS hospital like this one. We do him no favour in responding – we are simply fulfilling our contractual obligations. But let that pass too, and consider the man's health, shall we? As *doctors*. Now, I gather there is a possibility the hernia can be reduced by conservative methods, but it's clear that ultimately surgery will be the answer. You are refusing to operate – or to allow any other surgeon on your firm to operate, unless he has a blood test for HIV, so – '

'As I have every right, and indeed the duty to do so,' Lemon flared. 'What sort of surgeon would I be if I had so little concern for my own and my immediate staff's wellbeing that I'd expose myself and them to this loathsome disease and thereby expose future patients? Don't forget that chap in the West Country who picked this up somewhere when he was operating and then died of it and they had to go seeking out his patients to see who he'd infected and – '

'Rubbish,' Levy said crisply. 'If you use a halfway professional aseptic technique you should neither give nor get any infection any more than that poor chap did. You shouldn't believe all you read in cheap newspapers! None of his patients, as I recall, in fact suffered at his hands. I do agree, mind you, that you've had a poor record in that area – rather more infected wounds on your wards than in most other surgical wards last year, weren't there?'

Lemon's face mottled with an ugly colour. 'That is an outrageous suggestion! How dare you imply that – '

'I imply nothing,' Levy said wearily. 'I am just pointing out that the basis of good surgery surely is to use properly constructed barriers between patient and staff to ensure no passage of infection, either way. Actually, from all I know about the virus – and I have made some small study of it, unlike so many that I know – I can assure you that the patient, should his immunity be in any way compromised, will be at far greater risk from you than you will from him. But that is beside the point. He is not, as far as we know, HIV positive. So there is no reason why – '

'The man refuses to be tested!' Lemon shouted. 'So of course he's positive, and he damned well knows it! That's why he refused. That should be clear to the meanest intelligence.'

Levy raised his brows. 'I fail to see how you can draw such a conclusion from the evidence. He is, I gather, in a permanent faithful relationship and has been for many years. Therefore he is in a low risk group and – '

'Relationship! Relationship – faugh! To use such words for the sort of disgusting practices these scum get up to – you make me sick, Levy. You and all your kind! I will not tolerate this sort of practice in this hospital and so I tell you! Dean you may be, but I am not a negligible person here! Either that man accepts a blood test and agrees to abide by our decision about surgery on the basis of the results, and goes elsewhere if necessary, or – ' and he stopped and glared at Levy.

'Or what?' Levy said softly. 'Are you suggesting this is a resignation matter?'

Lemon was silent for a long moment and then snapped, 'No, I am not. I'm not going to be driven out of my own hospital by you subversives and – '

'One of these days you'll use this ridiculous language in front of witnesses, Lemon,' Levy said and smiled sweetly at him. 'And then I'll be forced to take you to law, you know. You really shouldn't indulge yourself this way. You'll find it becomes ever harder to control your tongue, you see, when there are other people about. Now, just you listen to me. I am no subversive – though why I bother to argue with someone who is certainly not fully accessible to reason I'm not sure – but as I say, I am not subversive. But I am concerned about the welfare of every patient who comes to this hospital, and who needs treatment. This man needs treatment. I am also concerned for the rights of every patient who comes here. This man has the right to refuse a blood test which could compromise him in other areas, outside the hospital. He has financial arrangements to make, and since the world of money is littered with people who are just as bigoted as you are, Lemon, there is no doubt that he will be refused the mortgage he needs for his business if he has a test and it is in fact positive. Also, if he is by any remote chance positive, his life will become a great deal more stressful than it is at present. He has made the perfectly valid choice not to be tested. I support his right to do so, and assure you that you are not at risk, as long as you practise safe and good surgery. If you can't accept that, then we will transfer the patient to another surgical team and – '

'Oh, no you don't!' Lemon said. 'It would be the easy way out, wouldn't it? The way you people use to slide your revolting methods and ideas in. That man was admitted on my take-in from A and E and he is therefore *my* patient. You will not transfer him for devious reasons of your own – '

'Ah! Excellent! You accept the responsibility for his care then? You will operate, since that is his need, and – '

'No, I will not!' howled Lemon. 'Not till he's tested. I've made myself as clear as crystal on this – '

'What you are making very clear is your wish either to see this man die for want of adequate treatment, or his discharge untreated from this hospital. Either way that doesn't seem to me to be the sort of care I would give to someone I designated as my patient. You're making it difficult for me not to take this matter further, Lemon.'

'You've already made the point that we have no witnesses to this conversation, Levy,' Lemon said and suddenly grinned. It was a distorting grimace, but Levy kept his eyes courteously on him. 'So it's your word against mine. And everyone knows what a subversive you are – '

'Such an odd word,' Levy said. 'I'm not sure you're using it in quite its proper context. I might as well call you a fascist, mightn't I? Or a closet homosexual who hasn't the insight to understand that his hatred of this group of people is based on – '

'Oh, very clever,' Lemon said and marched to the door. 'Very clever! I've heard you on this sort of line before. Whenever anyone objects to anything you say it's because he has a hidden desire for it. When I tried to get that Rosen woman's ghastly clinic out of here you were just the same – you and her together. Yes, well, it isn't surprising, is it? Believe me, Levy, you won't have much more time to carry on in this way. I'll see to it you start running this hospital as a decent place should be run, or get out. The latter for choice. Meanwhile, I'm telling you, I and my staff won't operate on a man like this until he's HIV tested. And nor will I stand by while anyone else in this hospital is coerced into doing so.' And he slammed out of the room and left Levy sitting at his desk staring after him.

After a long moment he sighed and pulled his list of internal phone numbers towards him. Lemon was getting worse. He'd always had a tendency to rigidity, even twenty years ago when they'd both been senior registrars at St Kitts. Levy had thought then that he had some deep-seated anxiety, for he never showed any signs of interest in anyone of either sex, devoting himself entirely to his work and to his church, and there was no doubt that he'd made himself into a superb surgeon as a result of that hard work. He had no distractions, no friends, no wife, no children to worry about (and Levy let his mind slide on to the matter of his son Joel and the way he had only yesterday wrecked the family's second car for the second time in two years, and immediately, with a strong effort of will, slid it off again) so why shouldn't he be superb? What else was there to fill his life? But now his rigidity and *idées fixes* were approaching paranoia. It might be time to talk to Barbara Rosen about him and consider what they should do. It was always hell to have to cope with a colleague with psychiatric illness; it had been dreadful three years ago when Bragg the anaesthetist had finally tipped over into total drug dependency and they had had to get him into care and out of the place before a disaster happened. Lemon was far more of a problem because he still had enough control to avoid spouting off too much, or too obviously, in a group. It was only when he had just one listener that he really allowed himself free rein.

And, in all fairness, there were people who would not see this latest anxiety of his as anything but reasonable. The BMA meetings he'd been to recently had been starred with discussions on the matter of HIV testing of surgical patients; there would be people right here at Old East who would defend Lemon's stance and go ahead and test a man such as Slattery without his consent anyway, getting the blood ostensibly for other purposes. Thank God Monsarrat had been able to resist his chief's demands and had come to him (though, Levy thought wryly, I wouldn't like to be in his shoes in the future when he has to deal with Lemon) so at least there was time to do something about the situation. But what? That was the problem.

He ran his finger down the list of phone numbers and then stopped. And after a moment picked up his phone and dialled.

'Who?' Kate said and slipped off her mask, glad to get the wet folds away from her mouth. The bacteriology people from the path lab were testing a new design of mask to see just how much infection was stopped by a layer of water-impermeable film between the fabric folds, and this one was clearly very efficient. The inner side was sodden and her face was sore and reddened from the constant wetness left there by her own breath. It had made the operation even harder than it should have been, that personal discomfort, and now she grimaced with relief as she peeled off her gloves and then her gown and dropped them all into the skip to be dealt with by the theatre orderly. 'Who did you say?'

'Professor Levy,' the staff nurse said. 'He rang down just after you'd started and said would you come and see him. Or he'd come down here if you'd rather.'

Kate peered up at the theatre wall to see the time. 'It's after five,' she said slowly. 'And I want to see Hynes back into the ward . . . Ask the Professor if he wouldn't mind coming over. I'd rather not change and then have to change back again. I'm sure he'll understand. Did he say what he wanted?'

'No, Miss Sayers. Just that he needed a word. I'll ring him, then – '

After she'd gone Kate stood for a moment looking round. The theatre itself always seemed to her so exciting a place: the glint of chrome and polished white tiles and glass; the smell of it, ferociously clean and disinfected; the smooth perfection of the design of the walls, all curves at top and bottom to prevent the harbouring of dust and with flowing lines to every door and

118

fitting. Before a list it looked rather intimidating, with its neat rows of bowls and trolleys covered to protect their collection of shining sterile instruments, the gloves and gowns set ready, the emptiness of the smooth table under the great eye of the lamp; but afterwards, as now, it was a comfortable sort of place, rumpled and messy like, she thought suddenly, a woman after sex. And then grinned at her own silliness. As though the clutter of bloody swabs still hanging from their counting board, the tangle of soiled green linen on the table and the puddles of blood and water on the floor looked in the least sexy: of course they didn't. Yet still there was that violated feeling to it all; and she liked it.

And just what does that say about my own attitude to sex? she wondered briefly as she turned to the door. Do I see it as dirty and messy, a violation and a spoiling? Well, maybe I do. It sure as hell isn't rosebuds and singing birds. And she frowned at the memory of last night and Oliver's urgency that had been so unlike the way it had used to be between them. Where was the peace and the time and the, well, contemplation, they had once shared? Now it was all rush and – no, she wouldn't think about it. And she pushed open the big double swing doors and went padding out in her soft white theatre sneakers, pulling her close-fitting cap from her head at last to let her hair fall free and to feel the bliss of cool air on the back of her neck.

It had been a dreadful case, simply dreadful. The outcome was good enough, she was sure of that; her registrar, who had been decidedly white about the lips as he had watched her knife slide round the penis and down into the groin to encircle the scrotum, had volunteered that at the end.

'He'll look like – well, as normal as it's possible to look, won't he?' he'd said. 'Never mind the function, just take a look.'

And she had lifted her brows and said, 'Well, that's what he – dammit, she – wants. Only the look of it. Doesn't care about the function at all.'

'Well,' the registrar had said, looking down on the exposed crotch area now that the towels had been removed. 'If I didn't know, I'd say this was a woman. Slightly flat about the mons perhaps, and not too lavish about the labia, but a woman all the

119

same. I'll be interested to see how it settles down once the stitches are out. How long will he – she need the catheter?'

'Hard to say,' Kate said. 'We have to make sure the urethral stump remains patent, of course. Don't want any granulation there. I'll try her without it after twenty-four hours, and if necessary recatheterise. Look, will you see him to the ICU – '

'Her,' the registrar murmured and Kate flashed a grin at him.

'Hell, yes. It won't be so difficult now, though. Yes, will you see *her* to ICU and make sure the nurses know the level of fluid input we want? And write up the rest of the post-op drugs, will you? And the antibiotic too. I want a wide umbrella here. That area of the bladder wall behind the prostate gave me a nasty time.'

'More blood too?'

'Oh, yes. A good deal. My God, that one did blow, didn't it?'

'Didn't it just,' he said appreciatively. 'I can remember learning the internal pudendal arterial branches and the perineal and so forth, but I never thought to see what they could do when you nipped them – '

'I had to,' Kate said, needing to justify herself to this young man. 'How else could I get the tissue of the penis away without interrupting the artery? And I could hardly clamp it too soon – not till I knew how much tissue I needed to save. Exsanguinate it too long and I'd have had no leeway for the vaginisation, would I?'

'I was fascinated,' the registrar said. 'But I'm glad it was you and not me – ' and he had gone and left her standing there to worry about whether Hynes had lost so much when that dramatic burst of pulsating bright blood had flooded her operating area that he would suffer undue aftereffects. But then she took a deep breath and shook her head at herself. If the anaesthetist had been worried she'd have cause to be, but he'd been serene about the whole thing.

'A healthy chap,' he'd said. 'He'll survive the operation well enough, that's for sure. Whether he'll survive the effects after that – well, that's another thing. Can't say I approve of this, and that's a fact.' And he too had gone stumping off to leave her alone in the theatre with the detritus of her operation. And she'd been grateful. She had needed time for herself.

But, it seemed, couldn't have it. What on earth did the Professor want? She had few dealings with him, since he was a physician, but those she'd had had been amiable enough, so she had no reason to fear this summons, but all the same a prickle of apprehension made itself felt beneath her ribs and she thought – It's like being at school. Just hearing the Head wants to see you makes you feel like some sort of criminal.

She put her head round the door of Sister's small office, where she was sitting over her post-list cuppa, gossiping with one of the junior housemen.

'Sister, I'll take the notes with me to ICU and write them up there. I believe Professor Levy will be looking for me. Will you tell him that's where I am if he comes here?' And she nodded at the houseman, who was a little embarrassed at being caught with Sister, who was famous for her cheerful disposition and sexual generosity towards good-looking young men, and went on her way. She'd be late home tonight; there was no way she'd leave Old East until she was sure Kim Hynes was fully conscious and there was no unwonted bleeding.

And just as well, she thought then. To see Oliver tonight after last night's discussion – well, it hadn't been quite a row, had it? – about Sonia would be little pleasure. Home at midnight and straight to bed was the likely pattern of the evening and it was just as well.

The Intensive Care Unit was as usual very busy and, as she walked into the hubbub, the beeping of the monitors and the hissing of oxygen and the general sense of urgency, she felt her muscles tighten. This was really where the patients' wellbeing was made or lost. The doings in the theatre were dramatic and important, of course, but the emphasis there was on drama. Here it was long painstaking watchfulness over the bodies brought tubed, wrapped, strapped and empty, it often seemed, of any human spirit, to be protected and tended and slowly brought back together. Not till her patient left this extraordinary place could Kate feel her job was even halfway done. The operation didn't end until the patient was back in bed in the ward.

Professor Levy was waiting for her, looking a little odd in a cap and mask and with a gown over his neat dark suit. There was no real reason why all visitors should be shrouded so, but Sister

121

ICU liked to express her authority by demanding such a ritual, so everyone obediently swathed themselves; and Kate wanted to laugh as she looked at the dapper little figure of the Dean standing there meekly waiting for her. But all she did was smile and say, 'Good afternoon, Professor. I'm sorry I couldn't come over to the Medical School – '

'I was grateful to get out of it for a while,' Levy said. 'I always am. Hate offices. Not too keen on these ICUs, mind you, though they've done wonders for a couple of my more extremis patients in their time. My dear, I need your help.'

'If I can, of course. May I just see my patient first?'

He followed her across to the high bed on which Hynes lay, her head still shrouded in a helmet of fabric and with tubes running from her nose and mouth to the oxygen tap beside the bed and to the suction machines. At the other end of her, people were busy checking her blood drip and the drainage from her bladder and her wound, and Kate took up her charts and read the last collection of information obtained from the various monitors and then took her pen from her pocket and wrote steadily for some time, while Levy stood quietly watching the patient and showing no restlessness at all. And Kate was aware of his quietness and was glad of it. A comfortable man to have around.

When she had set the chart back in its slot at the foot of the bed and leaned over Kim to see if she was ready to talk yet (and she wasn't) Levy said quietly, 'That your patient for Dr Rosen?'

Kate nodded. 'How do you feel about that?' she asked, watching him sideways.

He smiled, and though she couldn't see his mouth behind his mask, his eyes narrowed agreeably and she thought – I like people who smile with their eyes. Even more comfortable to have around. 'If Barbara said she agrees, then I do. We've talked interminably, she and I, half the night sometimes, about her work. Any arguments I've ever had on the matter have long since been demolished. And you?'

She shook her head. 'I have to admit I still get doubts. I did this afternoon when I started. It was – ' She stopped and saw it again in her mind's eye; her own hand so smooth and brown in its thin glove that it looked robotic and detached from her body, and the

122

knife, neat and small and so seemingly innocuous between her first finger and thumb, watched it in her memory as it hovered over the shaven skin and then descended to make the first long curving incision. She saw the golden-painted skin part and the edges curl back to show the bubbles of subcutaneous fat, creamy and sweetly pretty in the glare of the lights and watched it become starred with little flowers of bleeding points. She saw the penis and scrotum again, so aggressively male and yet so helpless in their stillness and watched her knife curl round to circle them with that red-starred fat; and then took a sharp little breath in and turned and looked at Levy. 'It was difficult,' she said. 'Not the sort of surgery I enjoy. Somewhat – destructive.'

'Most surgery is an insult,' Levy said and again his eyes narrowed agreeably. 'And now I need you to insult someone else for me. This time not only the patient.'

'Oh?' She was wary. Levy had a well-earned reputation for being manipulative. Whatever Levy wanted, usually, Levy got; he charmed his way into people's good books and once he had what he wanted smiled his way gratefully on to the next person. Was it her turn now to be involved in some of his politicking?'

'I'm being political,' he said disarmingly and she blinked at his perceptiveness and then blushed a little beneath her mask. Wretched man!

'Well?' she said carefully. 'I don't step outside my speciality much yet, Professor. I haven't been in it long enough to do that.' And it was her turn to smile disarmingly.

'I came to see you because you are competent and sensible but, I think above all, brave. You do what you think the patient needs, rather than what you want.'

She creased her forehead. 'But that's what it's all about,' she said after a moment. 'The patient's needs – '

'Ah, but there are many surgeons who say the patients only know what they want. It is the surgeons who know what they need.'

Her face cleared. 'I see what you mean. Well, I'm not that arrogant. I hope.' And then she laughed. 'What do you want me to do? I'm happy to listen.'

'You're very sensible,' he said. 'But then, it's a function of youth to be sensible. Listen, Kate – ' And she felt a moment of pleasure as he used her first name. They'd always been on pleasant acquaintanceship terms but this was suddenly intimate. And she liked it. 'Listen Kate, I've got the very devil of a problem. It involves Goodman Lemon – yes, well may you look alarmed! There will be ructions. But the patient, you see, is the one I'm concerned about. I'm sure we can find good reasons for a man of fifty-seven to need a genito-urinary consultation. And if he then needs urgent surgery? Let me explain what the problem is. And I hope you'll be the one who can solve it for me. And, of course, for the patient.'

And he took her by the elbow and led her to the little office Sister had at the far side of the ICU and began to explain it all to her.

Chapter Thirteen

At half past six Sister Sheward gave up all hope of getting to her concert at the Barbican. She should have gone off duty at half past four but she'd been willing to stay until seven at the latest, to see Mr Holliday settled after his physio and the late appointment in X-ray. But what with all the fuss over Audrey Slater and the Minister as well as that silly first year getting his trousers into such a twist over Joe's attack of breathlessness, it had been one hell of an afternoon; and when at six-thirty Laurence Bulpitt had arrived and told her he had to go through a long appraisal examination with Holliday that she and only she could assist him with, she admitted defeat. She sent her staff nurse from the second shift to phone and leave a message on David's machine to the effect that she was involved in an emergency and couldn't get away, and pulled the curtains round Holliday's bed with as quiet a hand as she could. No need to display her irritation with loud clattering behaviour. It helped no one, after all.

'I do hope I'm not causing problems coming at this time,' Bulpitt said and flashed her a wide smile. 'But I've been hectic today and tomorrow will be worse, so this really is the only time I can. And I have to admit that my wife's dinner party doesn't really attract me that much. Now, Mr Holliday – ' And he transferred his wide smile to the patient.

'Not at all, Mr Bulpitt,' Sister Sheward said, trying not to speak through clenched teeth. Convenient for him of course; was there ever any consultant, even the best of them, who didn't put his own convenience first? Even Neville Carr was famous for coming in to do his round before breakfast, on the grounds that he found it so much easier to get in through the traffic early, and never mind the havoc it created on a busy ward. Why should Bulpitt be expected to be any different?

But Bulpitt hadn't waited for her rejoinder. He was bending over Mr Holliday with an ophthalmoscope in his hand and peering at the old man's eyes while he murmured at him and she stood and watched him and straightened her tired shoulders. This shouldn't take too long; maybe she could just make it? Was it worth phoning David again?

But it was after seven when at last Bulpitt let her pull the covers back over Holliday's skinny old legs and led the way down the ward back to the nurses' station, and by then she had forgotten her irritation and her ruined evening, for there was no doubt that what she'd learned had been fascinating.

'I must say the change in the tremor's very marked,' she said and Bulpitt nodded, not taking his eyes from the charts on which he was writing.

'That was the most obvious change,' he said. 'I agree. A little coarse tremor when I tired him, but otherwise, much better. Hardly any pill-rolling movement, and he managed that glass of water as elegantly as you like. Had to be fed all the time before, you know.'

'Yes,' Sister said. 'His wife told me.' She grinned then, suddenly cheerful. 'And heaven help me but I've got a fair brace of determined wives on the ward at the moment. What with Joe Slater's missus stirring up the Minister, and then Mrs Holliday laying down the law on what we have to do for her husband – '

'The Minister? What happened?' He was all ears now and humped himself up to sit on the edge of the desk and stare at her. 'Do tell.'

Sister laughed now, seeing the whole episode in her memory. 'Marched into him pushing the tea trolley, didn't she? I'd let her take the teas round as a bit of therapy really, because she was so low, and she simply went up to his bed like an avenging fury and made him put down the phone he was using and stood there and harangued him for five minutes flat out about the awfulness of his being there and three beds being thrown out of the section to accommodate him and she having to take her sick husband home with not enough help to look after him when his chemo was finished. Oh, she laid into him, well and truly!'

'And where were you at the time? Not stopping her, I take it?'

She opened her eyes wide. 'How could I? I was busy hanging on to the secretary who was there with him, telling him all about it, so that he couldn't go and interrupt her. I mean, I was too busy and so was he. There was no sign of his private nurse, of course, and the detective as it happened had gone off to pee – oh, she did very well in the time she had. I was proud of her – '

'But you're not usually backward in coming forward with your praise, Vera,' he said and she glowed a little at the use of her first name. Everyone was supposed to be so egalitarian these days and often they were, but the consultants generally used the 'Sister' label out of extra politeness; yet politeness was the last thing Vera Sheward ever wanted from her consultants. 'If you felt that strongly about having him on the ward, why didn't you say so and stop him coming in? And now he is here why didn't you – '

'He's a patient of Agnew Byford,' she said and after a moment he made a small grimace and nodded.

'I take your point. That does make it . . . So you let Mrs Whatshername do it for you.'

'Why not? She's a capable lady with a tongue in her head. And her complaints would carry more weight than mine. She's a patient, you see, a voter. To Saffron I'm just an employee of his NHS. He oozes charm at me till I feel sick, but he pays me no real attention. But Audrey Slater – that's different. The voice of the voter, you see? It certainly seemed to be like that anyway.'

'How?'

'Mr Saffron asked me to arrange for another bed for Joe. Not to send him home.'

'Just like that!' Bulpitt said. 'Oh, isn't life grand! The noble Minister of Health, comfortably getting over his bit of angina in a showy NHS bed when he's perfectly well able to get himself tucked up out of the way at a glossy place, like the Wellington or wherever, has only to ask for a bed to be made available and it is – '

'Who said so?' Vera said sharply. 'I didn't!'

Slowly he grinned again. 'You refused?'

'Didn't refuse – of course not! I just told him the truth. That I just don't have that sort of clout. I ought to but I haven't. Told him that when people come to me and say they have to use my beds and move out three patients to make room for an important one I have no way of objecting – '

'You're a bloody marvellous liar! You reign over this ward like a duchess and well you know it. You let me bring my patient here – and Carr, too. Dammit, the Slater man wouldn't be here at all if you hadn't agreed to – '

'But Saffron doesn't know that, does he? I told him I couldn't do anything about it – that it was up to him really. That with all the cuts there'd been in the area and the fuss over the rumours about closing the hospital altogether people were very miserable. I pointed out the marchers outside in the courtyard with their banners – not that he could have missed them – and took Mrs Slater away and left him to stew in his own juice.' Again she looked reminiscent. 'Dreadful way to treat a cardiac patient, isn't it?'

'Dreadful,' Bulpitt said cheerfully. 'Quite dreadful.'

'Except that he's really getting on very well. If he were anyone else it's my guess he'd have been out on his ear two days ago. But Agnew Byford won't let him go in a hurry. He's worth his weight in – '

' – knighthoods,' Bulpitt murmured and they both laughed. Byford's hunger for public recognition was one of Old East's most enduring pieces of folklore. 'But we could do without too much fuss, frankly. If Saffron starts a drama over the bed availability and finds out how we poach Byford's beds – has he told Byford yet?'

She shook her head. 'He's away – operating in a private hospital in Swindon or somewhere. I heard him telling Saffron all about it before he went. Life saving isn't in it, believe me. You can see Saffron thinks he's being looked after by the Angel Gabriel crossed with a reincarnation of Aesculapius at the very least. Oh, he'll tell Byford fast enough when he gets back – '

'That's a pity,' Bulpitt said. 'Because I was hoping to use your services again, Vera.'

She frowned. 'Mr Bulpitt, you told me this was a one-off! Just this case, you said, because you had some suitable foetal material – '

'That was fully my intention. But when we got the foetus and had a look at it, we found there was a sizeable amount of available tissue. It was a twenty-six-week infant remember, so the substantia nigra was excellent.'

'Substantia nigra – ' Sister said, struggling to remember her neurology lectures, and angry with herself that she had to make such an effort. 'Is that all you can use?'

'Well, yes, but there was a good deal there, as I say. And Fay Buckland made sure the uterus was removed intact so the foetal head was protected even more. A really good specimen, and I was delighted to get it. And now we find we can store it too. I used what we needed for Holliday and the rest is in a tissue medium with antibiotic waiting to be disaggregated and made into a cell suspension. We can't do that till just before we inject it but of course I have every confidence we've got enough of the material there to use on at least three more patients. So I was going to ask you, once we transfer this chap back to my wards – and going by his immediate reaction to his operation, which was excellent, indeed remarkable, he'll be able to bloody well walk back – if I could bring down a couple more? I wouldn't bother you, Vera, really I wouldn't, if I had any nurses halfway as good as you to rely on, but my ward staff are a dead loss.'

'You ought to go and see them in the office about that,' Vera said reprovingly but basking in his praise. 'You can't just pinch Byford's beds – '

'Carr does,' Bulpitt said and she burst into laughter.

'Honestly, you're all the same, you men,' she said. 'Like kids – 's'not fair, 's'not fair – he did it first – he did it first – '

'And why not, if it works?' Bulpitt slid to his feet. 'Dear *dear* Vera, let me do it, hmm? It seems a great pity when we've got such good results from the one we've done not to have another go. The Birmingham lot are beavering away as well, in spite of all the silly headlines.'

'Headlines? I read about this in the *Lancet*. Have there been headlines elsewhere?'

'Here and there,' he said dryly. 'A hell of a lot of silly comment one way and another. You'd think we were transplanting whole brains the way some of the papers and TV programmes went on. Like mad scientists in the movies, making monsters. Such stuff! Yes, there's been a good deal of fuss, and that's one of the reasons I want to replicate the Birmingham work. We've all got reputations to make, you know, every one of us – '

She sighed and looked at her watch. 'I've put in three hours overtime today, do you know that?' she said conversationally.

'And I was supposed to be hearing Stephane Grappelli at the Barbican tonight. Ah, well, there it is. Send your patients down, Mr Bulpitt. But whatever you do don't get me involved with the politics of it all. Bad enough Byford will be going potty when he gets back and Saffron tells him about Audrey Slater. Just let me go home now, will you?'

'Of course!' he said and reached out and patted her arm. 'I'm a selfish devil – you should have said – '

'And it wouldn't have made the slightest difference if I had,' she said tartly. 'Would it? Not with your wife's dinner party to dodge.' She couldn't resist that. The patting of her arm had been so damned patronising and not at all what she would have preferred from him.

He laughed, a little awkwardly this time. 'That really had nothing to do with it,' he said. 'I'll have to put in an appearance anyway. I really did have to go through that check-up with Holliday. And surely you were interested?'

'Oh, of course.' She walked round the desk to the other side to check her records were all ready to leave. 'Um – you – er, David.' She peered at the first year who was standing on the far side collecting the temperature charts to be filled in by the senior nurse on duty. 'Pass me my bag, will you? Thanks. Of course it was interesting, Mr Bulpitt. To see that sort of progress in a Parkinson's – nil tremor, able to hold his own glass, much reduced rigidity, it's all great. But really I am very tired now, I want to go off duty.'

'On your way then!' he said and reached out one hand as though to pat her again and then seemed to think better of it. 'I'll see you tomorrow then, and arrange to swop Holliday for one or two of the other old Alzheimer's we have. It won't be so easy to measure any change with that but it'll still be useful, I think – good night, Sister!'

David went to supper at eight, already tired, and irritated that he'd been sent to first supper. That meant he'd have to go back to the ward for another half-hour before going off duty at nine, instead of being allowed to go to second supper and straight off. That would have been much nicer – time to get a drink at the pub over the road and a sandwich. Much nicer than the eternity of spaghetti that was all there seemed to be on offer in the dining room tonight.

Gloomily he piled his plate high with the despised spaghetti and found a corner table. He was dying for a cigarette, but it was now practically a week since he'd had one; well, almost. You couldn't count the couple he'd slipped in when other people had given him them. Certainly he hadn't bought any since that afternoon Joe Slater had been admitted and Dr Carr had said – and he slid away into thinking of Neville Carr as he pushed the spaghetti into his mouth; and managed to forget all about his yearning for a cigarette.

By the time he'd got to the tinned-fruit-salad-with-tinned-cream stage the others had come in, and he sighed as he heard Sian's strident voice at the hot plate complaining about the shortage of grated cheese for her salad. If only they didn't all keep on finishing up on the same shifts, he'd be able to dodge them. It would be so much nicer to be on the same shift as Peter; he always had a funny tale to tell of some sort. In hot pursuit, he was, of the staff nurse on Psych. Nurse Melons he called her because of her boobs, and she didn't seem to mind, even though he was just a first year. And David sighed and shifted his chair a little as Sian, followed by Suba and a second year he didn't know, came over to his table. There was no rule that said they had to sit together, dammit; why did they always make a beeline for him?

'You look as happy as a wet weekend,' Sian said as she sat down with a thump. 'Can't be that bad, surely.'

'How do you know?' David said. 'We're run off our feet on Male Medical! We've got the Minister of Health in the ward, that's all, so how can you know what it's like? You and your piddlers – '

'Garn! You're not having anything to do with the Minister of Health,' Sian said and began to eat voraciously. 'Everyone knows they've got private nurses for him. We had a meeting at the Union about it, all this about him being in on the NHS but really having private nurses from an agency. He's not going to get away with that.'

'It still makes a lot of extra work for us,' David said. 'All the beds shoved together so close because of three being thrown out of his section and all these extra patients that aren't really ours – '

'What sort of extra patients?' Sian cocked her head at him sharply. 'Is this something the Union ought to know about? We don't have any members on Male Med at the moment – what's going on there? You tell me.'

'Why should I?'

'It's your duty,' Sian said after a moment. 'Nurses have a responsibility to – '

'Bollocks,' David said and grinned at Suba. This was better. Having a go at Sian was rather cheering. 'I don't give a piss for your Union – '

'I hope you don't swear like that on the ward,' the second-year girl who had been sitting murmuring to Suba looked at him. 'And I'll teach you to mind your tongue here. Some of us are ladies, you know.'

'How can you tell?' Sian said and reached for her coffee. 'All look the bloody same to me.'

'It takes one to know one,' the second year said smartly and giggled, clearly pleased with herself. 'I won't waste my breath explaining to you, of course.'

Suba, always the peacemaker, smiled at David. 'I'm sorry you're so busy,' she said. 'It's horrid when it's like that, isn't it? No time really to think about what you're doing. We've been a bit like that, so many operations and all that.'

'Yeah, well, I think one of yours is what's made us extra busy,' David said and leaned back in his chair. It had been interesting listening in to what Sister and that consultant were talking about; not that he'd understood most of it, but all the same it was interesting. 'Didn't you say Fay Buckland was the name of the consultant on your ward?'

'Yes,' Suba said. 'Miss Buckland. She's very nice, bit sharp to talk to, but likes to tell you things. I was ever so silly, passed out in the operating theatre when she was doing a case, and I felt so stupid – but she came out after when I was sitting getting over it and explained all about why. I knew really – vasovagal, wasn't it? And standing still where it was so hot and feeling so – well, anyway I did know. But she explained and it was nice of her.'

'Well, she may be nice, but she's made us extra busy,' David

132

said. 'We've got this patient who had a brain operation, you see, and – '

'But you're on Male Medical,' Sian said.

'What of it?'

'They don't do operations on medical wards.'

'That's all you know. We've had an arterio-what's-it done on Mr Saffron, and now we've done this transplant thing on Mr Holliday – '

'What transplant thing?' The second year sitting beside Suba was all attention now, sitting very upright. 'What are you on about? What's this got to do with Fay Buckland?'

David sighed in a rather theatrical manner and leaned forwards resting his elbows on the table and propping his chin on his fists.

'It's all very easy really. We've got in the ward one of these people from Neurology, Parkinson's he's got. All shaky you know, and stiff as a board and can't feed himself or anything. Well, he couldn't, that was the thing. Not when he came down to us. But then he had his special operation with foetal substantia – well, whatever it was – and now it's all different. Feeds himself all right, holds the cup and doesn't spill it, it's really something. And I heard the consultant talking to Sister and saying something about Miss Buckland finding him the stuff to do it with.'

'I knew it!' The second year was as red in the face as though the dining room was a Turkish bath, and her eyes were glittering with excitement, and timidly Suba leaned forwards and tugged on her sleeve. 'Don't, Shirley,' she murmured. 'I mean, it's not something to talk to David about – '

'What operation did he do? Did he say exactly?' Shirley ignored Suba completely, concentrating entirely on David.

He stared at her. 'I told you he was talking to Sister. I was just there, like. Sorting out the temperature charts.' That sounded important, so he said it again. 'I was just sorting out the temperature charts. I was busy and they happened to be there talking.'

'It's what I told you about, Suba, I saw it in all the papers! Didn't you? How they take these aborted babies and use their brains to put in old people to make them young again? Oh, it's wicked, it really is wicked – '

'It's nothing to do with making him young again,' David objected. 'Not as I understood it. It was to stop the shaking and the stiffness. It's made Mr Holliday much easier to look after, I can tell you that much. But he's no younger. There's no operation can do that. He's ever so old – nearly fifty.'

'Take no notice of her,' Sian said. 'She's got a bee in her bonnet about abortions, this one. Never talks about anything else. It's very boring.'

'It's more boring to be a baby that's killed by an operation,' Shirley retorted. 'It could have been you if your mother had been wicked enough. The way so many are now. It's not having a bee in your bonnet to take a care for babies being murdered. You're the one with the bee, you and your Unions.'

'That's for living people, not ones that haven't even begun to be born,' Sian said. 'Some mothers just can't look after babies and it's better they have abortions than have any more unwanted babies.'

'All babies are wanted – ' Shirley began but David made a face and got to his feet.

'Sorry I ever mentioned it,' he said. 'The way you go on. Anyway, it's nothing to do with you. It's a patient on our ward, not yours.'

'It's everything to do with me,' Shirley said hotly. 'If they got the brain they transplanted from a baby they killed in a woman on our ward it's very much our business. Anyway, it's nothing to do with whose ward or anything like that. It's to do with all of us – all humanity.' And she opened her arms in a wide theatrical gesture. 'So I shall have to deal with it.'

'*You* have to?' Sian stared. 'You really are full of yourself, aren't you? Who do you think you are? And what can you do, anyway? You're a – '

'I'm someone who cares,' Shirley said and got to her feet. 'That's who. Someone who cares a lot. And what I can do is pass this information on to the people who can do something about it. David – that's your name, isn't it? You tell me: what else was said about this case? And what – '

'Mind your own business,' David said uneasily, poised to go. Gossiping when you were off duty about patients on your ward

134

— it was all wrong. The Pawn had warned them of that in one of their first lectures on nursing ethics. 'It's nothing to do with you.'

'But it *is*, if it was one of our patients who had the abortion, isn't it?' Shirley was wheedling now. 'Go on, David, tell us.'

He hesitated for a moment, but only for that. It was very agreeable, after all, to have information others wanted, exciting to be able to impart news.

'Well,' he said. 'It was a twenty-six-week foetus, I remember that. And he said the uterus was intact so the foetal head was protected — does that help?'

'Oh, yes,' Shirley said and breathed in hard. 'Oh, yes! It won't help Miss Buckland and your consultant, whoever he is, but it will certainly help us.'

'Us?' David said uneasily.

'Not you, ducky, and never you think it,' Sian said. 'You've really gone and started something now. She belongs to that group that spies on hospitals and then makes a great fuss when people have abortions. That's who you've helped. Did you want to?'

Chapter Fourteen

———————∞∞∞———————

'It's out of the question,' Prue said. 'It's the craziest idea I ever heard.'

'Why?' Ida stared at her sullenly. She hadn't expected this response at all. When she'd first had the idea, the night they'd brought Prue Roberts in and she'd heard all of them talking and found out about it, it had just come into her head like someone had come and put it there on purpose. Not like an idea of her own at all, just something someone else gave her. Providence if you like. It was meant. And here was Prue being so silly about it even though Ida had taken such care to time her little talk so sensibly, and even though it was obvious it was the answer for both of them. Why not? And she asked again, trying not to sound annoyed, knowing how important it was to be relaxed and calm. 'Why not?'

'Because – well, because.' Prue looked flustered and tried to turn away from her, but it wasn't easy, for Ida was sitting as close to the bed as she could get, and Prue was fixed by the drip still running into the back of her hand.

'But what else can you do?' Ida said, all sweet reason. 'I mean, you've spent all that money and you owe for it, don't you? I know they done it all wrong, and it didn't work but you still owe for it. Them people – they don't just give you your money back, you know, when they make a cock-up. But you're in a different state over it, aren't you? You borrowed it and you said you had to give it back – '

'Jerry won't push me,' Prue said uneasily and again tried to turn on her side away from her but Ida held on to her hand the way the nurse had shown her the night Prue had been admitted and been so restless and the nurses too busy to sit with her themselves. So Prue had to listen.

'You told me he said it was just a loan. That he needed the money back. And then you said if your Gary ever found out he'd murder you, and take the kids away from you. You said that. So

136

why not do it like I said? It'll be the best way. You said your husband won't be back for ages. Well, with a bit of care no one'll ever know. Your kids are too young to notice and if I get you some nice clothes, big coats and all like that, who's to know?'

Prue had stopped trying to avoid her eyes and was staring at her. Her face was a little pinker than it had been, still pinched and with the eyes looking watery and red-rimmed, but she didn't look like a pallid wax candle the way she had and Ida nodded approvingly at her.

'That's right, love,' she said. 'You just listen to me. You'll see I'm right. We can fix it easy, and my Tony'll never know, and he'll be happy and so will you and so will your poor little baby – '

Prue's eyes brimmed and Ida looked over her shoulder anxiously, scared there was a nurse around. She was supposed to be helping with Prue, not making her cry.

'*I* nearly killed it,' Prue said huskily. 'Nearly killed the poor little bugger – '

'You nearly killed yourself, that's what it was,' Ida said. 'That baby's fine. I made sure of that after I heard 'em talking. I can always find things out, I can, and I can tell you those people you went to, they never did your baby no harm at all. I heard Miss Buckland say. "No harm to the pregnancy," she said. They just made you bleed something awful, but she's repaired it, she said, and the pregnancy's all right. So you see – '

'It can't be. Not when I bled so much. I've been counting the bags of blood they give me. Seven it's been. Seven pints of blood I've had. The baby can't be all right, not after that.'

'Well, Miss Buckland says it is, and there you are. They wouldn't say so if it wasn't, would they? You had the scan anyway. That's what they did this afternoon, the scan.'

Prue closed her eyes. 'Is there anything you don't know?'

'Not a lot.' Ida sounded complacent, accepting the compliment. 'I keeps my eyes to the ground and my ears to the fore, know what I mean? And I think about what I hear and make sense out of it. You got to do something, stuck in here – '

'It's time you went home, isn't it?' Prue opened her eyes again and stared at Ida almost desperately. 'You said there was nothing more could be done. Time you wasn't here, if there's nothing they can't do.'

'I didn't say that.' Ida had gone a dull red. 'Not at all. I can have some more tests – she's going to see if I'm right for a test-tube baby, that's what she's going to do. They've got a project, Miss Buckland said, experimental and all that, but a project. And because I'm willing to be a guinea pig they're going to let me try. That's why I'm still here – '

'So if you're going to have a test-tube baby why did you say what you said?' Prue still had that desperate air as she stared at Ida.

'I never said I was having one. It's not that easy.' Ida looked down at her hand, still fastened on Prue's wrist. 'Miss Buckland was very straight with me, very straight she was. It's a one in a million chance, she said. It probably won't work. But I can have a go and she's willing to try for the research. So there's no promises.'

'But suppose it works? What about me then?'

Ida leaned even closer, a smile spreading across her face and making her eyes glitter. 'You'll do it then – '

'I never said so!'

'Well, why ask that if you aren't considerin' it? Eh? Why ask? Anyway, I can tell you it won't be no problem. I'll just tell Tony I had twins – '

'You're mad,' Prue said flatly. 'You'd never get away with it.'

'And how are you going to get away with the state you're in? Owing all that money and your old man abroad – what'll you tell him when he gets back, eh? Bet he'll be pleased when you tell him. "Here, Gary, I got in the club, didn't I? And I tried to get rid of it, borrowed money and will you give it back to Jerry – you know, the fella I went around with before you what you hates so much – give him back the five hundred quid what I owes him and by the way it never worked, and I can't get the money back, even though it never worked – " Can't you just see it?'

Prue was crying now, tears sliding down her cheeks in oily drips but Ida didn't care any more. The nurses were on their tea break, half of them anyway, and the rest were busy with that Mrs Walton down the other end who was still so poorly after her operation. No one would notice.

138

'And here I am with the best idea you'll ever get to sort it out,' Ida went on remorselessly, 'and you turning it down.'

'It won't work,' Prue said huskily. 'It's crazy.'

'It'll work. You can have the baby at your flat, can't you? Or if you like I'll find another place you can go, a nursing home or something. I've got the money, you know. My Tony keeps me short of nothing. I got the money, plenty of it. I'll pay off your Jerry and all the other prices that come in too. All you have to do is what I tell you. It's no trouble to you at all.'

'But it won't be yours!' Prue said. 'What's the good of it if it won't be yours? What good is it to your Tony if it isn't – '

Ida's fingers tightened on her wrist and Prue whimpered and tried to pull her arm away, but Ida held on. 'You ever say a word about it to anyone, anyone at all and you know what'll happen,' she said, and her voice was thin and low but very clear. 'It's just between us, whatever happens, just between us. I can make it all come right, and it's up to me to see it does. And if I do the work then it's the same as if I had it. I've tried everything else and this test tube won't work any more than any of the other things did. I know that. I'm not daft. So, I've got to do what's best for me, don't I? And if at the same time it's best for you, what are you making such a fuss over? Do you want more money? Is that it?'

'I don't want any money,' Prue said and then stopped. 'I mean I'm not selling nothing.'

'Of course you're not. I wouldn't ever say such a thing. But if you want more money as well as what I'm going to have to pay out for clothes and for Jerry and all that, well, if I got to, I got to – '

'I owe a good bit,' Prue said and looked down at her wrist where Ida's fingers were still clamped. 'Nearly a thousand quid, it is.'

'Christ,' Ida said. 'A thousand? What with – well, I can go to two and a half altogether. No more than that. So that should just about cover it. Will you do it then? Will you? I can't see what else you can do. You can't go back to that bloody botcher and get him to try again, can you?'

Prue seemed to shrink into her pillows. 'I couldn't go back – '

'And there won't be anywhere else you can go. I've been around and I know. I'm not stupid, not like some I know. You're too far gone, aren't you? That's what went wrong. You're too far gone. None of the charities'll touch you, not after all that fuss about changing the law and all.'

'I didn't know,' Prue said and there was a little whine in her voice now. 'I never show much and I didn't know. But I kept on being sick and – '

'Well, never mind. We can do it. If you do what I tell you. So say you will, eh? It'll be the best thing you ever did, honest – '

And she leaned over and kissed Prue's cheek with a loud smacking sound, sealing the bargain. But Prue just lay there with her oily tears sliding down her face and said nothing.

'I like it,' Radlett said. 'We could call it, *The NHS, are we* – '

'I've already got a title,' Oliver said hurriedly. '*The Unkindest Cuts of All*. Hmm? Seeing it's cuts in the services we're on about. And the tape the old man made, he talks about Maggie's cuts all the time, doesn't he?'

'We could edit that out – ' Radlett looked sideways at him and then sighed. 'No, I suppose not. Well, OK for a working title. *Unkindest Cuts* it is. Though why you should imagine our lot will understand a Shakespeare quotation I'll never know. They aren't the brightest, you know. We're not bloody Radio Four.'

'They'll understand,' Oliver said. 'If I have to spell it out. OK. I'll need some back-up here. Editing channels and someone with a bit of common sense who knows how to use a razor blade – '

'No way,' Radlett said firmly. 'This is all yours. You can put in a couple of extra expenses if you like, but extra hands you don't get. Do you own bloody editing. If the story's worth doing, it's worth doing all of it.'

'You're a mean bugger,' Oliver said equably. 'You'd think you were spending your own money.'

'The way the bastards upstairs get on my back I might as well be,' Radlett growled. 'So are you on or not? No in-house help at all. Just the use of a Uher. You can take one out and keep it – don't have to hand it in again every day – '

'Big of you,' Oliver said sardonically.

' – but make sure you account for every tape. They cost

money, those tapes. And be sure your exes are legitimate, too. I can't manage that much over the odds, even for a – '

'Watch it,' Oliver said ominously and Radlett lifted his brows at him and turned to go.

'You may not like it, but a star is what you're supposed to be,' he said curtly. 'Anyway, just take it easy. I can slot in an hour one-off by the way, or – '

'I'd rather have a short series. Give me a string of four halves, OK? Then I can spread it a bit further afield than just this business of the one old man losing his operation. There have to be other stories in other hospitals – '

Radlett shook his head decisively. 'Not this time around. Keep it to Old East. That's the representative London story – you know the sort of thing. Cover a lot of hospitals and all you get are single whinges that they can explain away. But you uncover a lot of stories in one place and it makes it a lot harder hitting.'

There was a little silence and then Oliver nodded. 'Fair enough,' and he grinned as the old man went away. He deserved his job, after all, he thought, watching him go slouching down towards the news desk and its clatter of telephones and computer screens. Still got a nose for the way a feature works best.

He stretched and then went padding over to the coffee machine to fill a plastic beaker with the thick black brew. It was a symbol of what had happened to him, he sometimes thought; he actually liked the disgusting stuff now, though he'd hated it when he'd started here. Twelve years, he thought then. Twelve years ago, before Sonia, before Melissa and Barnaby, before Kate – and he went back to his desk and sat there nursing the plastic beaker as he sipped at it, staring over the rim with blank unseeing eyes.

What on earth was he to do? He wanted Kate, of course he did. There were times when he knew that without her nothing would be worth anything any more, even if Sonia disappeared in a puff of smoke and left him the children without any problems. If Kate weren't there as well, life would be hell.

And yet, and yet – and he closed his eyes against the image that had risen into his mind, of Sonia, sitting up in bed with just the duvet between them, staring at him in that hard direct way she had always used and daring him to deny that he could still be

141

used by her in any way she wanted. He could have beaten her for the easy way she had made him react to her the last time he had gone to see her, the night he and Kate had gone to dinner with Esther and that boring husband of hers. Had that been why it had happened? Because he was bored by Richard and irritated at Kate for making him spend an evening in his company? Had he let Sonia get him into her bed just because of that? Surely not. Could he be so childish, so feeble, so −

'Yes, I could,' he whispered into the plastic beaker and the surface of the coffee stirred beneath the puff of his breath and sent its sickly smell up into his nostrils. 'Yes, I could.'

But it hadn't been just boredom. Because the evening hadn't been that bad, after all. There had been Esther and she was fun, a good friend to Kate and therefore to him too. Or at least so he hoped, though sometimes he had caught her looking at him with a considering stare and had wondered just what she said to Kate when the two of them were alone together. Did Esther advise Kate to drop him, to go away from him, to do without him? It would be good advice, for what good was a lover who was still tied up in knots by his bloody ex-wife? Who couldn't make the courts understand what was happening to his children at her hands? What good was he to anyone?

'I'm a good reporter,' he whispered then. 'A good reporter,' and then drained his coffee and chucked the beaker into the overflowing waste bin. He had four twenty-five minute programmes to plan out, and the sooner he made a start on it the better. There were people to be called, appointments to be made and ideas to be thrashed out. And he'd better start by getting some hard facts into his head.

And he reached for the phone to call his old mate Jimmy Rhoda on the *Globe*. It was a bloody nuisance always having to go outside the station to get access to a decent newspaper library. He'd been telling them that here for years, that they ought to keep a decent newspaper-type morgue but they ignored him, of course. Just kept tapes of past programmes, as though they were any use. That was the trouble with a station that worried itself as much about pop music as about its talk output. But Jimmy would help him out. He always did, and why not? Oliver had helped him out a good deal in their early years together at the

Beeb. And he sighed and keyed Jimmy's number on the phone
and settled down to some real work.

'Koestler,' Jimmy Rhoda said to the chief sub. 'Thou shouldst be
living at this hour. That's the guy. He said it all.'

The chief sub stared at him owlishly and said nothing, turning
back to the console of his computer, hitting the keys with a stub
of a forefinger to send columns of words crawling up the screen
in front of him.

'Why do I say that, do I hear you ask?' Jimmy said and sat on
the desk beside him. 'Yes, I thought I did. Well, I shall tell you.
Gladly. There's this chap Oliver Merrall — Ah! I detect a
response from you? The king of the call-in shows, you got it in
one. We started at the Beeb together fifteen years ago, straight
out of university, damp and pearly about the ears and dripping
with integrity we were. Happily I saw the light and jumped into
this illustrious pile of shit while he went off to beguile the
airwaves even further with a voice he used to practise with every
night in bed. A serious chap, old Oliver — '

'Have you got any copy to put in?' the chief sub growled. 'I'm
locking up your pages at half past six and — '

'Listen to me, you old bastard!' Jimmy said. 'I'm telling you
something sensible if you did but know it. Oliver rings me just
now, will I dig around in the morgue for him, get some stuff on
NHS troubles and especially Old East, the hospital in Shadwell.
Right. And here in my hot little hand, what do I have?'

'Your chopper most of the time,' the chief sub muttered and
went on stabbing at his console.

'Vulgarian. Of course. But what else? A letter, no less!
Someone has sent the editor a letter. It's from a patient in — wait
for it. Old East.'

'So?'

'So this patient has a story to tell! For a consideration.'

'Oh.' The chief sub looked bored. 'Another one of those "I'll
tell all for a million, settle for half if you insist, send a cheque." '

'Something like that,' Jimmy said. 'Something like that. But
it's a good tale. At least the way it reads in this letter it's a good
tale.'

There was a little silence between them as he sat and reread the letter and the chief sub sighed noisily after a while and said, 'Are you going to tell me or not? If not, get your arse off my desk and leave me alone. If you are, tell me and then get your arse off my desk and leave me alone.'

'Mm?' Jimmy Rhoda said and then grinned and ruffled the chief sub's thinning hair with one hand. 'I don't think I will after all. It's a nice story and I want to try it on the Ed. If she goes for it, then I'll follow it up. If she doesn't then I'll try it for the *Herald* diary – '

'One of these days they'll catch you at your little games,' the chief sub said. 'Selling stuff to the bloody opposition.'

'Yeah, well, one of these days,' Jimmy said and went back to his own desk, whistling between his teeth. First he had to get the stuff out of the morgue for old Oliver. That would be a pleasure, because he was a good guy, and anyway he was entitled to his payment for the lead he'd dropped in his, Jimmy's, lap. It might turn out to be nothing or it might turn out to be a real Koestler coincidence of the best kind. There could well be something worth sniffing out at Old East, and I've had two prods to send me on my way. Can't be bad.

It took just ten minutes to sort out with the library what Oliver wanted and then he punched the number nine on his phone for an outside line and keyed another number.

'Old East?' he said at length and smiled into the receiver. 'I'm just checking about visiting times in the ward where a friend of mine is. Kim Hynes. Can you tell me the name of the ward and what time is all right to visit? Hmm? Yes – yes. Ah – thank you so much!' And he hung up and sat there for a while with a pleased grin on his face.

Chapter Fifteen

The day had started badly on the ward: by the time Esther got on duty they were already at least half an hour behind so she walked into a state of barely controlled uproar that did nothing at all for her already unreliable temper. And when the night staff nurse told her, sweating a little around the ears and with her hair in a tangle on her forehead so that she looked more like an anxious Old English sheepdog than ever, that Jenny Caversham's fistula had clotted at around six a.m. and that while they were dealing with that, the old man, William Prior, who'd been admitted as an emergency a week ago and who had been nothing but trouble since he got in, had needed a new shunt made during the night because his Silastic tube had displaced and he had started a terrifying arterial bleed, she hit the roof.

'You idiot,' she roared. 'Didn't I warn you to watch that man like a hawk? The way he behaves it was inevitable he'd shift the bloody thing if he wasn't supervised. I told them he was a bad candidate for a shunt anyway – should have had a subclavian catheterisation – I suppose he was on his own, hmm? Was that it?'

'I'm sorry, Sister,' the staff nurse stammered, almost in tears. 'So sorry, but it was Jenny, you see. She was very disturbed and woke the others, and then Kim Hynes got agitated too and we were running from one to the other and – '

'Oh, forget it,' Esther said savagely, 'and let me get it all sorted out. Who's here to deal with Jenny?'

'Miss Sayers is on her way,' the staff nurse said. 'Sister Russell said she'd send for her, and there's the new houseman – I can't remember his name – '

'That's all I need,' Esther said and kicked off her shoes to put on her ward pair. 'A half-witted houseman who doesn't know one end of a dialysis catheter from another and – oh, go off duty, for heaven's sake, girl – you look ghastly!' And she felt a moment of guilt, for the girl did indeed look exhausted, and justifiably so; she knew from her own experience what hell her ward could be when things went wrong. Somehow problems always happened in clusters like this; never one thing at a time that people could cope with.

Just like home, and she scowled as she went hurrying up the ward to check on Jenny Caversham. Richard had been perfectly ridiculous this morning, expecting her to go all that long way round to deliver his bloody sandwiches to the Gants Hill place and being thoroughly impossible when she had of course refused; then the kids had been in a whining mood, losing socks and swimming gear and heaven knows what else besides and on top of all that Richard had started on yet again about it being time for her to stop all this stupid nursing lark and start working for the family business, so inevitably she had lost her temper. And now this. She'd deserved a peaceful happy ward this morning, not this shambles; and her eyes were hot with anger and self-pity as she reached Jenny's curtained bed in the end section and marched in.

The young doctor standing there looked up anxiously and then his face cleared as he saw her.

'Thank heavens it's you,' he said fervently, and looked down at the patient. 'We'll get this sorted out in no time now, Jenny. Sister's here.'

Jenny, who was lying with her eyes tightly closed the way she always did when she was alarmed, said nothing, but she managed a twist of her mouth that Esther knew was a welcome and for a moment her spirits lifted a little. At least here they were glad to see her, and weren't always complaining the way they did at home –

'Kate's on her way?' she said as she began to check on the tangle of tubes and connections to the machine that ran into Jenny's left wrist. 'How's it going now?'

'She's coming,' the houseman said. 'I'm afraid I woke her when I phoned, but I thought – anyway, she's on her way. It seems to be running though it's a bit slow. I've heparinised her and – '

'Did you get the thrombus out?'

He flushed. 'I tried, but – '

She nodded. 'OK. It's not the easiest of things to do. Just let me get there, will you?'

For the next little while there was silence as she worked her way through the various steps needed to get out the thick stringy clot that had stopped the easy flow of blood, and all the time Jenny lay with her eyes tightly closed, and the houseman watched, and when at last she had finished and the system was working properly again, Esther felt a moment of glow; for Jenny opened her eyes at last and looked at her and the houseman said softly, 'Oh, neat. Very neat.' It helped a lot to have that sort of approval.

The next half-hour was even busier as she harried her staff to catch up with the morning's routine, and when one of the orderlies serving breakfast burst into tears in the kitchen because 'Sister shouted at me for nothing', and she had to send for the domestic supervisor to get rid of the woman who couldn't be trusted to obey instructions and had been discovered giving a bacon and egg breakfast to one of the low-protein diet patients, all Esther's bad temper came flooding back. It shouldn't be like this. She should have enough nurses to do all that had to be done, and properly trained orderlies too. She shouldn't have to be such a slave driver to make sure the patients were properly looked after, and when Kate arrived, looking a little ruffled by her early call, Esther almost snapped at her instead of being glad to see her. Which made Kate, who had had a difficult morning on her own account with Oliver being somewhat distant, very snappy too. Altogether a bad start to the day.

And it got no easier. Kim Hynes, now allowed out of bed for a little while, flatly refused to cooperate with the nurses sent to get her on her feet, and burst into floods of hysterical tears when Esther tried to find out why she was being so obstructive. The noise she made and her copious tears – which though genuine enough as far as Esther could tell, were very obvious and indeed theatrical – upset all the other patients at that end of the ward, including Jenny, who began to thrash about and so threaten to dislodge her tubes yet again.

'Kim, for heaven's sake, be quiet!' Esther snapped at the heap of quivering pink silk that had thrown itself face down on its pillows and refused to be comforted. 'If you want to stay in bed and rot, then stay there. Just don't blame me if you get all sorts of complications from lack of exercise and the wrong breathing, that's all. I'm more than happy to let you make your own decisions – but for the love of heaven shut up and stop upsetting all my other patients. There's Jenny in a lather over you and if that leads to trouble with her dialysis again, I swear to you I'll be here to scrag you!'

Kim's shoulders heaved convulsively and the red-gold hair trembled as she banged her face into the pillow even harder, but she did lessen her noise a little and that gave Esther time to sort out Jenny yet again. She hated using tranquillisers more than she had to, but sometimes they were inevitable. And this was one of them.

By the time Jenny had settled to lie staring vaguely at the machine beside her Kim was sitting up in bed again, and as Esther passed on her way back to her desk she called in a weak voice, 'Sister – oh, please, Sister, do let me talk to you.'

Esther glared at her for a moment, irritated beyond measure by the way Kim looked at her with heavy pathetic eyes and a tremulous mouth. That the poor devil had problems and needed help was undoubted; right from the start Esther had been truly sympathetic to her unusual patient's needs, but the last few days, in which Kim had given in with luxurious abandon to a tendency to histrionics, had tried her patience sorely. It would have been much easier to snap at her now and march away but there was something about Kim's stare that was more than display. And she sighed and came to stand at the side of the bed.

'Well, Kim. Do you want to apologise for making such a drama?'

Mutely Kim nodded, gazing up at her with big appealing eyes. And Esther patted her hand and turned to go.

'Well, well. All forgotten then. Just try to be a little more aware of other people in future, that's all. And do as the nurses tell you. They're here for your health, you know, not their own – '

'Sister, don't go!' Kim reached out and held on to her and Esther looked down at her more sharply, for the hand was moist and a little shaky. She reached for the pulse and stood there with it thudding under her fingertips and then reached for the thermometer in its little cup on the wall at the head of the bed.

'And what have you been up to to get yourself so overheated?' she said as she slid the glass tube under Kim's tongue. 'Your wound's nice and clean and your output seems all right. Are you drinking enough?'

Kim nodded, still staring up at Esther with imploring eyes, and then as Esther took the thermometer from her mouth and twisted it to read it, she burst out, 'I'm so worried, Sister! Tell me what to do!'

'Worried about what?' Esther put the thermometer back in its cup. Only half a degree up; not enough to get really bothered about. It was excitement that had caused the fast pulse and the hot hand, not a fever. Something to be grateful for; the last thing they wanted was another bout of theatre infections. She remembered all too well what hell it had been the last time that had happened.

'I – it's so hard to explain. But – well, money, I suppose.'

Esther cocked an eyebrow. 'My dear Kim, aren't we all worried about money? I wish I had enough. I doubt you're that much worse off than the rest of us. You've got a good job, haven't you? And no one to depend on you? Or have you been spending too much on fripperies?' And she took one of the frills of Kim's pink silk bedjacket and slid it between her fingers. 'This must have cost a bomb.'

'It did,' Kim said mournfully. 'I thought when I bought it I'd have no problems – but the thing is, I got this awful letter. The day before yesterday.' Her eyes filled with tears again and she looked more woebegone than ever as she held the letter out to Esther. 'I mean, right after my huge operation a letter like this! What am I to do, Sister? What on earth am I to do? I'm desperate! I've got the mortgage to think of and the insurances and all that, and I'm behind as it is, and I'd meant to have a lovely convalescent week before I went back to work – oh, Sister, what shall I do?'

Esther had been reading the letter, and now she folded it and gave it back. 'Oh, Kim, I am sorry. Who is this Morris?'

'He's a shit, that's what he is!' Kim said hotly. 'He's always been after me, but I thought – I had old Mr Morris on my side, you see. This one's uncle. As sweet an old man as you ever met. Live and let live, that was his motto. He always said I was good at my job, he liked my stuff, so he said it made no odds to him what else I did and he let me stay on when I started my change. But now this! That bastard Ian, he's always been after me. Not like Mr Lew – '

'Well maybe it is as he says, Kim. If they're changing the sort of merchandise they're making and your designs just don't fit in – I mean, you're a very – well, you have a decided taste of your own, haven't you?' She tried not to look disapprovingly at the pink silk and its lavish lace trimmings. 'But surely you can go somewhere else? It might be better at that – '

'Somewhere they don't know about me, you mean? I should cocoa! Listen, Sister, the rag trade's like a village. A bloody village. Everyone knows everyone else's business, take it from me. There won't be a firm anywhere from Great Titchfield Street to Margaret Street and back who won't know all about me. And what's worse, more than there is to know. They'll tell such lies about me no one'll dare to take me on. I needed this job – oh, Christ how I needed it! I won't get another that easy – '

'Well, I'm not sure what I can suggest – '

'Do you know anyone that'd lend me money?'

Esther lifted her brows. 'Me? Where do I know people with money?' She made a face. 'My husband's a businessman, Kim, so I know how tough it is to get money even to run a business. Let alone for your own personal use – '

'I meant for my own business. I thought maybe – ' Kim stared up at her again, once more producing her pathetic look. 'I'm ever such a good designer, honestly I am. I understand what it is people like me need and there are ever such a lot of us. I thought, if I could borrow enough, I could start my own business, sell the stuff mail order maybe, to start with, and then get a shop of my own somewhere. I could pay it back in a year or two, I'm sure I could – '

'Listen Kim, if I had enough money to start a business, I might start my own,' Esther said and shook her head. 'I wish I could help, but truly – '

'Then I'll have to do it,' Kim murmured, and Esther said, 'Do what?'

'Oh nothing. It's just that – well I thought if I could get some money quietly I would. But there's another way I might be able to do it. It won't be nice, but there – '

Esther had reached the end of the bed, on her way back to her piled-up paperwork, but now she stopped. 'What do you mean?'

Kim wouldn't look at her now, just sitting there in bed with her head bent. 'It's nothing, Sister. Thanks for letting me sound off. I just thought – well, it's not important. Do you want me to get up now? I'll have a try if you do.' And now she did look up and smiled bravely at Esther, who stood for a moment longer and then said briskly, 'I'll send the little first year, Sian. She'll help you. And make sure you don't make too much fuss and disturb Jenny. She's resting.'

'I won't, Sister,' Kim said and smiled at her and she went away thinking – I must have a word with the social worker about her. See if she can sort things out. But before she got back to her desk she was waylaid by Mr Le Queux, complaining bitterly about the way his patient, Jenny Caversham, had been seen by Miss Sayers this morning after her dialysis had run into trouble. Why had she been sent for, and why had Sister not notified him and –

Esther sighed and readied herself for a long fifteen minutes trying to soothe him. It was the only answer she had found over the years of dealing with him; most of the time he was harmless enough, as long as everyone fussed round him, but every so often he found it necessary to jump on his highest horse and then it paid to coax him down with the most honeyed words she could find. Today it wasn't easy, because she was irritable anyway, but she had the wit and foresight to know that if she didn't make the effort she'd pay for it heavily in the future. So, she sent for coffee and biscuits for him and led him into her small office to explain.

Kate by this time had left the ward to do her outpatient clinic and Esther was glad of that, though she would have liked a chance to talk to her before she went, just to make sure they were friends again. It was miserable when they were snappy with each other; life was complicated enough without that. And Esther badly needed the chance to talk to her about Richard, and what she should do about his nagging. It would be so much easier to give in and become what he wanted her to be, a restaurateur with him. But she'd miss Old East abominably. Or would she? She really needed to talk to Kate.

But first, Le Queux, and she settled now to explain to him how she had told her night staff only to call him out if it was really essential to disturb him.

'I always say, sir, that it's a waste of time to make you come if we can deal with it without bothering you. Even for your patients. I mean, you have a list this afternoon and it would never do to lose your sleep before you operate, would it? You've told me that yourself. Well, clearly the staff nurse on last night understood that much but instead of checking with me about how to deal with the matter of Jenny's thrombosed fistula she called Miss Sayers. I think she gets mixed up, actually.' Now she played her trump card. 'I'm not sure she realises that Miss Sayers isn't – er – your registrar.'

As she had known he would, Le Queux bridled and then preened a little. He had fought tooth and nail, Esther knew, to block Kate's appointment to the junior consultancy. He'd wanted an older man, and one of his own kidney, a bad joke that had gone round the hospital like wildfire at the time. When Kate had got the post he'd been furious. Now to hear her described as little more than his registrar helped a lot and Esther watched him go marching self-importantly down the ward to start his round with a slight tinge of guilt. I really must call Kate and tell her what I did. She'll laugh, I know. I mean, I hope she will. Oh, damn. This is turning out to be a pig of a day.

But it still wasn't over. At half past twelve, just as they were up to their eyes serving the lunches with two orderlies short because of the loss of the stupid one this morning and the refusal of any of the others in the hospital to take her place, and a threat to turn the whole episode of the misplaced bacon and eggs into a Union issue, a patient arrived in a wheelchair from Psych accompanied by an anxious-looking young first-year boy.

'Please, Sister,' he said. 'Staff Nurse said I was to bring Mr Lloyd for his cystoscopy, and that I couldn't stay with him because we're too short-staffed and please when he's ready to come back could you call a porter and then – '

'What?' Esther roared. 'You're short-staffed? On Psych? And I'm supposed to – not on your nelly, young man. You phone your staff nurse and tell her from me that if she wants this patient to be seen here on this ward then he has to be accompanied by one of her nurses. I've no one to spare. Anyway, why isn't he being done in Outpatients?'

'They're having trouble with the examinees, Sister.'

Her own staff nurse looked up from the food trolley where she was trying to sort out the individual diets. 'I'm sorry — I should have told you. Miss Sayers called up to tell me. They've got the first-year medical students doing their vivas there, and they've sent over more than they expected from St Kitts, so Sister in OP said they'd have to do the cystoscopies up here instead of there. And she said — '

'Did she, by God!' roared Esther. 'Sister OP said that, did she? And why did no one think to ask *me* whether I could accommodate 'em, hmm? Answer me that.'

Staff Nurse went rather white. 'Well, actually, Sister, I said — you were up to your ears with Mr Le Queux and I knew you wouldn't want me to interrupt, so I said it'd be all right. We've got the treatment room free this afternoon. We did all the important jobs there this morning and I thought, by two o'clock when they want to start them, it'd be all right. I'm sorry, Sister. It's all my fault.'

There is nothing of course that makes anyone angrier than being offered an explanation and apology and having all reason to complain thereby removed, and Esther was no exception. For the next ten minutes she harangued her staff nurses, snapped at the young male first year from Psych and thoroughly indulged her own bad temper, and that seemed to get to the old man who had been sitting happily slumped in his wheelchair. Suddenly he began shouting in a loud strong voice and waving his arms about; what he was shouting no one was able to work out, though the nurse looking after him seemed to cope well enough, bending over the old man and muttering in his ear, but it added to the fluster that had attacked the ward since early morning and for two pins, as Esther told her staff nurse wrathfully, she'd go off sick right now, this very instant —

At which point Kate arrived from OP and went straight up to Esther and said coolly, 'I'm sorry not to have phoned you sooner, but I have to tell you I've agreed with Professor Levy to take a

153

patient over here from Male Surgical. I hope that won't make life too tricky, Esther, but I knew you'd manage somehow. He'll be over here in a half-hour – I have to cystoscope him and then maybe operate. I'll explain it all to you later – it's a rather tricky situation.'

But the damage was done. That was the point at which Esther really lost her temper.

Chapter Sixteen

David went off the ward to go to the special lecture for the first years with a sigh of relief. It was tiresome to have an extra lecture chucked at them like this instead of waiting for their usual study block but the Pawn had said it was a vital one on Medical Ethics and this was the only time the professor could fit it in, so there it was. The first years had to be there or else. Of course, he'd muttered and moaned with the rest of them when it had first been posted on the board and their clinical tutors had warned them what would happen if they missed it, but now he was glad. Life on Male Med had been absolute hell all morning. Getting away had a lot going for it.

'I've had the worst morning ever,' Sian announced as she caught up with him in the yard on the way over to the nurses' lecture theatre. 'I thought Esther Pelham was all right, but this morning, Christ, what a bitch! Never stopped bawling at everyone long enough to catch her breath.'

'Do you call her Esther to her face?' David said, momentarily diverted. 'You made such a fuss over the business of names before we started but I'll bet you're the same as the rest of us now and call her "Sister" – '

'I never talk to her at all if I can help it,' Sian said. 'Bitch that she is. Some poor orderly on our ward, been there donkey's years, she has, got such a lathering over accidentally giving a patient the wrong breakfast, you'd think the sky had fallen in. Chicken-Licken wasn't in it with Esther-Lester, believe me. I told her, the orderly, go to the Union, I said. She can't go on at you like that, not when no harm's been done anyway. The fella never ate it – Sister saw and shrieked so loudly, poor bugger lost his appetite altogether – '

'But maybe it would have been awful if she hadn't noticed. Was he an operation case, then? If he had been and he'd eaten it and then had an anaesthetic and choked to death, the orderly could have killed him, couldn't she?'

'Oh, balls,' Sian said a little uncomfortably. 'It wasn't like that. He was just a kidney on a low-protein diet. It wouldn't have – '

'What did she give him?'

'Bacon and eggs, and – '

'And you told the woman to go to the Union?' David jeered. 'Honestly, Sian, you really are the pits. She ought to be chucked out, not protected. She's dangerous – '

'Why?' Sian flared at him. 'Just because she's an orderly it doesn't mean she can be walked all over. She's got rights too, you know, and these bloody sisters who think they know it all – '

'They know more than your stupid orderly, that's for sure,' David said. 'Listen, if you're looking for Union fights, you ought to be with me. We've had a much worse bloody morning than you have. What's going on makes me so mad I could spit. I think the Unions are a waste of time, but even I'd complain over this Saffron business – '

'We have,' Sian said. 'Much bloody good it's done. He's a real twister, that one. If we make any fuss about him being on an NHS ward, then they open their eyes wide and say do we want him to go to a private ward, and if we say it's all wrong he's got private nurses, they say it's so that the other patients won't be put out or suffer, and that anyway it's because of security, on account he used to be the Northern Ireland Minister. Whatever we say they come up with a fancy answer. But don't think we're not trying. Look at that!'

And she pointed at the demonstrators outside the Medical School who could now clearly be seen, still waving their home-made placards and banners as they marched dolorously from front to back of the building. 'They're there specially so Saffron can see them from his window. The best thing you can do is make sure he does – '

'Oh, we don't get anywhere near him,' David said. 'There he sits up at his end with everyone fussing over him but *we* never get near him. We're not important enough.' He laughed then. 'Mind you, one of the visitors did and there's been no end of a fuss ever since. She nagged Saffron because we can't keep her husband in a bed any longer even though he's dying, poor devil, and so Saffron nagged Sister and his consultant and the consultant's

156

been on at Sister for letting the woman get near him and she got mad at the consultant and they've been fighting and in the middle of it all we've got other patients on the ward who shouldn't be there and he's found out – oh, it was rich this morning. I wish you'd seen it all. You'd have loved it – '

'Mr Saffron,' Vera Sheward said firmly. 'There is nothing I can do about this. This is an open NHS ward and not a prison. If patients and their visitors wander about then there it is. They've every right to. I can't lock them out of half the ward, can I?'

'I don't see why not.' Saffron sat bolt upright against his pillows, staring at her with eyes mostly hidden by the reflection of the light on his thick glasses. That made Vera uneasy; it would have been easier to cope if he didn't give back that blank cartoon character sort of glare. 'And it is not half the ward, is it? Merely a segment of it. But let that pass. I am simply making the point that some privacy is not an unreasonable request. If you were doing something to a patient behind a curtain, you wouldn't allow any other patients to come wandering in, would you?'

'Of course not. That's the purpose of curtains. Of course, if you're saying you want your bed permanently curtained – '

'Sister, you know I am not. I am asking you, simply, to please leave me in peace here. To tell your patients not to come into this section. A plain enough request, I would have thought.'

'This section is part of my ward, and therefore available to *all* my patients,' she said stubbornly. 'And I can't possibly ban people from it. If a physio tells patients they have to walk three lengths of the ward two or three times a day – which they often prescribe – then that is what they must do. To make them reduce their exercise simply to accommodate a special patient who is being given unusual status – '

The colour in his cheeks seemed to increase and she felt a moment's unease. He wasn't her patient, of course; that had been made manifestly clear to her by the private nurses who had been brought in. She could feel the furious glare of the one now standing at the far side of Saffron's bed, even without looking at her. But one of her own patients or not, the man was ill; he was in here for investigation and treatment of cardiac insufficiency and to harangue him as she had been was hardly fair. But

157

dammit all, she'd had Byford on her back most of the morning, complaining at her. She had every right to give the man back some of the trouble he was causing – but she bit her tongue now.

'Well, Mr Saffron,' she said, peaceably enough. 'I'll do what I can. But I hope you have some clearer understanding now of what life is like for so many of our more ill patients and their families. No one is trying to make things hard for you, but – '

'Some success is being enjoyed all the same,' Saffron said and rested his head back on his pillow. 'I've assured Mrs – what was her name? – I've assured her that I will see to it efforts are made on her behalf. I can't do more.'

'You'd better rest, now,' Vera said and turned to go. 'I'm afraid there may be some disturbance later this afternoon because we have a special case that will need to go down to the operating theatre, but we'll try not to cause too much upheaval – '

'Thank you, Sister,' the private nurse said icily and Vera flicked a glance at her and then went away, guiltily aware of the way Saffron was looking. Far from well. The sooner Byford finished what he had to do for him and let him go home to get over it all the better. And for a moment she felt a pang of real pity. He was not a pleasant man, Saffron, being pompous in the most ridiculous way and to a degree that had amazed Vera. Could the stereotyped notions of politicians be in fact accurate? He was also selfish and arrogant. But his life was clearly a difficult one, for even while he was here dealing with a potentially life-threatening illness the work did not stop. The steady traffic of secretarial and security people drove her nearly to distraction. What must it be like for the man at the hub of it all? She shook her head at the images that conjured up as she reached the end of the ward where Mr Holliday was sitting in a wheelchair waiting for a porter.

'Well, Mr Holliday!' she said cheerfully, at last pushing Saffron out of her thoughts. 'Do you feel as good as you look?'

'Better,' the man said after a moment, and she smiled even more widely for the change in his speech was marked. Without the rigidity of muscles which had locked his mouth and throat and tongue in a harsh grip his words, though slurred, were much more comprehensible now.

'And your physio – how does she say you're getting on?'

'Marvellous,' the man said and slowly smiled. It was a difficult grimace, and could have looked like a leer, but since for many years even that much had been impossible for a face locked in a Parkinsonian blankness, it was a major achievement and Vera felt her spirits lift as she looked at him.

'I know Mr Bulpitt's delighted with you,' she said and leaned over to wrap his rug more firmly round his knees. 'And I do hope the improvement is maintained or even increased. Keep in touch if you can – even after you get home. Let me know how things are – '

'Can you spare a minute, Sister?' Mr Holliday's eyes flickered as he shifted his gaze over her shoulder. 'Wife'll be back in a minute – need to ask you – '

Vera crouched beside him to hear him better. His voice was improved perhaps, but still difficult to follow.

'I don't mind waiting for her if you want her to explain,' she said kindly. 'Don't exhaust yourself – '

'No – can't talk to her. She gets annoyed. Listen, Sister.' He stopped and swallowed and automatically she leaned forwards to wipe his mouth with the towel kept tied to the side of the chair, and then stopped herself. It really was remarkable; before his operation he had salivated all the time. Now it was clear he could get rid of it all for himself. Remarkable.

'So tell me,' she said. 'What is it?'

'I'm worried about the woman,' Mr Holliday said and she peered more closely at him. He must have been good-looking once, she thought; a thin bony man with a well-shaped head, and good thick hair still, even though rather grey, and large dark eyes which lit up the wreckage of an interesting face. The patch of bald skin on his scalp where he had been shaved to make his operation possible gave him a rather endearing infantile air, and she wanted to hug him, to rid his face of the pathetic look that seemed to hang over its smoothness.

'What woman, Mr Holliday?' His wife perhaps? It wouldn't be surprising if he were frightened of her, come to think of it, Vera told herself. A small and very birdlike lady who looked at first sight to be a fragile creature, she was in fact a whirlwind of activity, much given to streams of chatter and sharp little actions

159

that pushed her helpless husband about his bed as easily as if he were a bag of laundry. Vera had to be very firm with her to prevent her taking over half the ward. 'Who worries you?'

'The injection,' he said and stared at her very hard. His voice seemed less capable now as he became tired. 'The woman what gave it me. Is she all right?'

Vera frowned. 'But it was Mr Bulpitt who did the operation –' she began but Mr Holliday closed his eyes in clear exasperation and then snapped them open to stare at her again.

'No – the stuff I had. The woman whose baby – is she all right?'

'Ah.' Slowly Vera straightened up and her knees creaked as she flexed her strained muscles surreptitiously. 'Well, she's fine,' she said after a moment, speaking heartily. Too heartily perhaps. 'You needn't worry about her – '

'I do,' Mr Holliday said. 'I worry all the time. Did she – does she know?'

'Know what?' Vera was hedging for time and knew it. She could see through the big double doors to the lift gates from which Mrs Holliday had just emerged and was standing talking with great vivacity to one of the nurses. Come on, woman, she thought. Come and get me out of this –

'Does she know about my operation?' Mr Holliday managed the words in a little rush, as though the only way to get them out was to push them out. 'Did she say it was all right?'

'But no one has to say it was all right for you to have an operation, Mr Holliday. Only you – '

Mr Holliday looked at her with such intensity that Vera felt her face redden. There was animosity in that glare now.

'You know what I mean,' he said and his failing voice made the words seem almost menacing. 'That woman and her baby – '

'The pregnancy had to end, Mr Holliday,' she said. 'I can't go into details, it wouldn't be right. But I can tell you that if the doctors hadn't operated she'd have died. They told me that, because I wanted to know too. Could have died before the baby was due to be born. It had to be done.'

He tried to nod but managed only a tremor. 'I know that, Mr

160

Bulpitt said. But did they tell her what they were doing? Did she get asked?'

The big double doors at the end of the ward opened and Mrs Holliday came bursting through them with her usual headlong rush, titupping along on her high-heeled shoes like an anxious sparrow, talking all the time.

' — so when I said, she changed it, so there's no need to worry, Reg. We've got the transport all fixed up and the home help and the laundry and Miss Allen's ever so good in the Social Services department, very kind and helpful, and says she'll see to it Mr Bulpitt knows all that is happening, now are you ready, dear? That's right then, all set to go and maybe we can get Sister to send her porter to see us on our way. Thank you, Sister, you've all been wonderful, really wonderful — '

Mr and Mrs Holliday disappeared in a backwash of chatter as she harried the porter along with Mr Holliday's chair and Vera watched her go with mixed feelings. If only the man hadn't waited so long to talk about it, she would have been able to sort it out, get Laurence Bulpitt to come and talk to him perhaps; but as it was — and she straightened her back and turned away as she saw Neville Carr getting out of the lift into which the Hollidays had disappeared.

He would want to spend some considerable time over Joe this afternoon, now that he'd had his last chemo, and there was the matter of his bed to discuss. Had Saffron really managed to arrange matters so that she was given the extra beds she needed, and could Joe stay a little longer? Maybe he had managed to get Byford to agree to get rid of some of his long-term patients; they really ought to be in a geriatric ward, and she'd been telling him that for heaven knows how long. If he at last had seen the light, she would have good cause to be grateful to Saffron after all . . . So, despite a rough morning, things might be looking up on Male Medical, after all, she thought, and went to meet Neville Carr.

Chapter Seventeen

'I'd rather not let him in,' Herne said and pulled his chair closer to Professor Levy's desk, trying not to notice that the Dean's office looked even shabbier than usual, if that was possible. 'But if I refuse it looks as though we've got something to hide. And they'll make more of that than they've any right to do. On the other hand if I do let him in, God only knows what some idiot of a porter mightn't come out with, and you can't trust these media people to know the difference between what porters say and what we say – '

'What porters say has been known to be more direct and to the point than anything that ever comes out of your offices,' Professor Levy murmured. 'Are you asking if – '

Herne scowled. 'Of course I'm asking,' he said, even though of course he had been doing nothing of the kind. 'The last thing I want to do is waste your time, let alone my own. I have a job to do here as well, you know.'

'Oh, well do I know it,' Professor Levy said and smiled sweetly. 'You've made it into a very important job.' At which Herne first bridled with pleasure and then frowned; it was impossible to know when this bloody man was being serious and when he was sending you up. 'Well, since you ask, I'd say let him in. He'll make his programme anyway. You can't stop him. This way you can at least put in your own sixpenn'orth.'

'Hmph,' Herne said. 'Well, I've got better things to do than talk to the wretched man. All he wants to go on about is cuts, cuts, cuts. As though Old East was the only place to be suffering.'

'As far as I'm concerned it's the only place whose suffering matters,' Levy said with a sudden flash of energy. 'And if you felt the same sort of partisanship it mightn't be a bad idea. Maybe you'd fight a bit harder for us. As it is you give the impression sometimes of acting more as an apologist for the DHSS than a person responsible for management here.'

'That's nonsense,' Herne said huffily. 'I simply have the sense to take a global view and don't pretend that the sun rises and sets in just one hospital. But that doesn't mean I don't care about this place. Of course I do. It's my job to care – '

'But it's inside the DHSS that your own career will grow, isn't it? Not here,' Levy said. 'Oh, forget it, Herne. I'm tired of digging over this old ground. Is that all? This chap and his programme. Was there anything else?'

Herne sniffed and bent his head over the sheaf of papers in front of him. This weekly meeting with the Dean of the Medical School was supposed to facilitate the smooth running of the hospital; as far as Herne was concerned it just gave the bloody man another chance to stir up trouble. The way he went on you'd never think there was a Region to worry about let alone an Area Health Authority –

'I'd be glad if you would stop encouraging those demonstrators to go on about things they don't understand. What do they know of NHS finance?' he said loudly then, and lifted his chin to stare at Levy. 'They have no right to be here and you should call the police and get them evicted from the hospital premises. *Your* section of the hospital premises, as you've pointed out to me often enough – '

'Why don't you tell them? You've as much right to do so as I have.'

Herne flushed. 'And have you call out all the medical students to join in and turn it into a complete circus? I'm not as green as that, you know.'

'I wouldn't dream of calling out the medical students, even if they'd listen, which is highly unlikely,' Levy said and then laughed. 'Anyway, they need no calls, believe me. I'm surprised they haven't joined in already.'

'They might as well have done.' Herne sounded savage now. 'The way they feed them with tea and buns – probably hospital property at that. Look, Professor, you know perfectly well that if *you* talk to these demonstrators they'll go away and the students won't come out unless they know you're in agreement with their being there. You've got the whole school eating out of your hand and – '

'How agreeable for a Dean,' Levy said. 'And rather rare. But I doubt if it's quite so clear cut, you know.'

'Do you? Well, I don't. And please believe me, these demonstrators are doing no one any good. The DHSS people see their presence here while Saffron's on the premises as a clear indication that we lack control over the place and – '

'Ah!' Levy said. 'I see now! They're after you, are they, because of it? That's why you want them out.'

Herne reddened. 'Well, of course they blame me! It's what I'm for, dammit, being blamed for everything. The patients and the unions blame me for the cuts, you and the rest of the medical staff blame me for the state of the budgets, with all of you wanting to spend like lunatics and to hell with every other department, and the DHSS says all of it's my fault no matter what happens. It'd serve you all right if I just walked out on the lot of you. I could go into the City, I swear, and earn a great deal more for half the effort.'

'You should,' Levy said. 'And I don't mean that unkindly. I think all you managers should get out of the NHS. We ran it all well enough in the past without any of you – a good matron and a few of her senior sisters and the medical staff and between us we kept the hospitals running like melted butter – '

'Yes,' Herne said and got to his feet. 'Those were the days when you had to send nurses out into the street with trays of little flags to sell and had fund-raising committees constantly running jumble sales and begging for cash for essential equipment like thermometers. Not that we're not getting damned close to having to be like that again. But your so-called good old days were cheaper, because they were before renal dialysis and Byford's cardiac transplants and ICUs and SCBUs and all the rest of it. This is nearly the twenty-first century, Professor. A little more modern thinking'd do you no harm. Nor those demonstrators either. Modern medicine needs modern economic thinking, not bloody demonstrations, if you'll pardon my language. I'll tell that man Merrall you'll talk to him, then. Good morning.' And he turned and went, leaving the Professor looking after him in some compunction. Poor devil, he thought. I suppose it isn't really his fault. And we do all go on at him –

Merrall came to see him that afternoon at two o'clock. He'd been very punctilious, making an appointment for the interview and arriving dead on time, and Levy looked at him with a slightly beady-eyed stare as he sat down at the desk in front of him and started to fiddle with his tape recorder.

'These Uhers are very good, sir, but they need to be handled with respect,' Merrall said. 'But that's it, I think – yes, it's fine – just a few words for level if you don't mind, Professor, and then we can – '

'But I know you,' Levy said and stared even harder. And then his face cleared. 'Of course! At the last hospital ball we had, Christmas. Didn't you come with Kate Sayers?'

'Er – yes – ' Oliver said a little hurriedly. 'I think that will do for level, then. Now, if I could just start by asking you – '

'I understood you were – how shall I say, pretty close?' Levy said and then smiled disarmingly. 'I'm a wicked old gossip, you know. I like to know all I can about my people here. And some said that you and Kate – '

'Well, yes,' Oliver said. 'But that has nothing to do with my being here. Doing this interview, that is. That is the result of a letter I was sent by a patient of Old East.'

'Oh?' Levy was satisfied now he'd placed Oliver accurately. 'Well, that's interesting. Which patient?'

'Would you know if I told you the name?'

'Very probably,' Levy said with some complacency. 'It's one of the things I'm famous for. I get to know the patients well, and not just my own. And I make a point of remembering names.'

'This one is called Ted Scribner and – '

'Scribner . . . Scribner?' Levy crumpled his face, thinking hard. 'That says nothing to me, dammit. Hubris, you see. Shouldn't have boasted of my memory's prowess.'

'You wouldn't remember this one, Professor,' Oliver said drily. 'He hasn't been in the hospital yet.'

Levy's face smoothed happily. 'Ah, well now, I feel better then! But you say he's a patient? An outpatient perhaps?'

'A waiting-list patient,' Oliver said pointedly and flicked a glance at the dial of the Uher. It had been recording all through and the needle was peaking exactly where it should. This would be a good clear recording. 'He's been waiting to come in here for a prostate operation for some time now. He's very unhappy, it seems. Tells me that he's exhausted because he wakes up six or seven times a night to go to the bathroom and that he has sundry

165

other discomforts I needn't elaborate here. And he's been told five times that there's a bed here for him to have this operation – and five times it's been cancelled. So you'd hardly know him, would you?'

'Oh dear.' Levy shook his head. 'It's dreadful, isn't it? It happens too much. I worry about it a great deal you know, and yet there is so little I can do. I'm just the Dean of the Medical School, one of the physicians here. I have to fight for my own patients as hard as any other consultant to get them in when they need to be to get all the care they should have. Over and over again I do domiciliaries – home visits, you know – to people I know ought to be in bed here at Old East. And what can any of us do? There simply aren't the beds. Our nursing strength is down because before the improvement in their remuneration we couldn't keep recruitment up, even here at Old East, which has a splendid reputation, and even now we're very short on nursing strength. Mr Merrall, I can assure you that if you and your listeners can find ways to improve the bed situation in this hospital no one will be more grateful than those of us who work here.' And he beamed at Oliver who looked a little nonplussed for a moment. But not for long.

'The reason this particular patient is so irate about the loss of his promised bed on the last occasion is because he believes that beds are being unfairly allocated,' he said smoothly. 'He tells me – ' and he glanced down at the open notebook on his knee. 'He was in a local pub the evening of the day he was supposed to be admitted and heard several of the young nursing staff talking. And because they spoke loudly he couldn't help overhearing the conversation and discovered that there was admitted that day he was turned away a man who was to have a sex-change operation.'

There was a little silence and then Levy said carefully, 'You say this man overheard this in a pub?'

'Yes,' Oliver said and held the microphone as invitingly as ever towards him.

'My dear Mr Merrall, you can hardly expect me to comment on information from such a source!' Levy said and his face showed no signs of the fast thinking that was going on behind it. 'I am frankly appalled that such conversations about our

166

patients should occur in public, and steps will be taken to make sure it doesn't happen again, but – '

'So you're refusing to comment simply because the source of the information doesn't please you?' Oliver cut in.

'Not at all!' Levy said and smiled at him. 'I have more sense than that, Mr Merrall. No, I need time to check on this story. I need to find out what the reason was for the withdrawal of an offer of a bed to this gentleman and also what other patients were admitted that day. By all means come and talk to me again, once I've managed to get the facts. But there is no point in mere surmise, is there? It's facts you want – you and your listeners. So come back later and you shall have them.'

And he folded his arms and nodded politely at Merrall and said no more, and Oliver, experienced as he was, admitted defeat and switched off the Uher.

There was a short silence and then Levy said explosively, 'Damn it all! Will we never teach these wretched children not to talk so much in public?'

'Are you saying it's true then?' Oliver reached for the Uher, but Levy shook his head. 'Switch on again and I say not another word,' he said. 'Of course I'm not. I'm not saying it isn't, however. This sort of talk generally is pretty accurate, damn it all. Why shouldn't it be? The nurses are at the bedside. They know what's going on better than anyone.'

'Wouldn't you know if there was a sex-change operation going on here?' Oliver asked. 'I can't believe you do that many.'

'No, not many,' Levy said and smiled again.

'So? Is there such a patient in at the moment?'

'There may be – but even if there were, what relevance would it have to your Mr Scribner?' Levy said. 'We've several hundred patients in here. Probably we had twenty or thirty admissions the day he was told his bed wasn't available. Am I to throw out all the other admissions in order to accommodate him?'

'But if it's true and there was an admission for a sex-change operation,' Oliver said doggedly. 'That patient would be in the Genito-Urinary Unit, wouldn't he? He'd hardly be in the Gynae ward. At least not at the first stage of the operation. Later, maybe – and Mr Scribner was to be admitted to Genito-Urinary – '

There was another little silence and then Levy said carefully, 'Something tells me you haven't discussed this matter with Kate.'

Oliver lifted his brows at him. 'Of course not.'

'Why "of course"?'

'Because the last thing I want to do is cause her any – look, I'm doing this story because I feel I must. Mr Scribner's letter to me was a very moving document. It's my damned bad luck that not only is the hospital involved one where a friend of mine works, but the same ward is involved. That being so the less I talk to Kate the better.'

'Mr Merrall, did Mr Scribner tell you who his consultant was?'

'Keith Le Queux.'

'Have you spoken to him yet?'

'Er, no. I wanted to be sure I had all the other facts clear first – '

'It's just as well. I take it you are assuming that if this so-called sex-change operation was admitted – and I make no statements either way at this point, you understand – you are assuming that he would be admitted to GU under Mr Le Queux's care?'

'Well, of course,' Oliver said. 'Scribner is certain that he lost his bed to this other case. So, it must be . . .' His voice trailed away and Levy watched with interest as the pupils of Oliver's eyes suddenly enlarged as the possibilities slotted into place inside his mind. 'Oh my God,' Oliver said.

'Well, yes,' Levy said almost apologetically. 'I think a little praying might be in order for you, Mr Merrall. If you value your friendship with Kate. Because you are quite right in your new realisation. I will now tell you that such a patient was admitted and is having treatment here. Under the care of Kate Sayers. So now what are you going to do?'

'You can't do nothing to stop me,' Ida said sullenly. 'And anyway, it's none of your business.' And she moved a little closer to Prue.

'Of course it is,' Sister said briskly. 'I never heard any such nonsense in all my life, telling me what happens to my patients is none of my business!'

'Well, what am I doing that's so wrong?' Ida said. 'I just said as

I'd promised Prue here I'd give her a bit of help, that's all. There's no harm in that, is there? It's not like I got a lot to do. Miss Buckland, she said go out for another month till she can try next time, and all I want to do is keep myself occupied. You heard what Miss Buckland said about not getting obsessive. Well, if I go and help Prue with her babies and all then I won't get obsessive, will I?'

'Is this what you want, Mrs Roberts?' Sister Morgan bent over to peer into Prue's pale face. She was sitting on the old blue chair in the day room, her knees held together carefully and her bag of things beside her, her head down so that her hair covered her face, and it was difficult to see her at all clearly. 'Mrs Roberts?'

'What?' Prue looked up now and stared at Sister. Her pallor had greatly improved; there was some normality about her now, but all the same her eyes seemed strained and there were lines there that didn't belong on so young a face. She looked closer to thirty-five than twenty-five, Sister Morgan thought and threw an urgent glance at her watch. It was almost time for Miss Buckland's round and she really didn't have time to waste this way.

'Look, let me get someone up from the Social Services department to talk to you,' she began, but both women jumped on that.

'No,' they chorused, and Sister Morgan looked from one to the other, nonplussed.

'Well, I suppose it's out of my hands,' she said at length, and pulled her cuffs down over her wristwatch. 'If you're determined, Mrs Malone, then that's an end of it, I suppose. As long as Mrs Roberts really wants you to go home with her – '

'Yes,' Prue said drearily and didn't look at Ida. 'Yes, it's what I want. She'll be a good help to me. The Social are bringing the kids back this afternoon and I'll need a bit of help.'

'Well, if you need any further advice, call your health visitor, you understand? And they'll be sending a social worker down from the Town Hall to see you, I dare say. Now, have you got your appointment card for antenatal clinic? Good, make sure you keep it, now. After all that's happened you'll need a lot of watching. And er – ' She moved a little closer to Prue and with a deft turn of one shoulder managed to exclude Ida Malone from their conversation. 'If you get – um – worried again, don't go doing anything silly. You understand me? You're all of twenty weeks and you can't go fiddling about. You're all right this time, but you've had a nasty go. It isn't the answer, believe me. If it was, you can be sure Miss Buckland – I mean, she's a very caring doctor and never refuses unless – well, anyway, no nonsense now, you understand?'

'Yes,' Prue said dully and after one last look at her Sister Morgan went hurrying away down the ward in a whisper of nylon uniform and a slap of rubber-soled shoes.

'She knows what you're up to, and she's going to stop it,' Prue said after a moment and shot a sharp little look at Ida. But Ida was staring at her with her eyes wide and glittering and showing no anxiety at all.

'Not she,' she said confidently. 'She's just going through the motions, like what they have to. She'll forget all about you the minute you walks out the door. That's what they do here, get all excited about you while you're in, but after you're outside it's a case of poof, that's the patient that was, who gives a damn any more? None of 'em. Your notes'll go back down to that record office and they'll send the cards and the records through to the antenatal and no one'll ever give a damn if you don't show up. It'll be a case of thank God we can go to lunch early, one patient less. Never you think otherwise, ducky. They don't care.'

'They do,' Prue said with sudden passion. 'They've always been ever so good here, they have. They'll notice if I don't keep my appointment, you see if they don't. They'll get in touch.'

'Oh, yeah,' Ida jeered. 'They'll get that there clerk to send a special card they got printed about "You missed your appointment, please make another" and that'll be that. No one'll notice if you don't make a new appointment. They'll reckon you've moved away, that's all, and bob's your uncle.'

'I'd rather have the baby here,' Prue said after another long moment. 'I had the others here. It was all right, it was.'

'It'll be better in this other place. Small it is, and real nice. Private.' And Ida nodded once or twice, full of satisfaction. 'Real nice, a private place. You'll have a good time there.'

'They won't let you take the baby away afterwards, anyway,' Prue said with sudden malice. 'None of these hospitals ever do.'

'I told 'em you was my sister when I booked you in,' Ida said. 'Did it on the phone I did, all right and proper. They took the booking, no trouble at all. I always had it in my mind I'd go there myself if I had a baby natural, only I never – well, anyway they took the booking when I said you was my sister. So they'll be no trouble. You just go in in twenty weeks or so, you have the baby and then I'll take you both home, like. Only *you* can go home and me and the baby you won't know nothing about. Least said, soonest mended.'

'You're mad,' Prue said and stared at her again. 'Do you know that? Stark ravin' mad.'

'Don't you be so full of your bleedin' self!' Ida said and there was so much venom in her voice that Prue shrank back into her chair. 'I got an idea that'll save your bacon and all you can say is I'm mad? There's bloody gratitude. I'm spending all this money on you – that coat you got on, didn't I get it fetched in for you? Didn't I? Don't you go saying I'm mad.'

'I mean you can't just take a baby what isn't yours and say it is,' Prue said, sulky now. 'That's what I meant.'

'And what'll happen if I don't? Do you want it?'

Prue closed her eyes and tried to think. She saw in the yellow tinted glow behind her lids the long passageway in the flat, with the pram crowded to one side and the clothes horse with the nappies on it at the far end, and then saw the bedroom with the two cots in it and the clutter of the sitting room with Danny's bits and toys everywhere and Gary shouting at her because of the mess, and thought of the way she felt whenever the baby cried and felt the tears slide out of the yellowness to wet her face.

'I don't know,' she said.

'I do,' Ida said. 'I know you. You don't want this baby, not really. You got two and they're all you can deal with. This one you wanted to get rid of. You still do, don't you?'

Still the tears slid down Prue's face as she sat there feeling the great cold lump in her belly and hating it, and thinking of Gary in the sand somewhere. And hated him and could say nothing.

'So, why shouldn't I help you, eh? I'm glad to. I want to. It'd be a blessing to you and I want to give it you, that sort of blessing, and I want the baby and it's all so *sensible*. Don't you tell me I'm mad. It's the only way to do it. And it's what we're going to do.'

She looked up to see the porter coming towards the day room pushing an empty wheelchair. 'There,' she said brightly. 'He's here. Time to go then. Come on, Prue. You'll see. I'll get you home and sort things out for you in no time. You'll see. It'll be the best thing you ever did.'

Suba looked up from the nurses' station as the wheelchair went by and said quickly, 'Goodbye Mrs Roberts. I hope everything goes well for you.' And never thought to say goodbye to Mrs Malone as well. But Mrs Malone was like that, she thought as the two women disappeared out of the swinging double doors. It isn't till afterwards you think of what you ought to say to her. And she bent her head again to Mrs Walton's notes, trying to read all she had to read before she went off duty. She had a lot to remember for the meeting tonight.

If she went of course, she reminded herself, then. If she went.

Chapter Eighteen

———————

'I'm not sure, you know,' Jimmy Rhoda said judiciously. 'Not sure at all.'

'Why not? It's true, every word of it.'

'Oh, I dare say it's true enough,' Jimmy smiled sweetly. 'Here, can I smoke in here? Of course I don't disbelieve you. It isn't that.'

'Then what is it? And it's better you don't smoke. Sister gets shirty enough when the patients do, let alone the visitors. And quite right too. Your body shouldn't get attacked with smoke and all that. Ought to treat your body like a temple, really. Be careful what you put in it – '

'Yes,' Jimmy said after a moment, and shoved his cigarettes back into his pocket, keeping his head bent while he did so, to stop his face being seen, knowing the expression that was on it. Body a temple? Jesus Christ! Wait till he took this little lot back to the office. They'd laugh for a week.

'So, what is it then? Why can't you – '

'It's not your story, you understand,' Jimmy said, and after a moment and with a very obvious gallantry leaned forwards and patted the long-fingered hand with its blood-red nails. 'It's not that I doubt. And it's very interesting as well as true. No, the problem is the money – '

'Oh?' Kim stared at him. 'What about the money? Isn't it worth it? Aren't I worth it?'

'I'm sure you are,' Jimmy said heartily. 'Anyone would think so. The thing is, though, will my editor? She's a hard woman – ' And he shook his head dubiously. 'A very hard woman.'

'A woman ought to understand,' Kim said. 'Oughtn't she?'

'Well, I dare say she would,' Jimmy allowed. 'But she has to watch the budget. And you're asking for a lot of money, you see. I can allow – on my own you understand, without going to the editor – I can go to a thousand – '

'A thousand?' Kim almost squealed it. 'It's worth a bloody sight more'n that – '

'I dare say it is, to you.' Jimmy was all sympathy. 'But the fact of the matter is my editor – '

'Then forget it. I'll go to someone else.'

'Not as easy as that.' Jimmy sounded really regretful. 'I mean you've told me now, haven't you? It's like, public. I can do the story from the other end, as it were. Come to the people here, say I've heard on the grapevine about this operation, want to do an article anyway, and then you'd get nothing – '

Kim's eyes brimmed in their usual ready fashion as she stared at him. 'You wouldn't,' she said, and her voice cracked a little. 'I mean, it's all I've got now. I told you. I've been sacked and I can't get another job that pays. A business of my own, it's the only way – and if you don't pay me and just do it anyway I might as well cut my throat and be done with it, because I've got to have money to start a business, haven't I? Without it I'm as good as dead.'

Jimmy shifted uneasily in his chair. 'Are you sure I can't smoke in here? No? Well – look, I'll do the best I can. If I can stretch it to, say, fifteen hundred, will that help?'

'I'd hoped for at least five thousand,' Kim said.

He shook his head firmly. 'Out of the question.'

'If I had three I could maybe do something. Start in my living room. But I'll need some machines, and someone to do some of the sewing. I'm a designer, not a seamstress. And then there's the pressing and the investment in fabric and trimmings and the packaging and then I've got to go out and sell it and you can't do that by bus, can you? I'd hoped for at least five thousand to cover all that. But if I had three – '

'Well, look, I'll put my own job on the line,' Jimmy said, sounding handsome. 'I'll make it two. Two thousand quid. You can't say fairer, can you? That ought to be a beginning. But you won't get more anywhere. If you get anything.'

'Oh, shit!' Kim said. 'You really have got me by the short and curlies, haven't you?' And then she giggled. 'Not that I've got much of those left, mind you – ' And Jimmy laughed too, trying not to show his jubilation at getting the story so cheaply. And pulled his notebook from his pocket and settled down to some real work.

Sian had been thoroughly annoyed when she'd been sent to clean the dialysis machine after they took Jenny off it. That was an orderly's job, and she said as much with some vigour when the staff nurse told her to do it.

'Really?' the staff nurse had said sharply. 'Is that so? Well, if we had an orderly, maybe we could send her to do it. And if there hadn't been that fuss over getting the Union involved over Mrs Aspinall making such a stupid ass of herself with that breakfast, maybe we could have got another orderly in her place. As it is, the Union refused and so we're short-handed with orderlies which means as usual that the nursing staff have to step into the breach. *You*. You're the ward junior, so you get the job.'

Sian had bristled. 'I'm not a scab. I don't do other people's work just because – '

'Matter-of-life-and-death,' the staff nurse said in a gabble, and showed her a tight-lipped smile. 'I'm as much involved with the politics of this place as you are, my friend, and I can tell you that if you refuse on such grounds I can make all sorts of problems for you because having the dialysis machine ready for the next patient that needs it is life-and-death stuff, as you'd know if you'd been on this ward a little longer than five bloody minutes. So are you going to do it, or do I have to send you to be disciplined? Sister'd back me, and the Union won't step in for you, believe me. Not on this sort of issue. They've got more bloody sense and it's time you got some too. Stirring up that woman like that – I could have killed you – '

So, Sian went to clean the machine, and took as long over it as she dared. She'd show that bitch where she got off, she thought furiously as she sluiced the tubes through in their special lotion. She'd show her –

It was a little while before she realised that Kim and her visitor had forgotten she was there, and had stopped talking in the low tones they had started with. Sian had drawn the curtains to do her job, partly to give Kim privacy but mostly to hide herself and her ignominy out of sight. If the other nurses came by and saw her they'd know what had happened and no one, least of all Sian, would want that. So there she had been for over half an hour now, fiddling with that damned machine, and Kim and her visitor were talking.

Listening to other people's conversations had always been to Sian something that was natural and perfectly reasonable. She had never understood the embarrassment some people showed when they were inadvertent eavesdroppers, and had said as much, often; and indeed had often been a deliberate eavesdropper. It was usually the quickest, simplest way of finding out what was going on, and knowing what was going on was lifeblood to Sian. Well, she would say reasonably enough to anyone who would hear her, isn't it to everyone?

So, now she listened with all the concentration she had, and felt herself get more and more angry as she did so. Not with Kim, though from the start she had disliked him. To see him make such a display of himself was disgusting to Sian, who anyway regarded with disdain any woman who wore red nail varnish and who curled and dyed her hair, and she had consistently refused to say anything but 'he' and 'him' when she spoke of the patient in bed seventeen. As far as Sian was concerned Kim Hynes wasn't much of a man and was certainly no woman; she would loathe any woman who looked like that and to see a man deliberately ape such style – Sian had actually shuddered. But now, listening to the smooth tones of the man beside Kim's bed Sian bristled even more. At him.

Bloody robber, she thought as she rubbed at the chrome of the dialysis machine. Bloody man, making even more of a fool out of that idiot. It's all wrong; I've got to stop him. And then the curtains billowed and there was the scrape of chair legs on the floor as the man stood up and prepared to leave.

Sian thought for a moment and then, as the man began a convoluted 'Goodbye', straightened her back and, moving swiftly, went across to pull back the curtains. Looking at the man, she felt obscurely, would be the first step to dealing with him and as the curtains rattled on their rail she looked sharply from one to the other of the two startled faces on the other side.

'I'm sorry, Kim,' she said brightly as Kim stared back at her. 'Did I disturb you?'

'Not at all,' the man said smoothly and smiled at her and Sian shifted her gaze to him. Small and rumpled was the first impression she got of him. And then saw a round face crowned with a fast receding hairline behind which grew a fringe of very dark hair, and the somewhat overcoloured cheeks of the heavy drinker. But he was in fact quite young despite that collection of attributes; not much over thirty-five, she hazarded. And then he grinned at her and looked even younger.

'I was just saying goodbye,' he said. 'I imagine visiting time's almost over.'

'There aren't set times exactly,' she said and looked back at him pugnaciously. 'Not for relatives. Are you a relative of Kim's then?'

'Just a friend,' the man said easily and grinned again. It really was quite a friendly face, Sian thought, and began to feel a little less angry. 'Everyone needs friends. Better than family, sometimes, eh Kim? Friends you choose, family you get lumbered with.'

'Ooh, original, isn't he, Nurse?' Kim said and glittered at Sian and Sian looked at that smooth painted face and then flicked her eyes back to the man now standing at the foot of the bed.

'I'll show you the way out,' she said abruptly. 'As you're going.' And moved forwards purposefully so that the man had to follow her.

'I'll be in touch, then, Kim,' he said over his shoulder and then followed Sian down the ward towards the double doors at the far end.

She turned on him with a combative stare as they went through them and could no longer be seen by Kim, who had been staring down the ward after them. Sian had been able to feel those heavily mascaraed eyes on her back, so intense had been the stare.

'Listen, mister,' she said in a low voice. 'I don't know what you think you're up to, but if you make trouble for any patients here, whoever they are, we won't put up with it.'

He looked down at her, amused, and his face wrinkled into a wide grin. 'Who won't?'

'I won't for a start,' she said fiercely. 'That poor devil – how long have you known him?'

'Never met *her* before today,' the man said smoothly and grinned even more widely.

'I didn't think you had. Then what are you up to? Who tipped you off?'

'What I'm up to is nothing that's bad, nothing that's illegal, and nothing that's any of your damned business,' he said, still equable, and still grinning at her. 'As for who tipped me off – bless you child, she did.'

'Don't call me child, you great – you – ' she spluttered and then took a sharp little breath in through her nose. 'Don't you bloody patronise me, mister. I don't go for it. It might do for you old-timers, but me, I'm a today person, know what I mean? So none of your nonsense with me. Our patients are here to be looked after, whatever they're like, and we don't want you newspaper people sneaking around after them – '

'Clever girl, got me in one,' he said approvingly. 'Not that it was difficult, I imagine. Seeing I was running an interview there – '

'And if you start any trouble for that poor devil I'll – '

'What will you do?' he said and she had faltered for a moment.

'I can alert the necessary authorities,' she said with all the dignity she could muster. 'There are ways of keeping you people out of here.'

'Now why should you want to?' he said, and leaned his back against the wall, settling down for a long conversation, his hands thrust deeply into his trouser pockets. 'Aren't we the free press, one of the bulwarks against injustice?'

'Oh, sure,' she said scathingly. 'So you lot say. Though what sort of bulwark you can build out of boobs and bums all over page three is anyone's guess.'

'Oh, that's what you get in the comics,' he said, still very relaxed and comfortable. 'Not on a *real* paper. I'm on the *Globe*. We're a paper – no tits and ass here. Sounds better in American, doesn't it? Not so cheap – '

'It's cheap wherever it is. And you're just as bad as the people who do it – '

'Now let's stop all this, shall we?' Still he looked as urbane as ever, but there was a little edge to his voice now. 'This is getting just a shade boring. So I'll put you straight, hmm? I got a letter from your patient Kim Hynes. She was asking for money. Says she'll TELL ALL, in capital letters, if we pay her enough. Pictures, grisly details, the whole bit. So, like any reasonable journalist, I came along to find out. Now you tell me: just how wicked is that? Where is the boobs and bums sinfulness in that? We haven't even published it yet. All I've done is listen to a sad tale of woe, and that's the end of it. Or it might be. The way you're going on makes me begin to wonder if there's more to this than meets the eye. You seem to dislike the woman from all you say. Very protective and all that, but you don't seem to like her much – keep calling her a poor devil – '

'He agreed to *sell* it to you, this story?' She stared at him, her forehead crumpled with disgust. 'Actually offered to sell to you for money? Ye gods, what a shit!'

'I said you didn't like her – '

'Her my – my left foot,' Sian said and reddened. 'That's a man, with a lot of mad ideas about what women are like. No woman would be so bloody daft – '

'My, but you're an intolerant little madam, aren't you? And I thought nurses were so sweet and understanding. Just shows how wrong you can be, doesn't it? Would it amaze you to know that there have been women in poor old Kim's situation? That women have had sex-change operations? Swallowed hormones to grow themselves beards and give themselves basso profundo voices? Because they have. I know one who went to the Human Rights court in Strasbourg over it – '

'Oh, what's that got to do with anything?' She was angry again now, and eaten with the embarrassment of having made a fool of herself. 'I still reckon it's a dirty thing to publish stuff like that for money and – '

He shrugged. 'People have to make their livings the best way they can. Kim Hynes lost her job because of the situation she's in and she's doing all she can to get enough together to start her own business. I'd have thought that was admirable, not a cause for this sort of reaction. But there, we of the press are maybe a little more open-minded than you handmaidens of Hippocrates.'

'Well, I don't just care about one patient,' Sian flared at him, her face red now with the confusion of feelings that filled her.

'There are others, you know, who get the dirty end of the stick because of the likes of Kim Hynes – '

'Oh?' He was still leaning negligently against the wall but seemed to have gone tight with interest. 'How do you mean?'

'Well, waiting lists and so forth – ' She stared at him and seemed suddenly to realise how indiscreet she was being. 'Oh, it doesn't matter. And it's none of your damned business anyway! Just keep out of my way, do me a favour. And if you come back here, watch out, because I'll tell Sister what's going on and she won't be a bit pleased. They don't like journalists here – '

'I'll bet they don't,' he said. 'Mind you, some of the people who use the place do. I saw the demo going on outside. I'm covering that too, seeing I'm here, so I suppose you object to that as well.'

'Don't you sneer at me! I most certainly do not object! I agree with them totally. It's all wrong what they're trying to do – close this place down. They have to be mad. It's all part of this bloody Government's policy of course – make the NHS a second-class service and turn all the hospitals into workhouses while the private set-ups make a bloody fortune out of those who are forced to pay – it makes you sick. Of course I agree with the demo – '

'Then you want that publicity, I imagine. Even in a boobs and bum paper? Not that we are at the *Globe*, of course – '

'Oh, blast you,' she said after a moment, and then, to her own amazement, laughed. It all seemed so silly suddenly, and he grinned back at her, cheerfully.

'Attagirl,' he said. 'Seen the light at last. Listen, when do you get off duty?'

'None of your business,' she said, on safe ground again now. Men who wanted to chat her up she understood and could handle. Men who sneered just made her feel ready to burst with rage.

'I can work it out,' he said and looked at his watch. 'It's nearly seven now, so you're on the middle shift. Off at nine, hmm? I saw the pub over the road – I'll meet you there at half past, get a few in and we can talk about the evils of the Government and the way they treat the NHS and say how we'd do it better. And you can put me in my place over the Kim Hynes story. What do you say? Give you your chance to put the world right – '

'I should cocoa! I can just see you printing what I've got to say, a junior nurse – '

'Never you think it, my love, never you think it. I can get quotes from professors and high-up brass till they come out of my ears. It's people like you, at the sharp end of the coal face where the nitty-gritty grows and the bottom line gets down to brass tacks that are really interesting. So, is it a date?'

'Not if you talk that way,' she said and turned to go back into the ward.

'I promise you not a cliché shall sully these ruby lips,' he said promptly. 'Half past nine then.'

'I'll think about it,' she said and disappeared into the ward, well pleased with herself. It would be quite fun finishing cleaning that bloody machine now, with something interesting to look forward to.

Chapter Nineteen

'You'll be happy to know, I'm sure, that your cystoscopy findings are clear,' Kate said and smiled down at Gerald Slattery. He was sitting up in bed very neatly, foursquare against his tidy pile of pillows in red-striped pyjamas carefully buttoned to the throat, and with his thin hair combed over his shining pink scalp equally neatly.

'I didn't think they'd be otherwise, to tell the truth,' he said. 'Seeing I hadn't had any problems with the plumbing. I told you I didn't – and I told that *lovely* black doctor – I still don't know why I had to go through with that. Not for a *hernia*. It's all been explained to me, you see.'

She avoided looking directly at him, keeping her eyes on his chart. 'We just thought it as well to be absolutely sure,' she said. 'How are you feeling this morning?'

'Sore,' he said. 'This lump's like a *billiard* ball where no one should have to have a billiard ball. And I can't pretend I'm not getting worried about it.'

'We're going to deal with it,' she said. 'I've listed you for surgery tomorrow morning. Is that all right with you?'

'Couldn't be better. At last. Anything's better than sitting round here waiting. It's like being in prison and expecting the chaplain to turn up *any* moment to let you know that the executioner's getting restless. Why the delay, if I may be so bold as to ask?'

Now she did look at him, consideringly. So far all the discussion about the pros and cons of this man's operation had been between herself and Professor Levy and whoever else he might have chosen to talk to. Kate had deliberately not asked him about Goodman Lemon's reaction to the way Levy had scooped this patient out of his ward and got him transferred to hers. She had enough to deal with with her own work without deliberately getting involved in the intricacies of hospital politics any more than she had to. But she was well aware of what was

182

likely to happen when Lemon found out what had been done, and wasn't the patient, too, entitled to know? He looked back at her with bright rather protuberant pale blue eyes, and she saw the intelligence there and the watchfulness and made up her mind quickly.

'Do you realise you've caused rather a fuss?' she said abruptly.

'Oh? In what way?'

'You refused some blood testing.'

'Ah, yes. I thought that perhaps – well, I'm entitled to refuse, aren't I? I'm not a *fool* you know, and I've eyes in my head and I can read. I've followed the arguments you doctors have been having. There's one lot leaping about saying they reckon they've the right to do secret blood tests on us without our consents, and the other lot saying it's unethical. Me, I agree with the *other* lot. But then – ' He looked up at her with his chin tilted a little and laughed. 'As the tart said, I would, wouldn't I?'

'Would you?'

'Oh, Doctor, *please*! I gave you credit for being – well, really! I mean, just look at me! Of course I'd refuse! Of course I *did*, come to that.'

'Just what are you refusing?'

'Oh, come on, Doctor! Don't treat me like a *baby*! I thought better of you, I really did.'

'I'm not trying to treat you in any way but what is best for you, truly, Mr Slattery. I just think we'll get on better if we understand one another fully. And we can only do that if we talk directly and not in circles. Now, you tell me what it is you fear and I'll tell you what the problems here have been. Fair enough?'

He looked at her for a long considering moment and then nodded. 'Fair enough,' he said and then leaned over to scrabble in his bedside locker and pull out a writing case.

'I'll need my documents, won't I? Right – here we are – ' and he brandished a newspaper clipping. 'All right. You begin.'

'No. You.'

'Ooh, you do *cheat*. All right then, I've nothing to hide! Look, I'm gay. Homosexual, you know? And do note how I pronounce it – homo as in tommyrot, not homo, as in oh-dear-no. It means I fancy my own sort better than the other sort. Nothing against *you*, Doctor dear, you understand, it's just the way I am. And my sort, God help us, have been struck by one of the bloodier plagues of Egypt and everyone's having *conniption* fits. Not me, though. Me, I've got my old Stewart. We've been together for seventeen years, a right old married couple we are, never strayed, either of us. Couldn't be doing with teaching someone new all our little ways, to tell you the truth of it. So, as I say, there we are. Nice, normal and married. Yes, *normal*! Don't stand there looking as though you've been stuffed. In our terms we're normal healthy ordinary chaps, with as much right to be camp as everyone else has to be boring. If we want to carry on like we live in pink tents, why shouldn't we? It's no crime — '

'I really only want to talk about your treatment,' Kate murmured. 'Do we have to have the whole lecture?'

'You told me to start first! Anyway, when all the fuss started we both agreed, Stewart and me, no tests. We aren't at risk, we're sure of that, and we know bloody well what'd happen if we do test and by some *mad* chance it turns out we've got a touch of the plague from before seventeen years ago. Who can say, after all? Better not knowing, that's our motto. And then we saw all this stuff in the paper' — and he waved the newspaper clipping in the air — 'about how doctors may do secret tests and put them on computers and we both said not on your nelly, *no* tests if we get ill. Not without we know what they're doing and why. And then, bugger me, if you'll pardon the expression, there I go getting this hernia and what can I do but keep my word to Stewart? No testing. So now what? You tell me.'

She nodded and stood looking at him as he stared down at his newspaper clipping. She had recognised it; an item that had appeared in one of the Sunday heavies about the row at the BMA between consultants and GPs, and she had been irritated by it then and still was. As far as she was concerned no one had any right or need to force a blood test for HIV on anyone. Even as a surgeon she wasn't concerned; there had been enough discussion of the fragility of the virus and the protection conferred against it by use of normal and necessary barrier methods of surgery in operating on these patients to reassure her. She had long ago decided that should the problem arise in any of her list all she'd do was put the patient on last, so that the theatre could be carefully cleaned and sterilised afterwards, and would herself operate with a no-touch technique. She'd done her first surgical house job as an orthop under a man who was so obsessed with infection control that no one was ever allowed to set a finger inside any wound he dealt with. All instruments and nothing but instruments was the rule. Even the finest needles were threaded with forceps to hold them and their thread. A difficult technique, but it could be done and could be learned. She could operate on most things she now dealt with in the same way, of that she was certain. So she had turned the page of the newspaper and given the matter no further thought. Till now, watching Gerald Slattery carefully folding his cutting and tucking it away.

'The day you were admitted the surgeon in charge was Mr Goodman Lemon,' she said abruptly.

He grinned at that. 'Sounds like a recipe for a farmhouse cake. I *adore* baking – you must give it to me.'

'If you knew him you wouldn't be so flippant,' she said sharply. 'He has – strong views on a number of issues.'

'And gays are one of them? Thinks we're the scum of the earth and so forth?' Slattery said and for the first time sounded bitter. 'Nice to be some people.'

'Yes, he's like that. And refuses to operate on people he thinks are – gay – unless they're HIV tested first. So we had to find a way to get you transferred to another surgeon since you refused testing. That's why the cystoscopy. I'm sorry you had to go through such a thing – '

'No harm done,' he said. He was staring at her now very fixedly. 'Nice to know I'm clear in there, I dare say. So you're not scared of plague rats like me?'

She reddened. 'I don't see you that way.'

'Nice of you. Tell me, does this cake recipe man refuse to operate on smokers and boozers? Or doesn't he worry about that sort of morality?'

She raised her brows. 'I'm not sure that – '

'It's the same sort of thing, really, isn't it? Self-induced disease and all that, hmm? We're treated like bloody dogs when we're ill because they think we've brought it on ourselves, but not the cancers of the lung and the hobnailed livers – oh, no. They've got nice *normal* weaknesses, not like us, who find ourselves loving the wrong sort of people. Or what the cake man thinks are the wrong sort of people.'

'I really can't discuss that,' Kate said. 'I want only to reassure you that under my care you won't have to have any test to which you object and I'll do your operation tomorrow morning. Are you happy to let me?'

'If you're happy to do it, I'm grateful. I don't want to feel worse than this. It won't get better on its own, will it?'

'It seems unlikely,' she said. 'We haven't been able to reduce it – to push it back.'

He grimaced. 'And don't I *know* it. Felt like a lump of dough I did, the way everyone kept kneading away at me. No fun at all, even though you'd think it would be. So you're not scared of me – that's interesting – '

She shook her head. 'No,' she said. 'I'm not scared. There's no need to be.'

'Why? Because you think you're cleverer than the cake man at dodging the bugs or because you think I'm not infectious?'

He looked at her very directly and his eyes seemed to glitter a little and she thought – He's terrified. All this show and under it he's scared silly.

'Both,' she said lightly. 'But most of all I don't think you're a risk to anyone. Not after seventeen years with the same partner. This is one of your new infections, isn't it?'

'I always said I liked women,' Gerald Slattery said and smiled at her widely, his teeth glinting in the sunlight. 'I always say to the others when they go on about women, and some of them do, I'm afraid, some of them do, you don't know *what* you're missing. Thanks, Doctor. See you with the knife then – '

'Yes,' she said. 'See you with the knife. Good morning.'

Esther stopped her as she reached the end of the ward, her head down as she went on thinking about Slattery. Should she warn the theatres now that she wanted to use a no-touch technique for the man's operation or deal with it in a more casual sort of way tomorrow when she got there? Would Theatre Sister fuss if she told her now? Would – the thoughts were sliding around in her head and hard to control, and being interrupted by Esther was to be welcomed.

'Prior,' Esther said as Kate stopped and looked at her. 'Have you been able to do anything about him?'

'Mm?' Kate did her best not to look stupid as she tried to remember what it was she was supposed to have done about William Prior.

Esther sighed a little theatrically. 'I knew you'd forget. You just hate having to transfer anyone, don't you? You said you'd call St Kitts, see if they could take him off our hands. You know old Davies likes you and does what you want when he can. Prior really is more of a social problem than a medical one – and medically he's bad enough.'

Kate sighed too, remembering. 'What's he done now?'

Esther giggled then, somewhat spoiling her image as a sensible ward sister. 'I wish you'd seen it. You know that chap who was admitted last night, query renal colic? He was fairly smashed – the pethidine you wrote him up for the pain knocked him for six – and couldn't really do anything much when it happened. But Prior was disconnected from his machine for a while – I thought he could go a night without and we'd see how stable he was – and though I'd set one of the nurses on to special him, she had to go off for a moment or two because there was a panic in the next bay, and old Prior got out of bed and decided that Mr Burles, the renal colic, was his wife. Or whatever. Anyway he climbed into the poor chap's bed next to him and got a good deal friendlier than Burles might have expected from a total stranger, and a bearded smelly old man at that. He's a banker or some such, apparently – very proper type. The nurse came back, thank God, and saw what was happening and got Prior out and managed to get him back to his own bed and then, clever girl, was able to persuade poor old Burles that he'd dreamed it all because of his pethidine – ' Again she giggled and Kate felt her own face crease.

'But it was a close run thing. He was all set to sue the hospital, the Area Health Authority and the entire damned DHSS come to that. It'd have been as interesting a case of rape to come to court as most, wouldn't it? Really, Kate, you'll have to do something about him. Prior, I mean. Burles is fine – seems to have passed his stone and after he has his pyelogram done this afternoon it's my guess we can send him on his way rejoicing. If a little ashamed of the quality of his dreams. But Prior! Will you call St Kitts, see if they'll take him into their unit?'

Kate shook her head. 'Sorry, Esther – I already did. As soon as we discussed it ages ago. They're chock-a-block, and anyway, they won't take any of ours because I never agree to take any of theirs. I mean, you won't, will you? So there you are. You'll have to manage the old man as best you can. Poor devil – '

'Poor devil he may be, but I'm worse off than he is,' Esther retorted. 'He's a bugger to deal with. Oh, well, I thought I'd have another bash. I'll nag the nursing office to see if I can get some extra nurses to help me out, seeing I can't get any joy out of you.' And she made a face and went bustling off to bawl at one of the hapless juniors down the ward who was standing chattering instead of working, leaving Kate to go on to her outpatient clinic still undecided about how to handle the theatre sister over Slattery's operation.

Oh well, she told herself as philosophically as she could as the rattling old lift took her down to the echoing basement where the outpatients waited in untidy noisy rows for her, whatever happens the man will be rid of his hernia. And that's what matters.

'And what the hell are you doing here?' Oliver said after one stupefied moment. 'You're the last person I'd expected to see.'

'You weren't supposed to see me,' Jimmy said. 'Damn you. Why can't you go someplace else for your morning coffee?'

'Why can't you?' Oliver hauled his Uher on to the table and sat down facing him. 'You're a sneaky sod, Rhoda, you really are. I ask you for a bit of information and you come straight round here sniffing round – '

'I bloody didn't!' Jimmy protested. 'Here, I'll get you some coffee. It tastes like puke, believe me, but it's hot and wet. Hold on.' And he went over to the counter at the end of the visitors' canteen and began to chatter at the large woman in the flowered apron standing behind the big urn as Oliver relaxed and stretched at the table.

Not a bad morning, he thought. An interview with Herne at last, and though the man had been unbelievably cagey, at least he'd said something; Oliver would be able to get enough of his damned pap out of the tangle of tape he'd provided to put in the finished programme and so stop anyone saying he hadn't given the management of Old East a fair crack of the whip. That and the stuff he'd at last got out of the Professor and the demo leader – interesting woman, that – and he was well on the way to having his first half-hour show and a certain amount of the second. Not bad after only a few days on the job. And still not a word of what he was doing to Kate. That was quite an achievement.

But he felt bad about it. They'd been together now at the Finchley Road flat for almost fifteen months and though there had been no-go areas, God knew – with Sonia in the background how could it be otherwise? – they'd never had to keep big secrets from each other. Not that this was exactly a secret, he told himself now as he watched Jimmy getting even more expansive with the flowered apron. This was work, and they'd never exchanged every detail of each other's working day with each other, so this could hardly be called secretiveness.

No? jeered a little part of his mind. Then why are you sneaking round so carefully watching out for her so that you can dodge her if you spot her? How can you say this job isn't involved with hers? That damned sex-change operation is hers; when are you going to interview her about it? And he grimaced as at last Jimmy Rhoda turned away from the counter to bring the two plastic cups of coffee over to him.

'I didn't bring anything to eat. All they've got are those roof-tile things they call chocolate chip cookies. Disgusting. Sugar?'

'No thanks. What are you doing here, Jimmy? Treated my call as a tip-off, did you?'

'In a way.' Jimmy dropped three spoonfuls of sugar into the plastic cup and stirred vigorously. 'Not on its own, you understand. I had another tip-off as well – '

'Another – ' Oliver stared at him over the rim of the cup. 'What sort?'

'Why should I tell you? You'll scoop me and then where am I?'

'Oh, shut up, idiot! I'm radio and you're a bloody rag. You know there's no competition involved. Different markets entirely. What tip-off?'

Jimmy looked at him for a long moment and then sniffed hard.

'Got to think about this. I need some more information before –
Look, if I cut you in on this, you cut me in on yours?'

'How?'

'Well, what's your angle? What story are you doing? Let's see
if there isn't meat enough on this bone for both of us and no
wires crossed.'

'You're so bloody literate you amaze me,' Oliver said. 'If you
mix your metaphors much harder you'll come out with alphabet
soup. You tell me what you've got, I'll tell you if it cuts across
me.'

'Like hell,' Jimmy said. 'Do I look as though I was born
yesterday? You tell me yours first – '

Oliver sighed. 'It'll have to be the usual trick then. Here – '
and he pulled his notebook from his pocket and tore off a sheet.
'Are you enough of a journalist to have a pen with you? Oh,
miracle of miracles – OK, I'll write down my angle, you write
down yours and we'll swop at the same time. Fair enough?'

'What else can I do?' Jimmy grumbled. 'Give me a pen that'll
write, for Christ's sake, this one's dried up. Ta.'

There was a little silence as they both scribbled and then when
both had finished and folded their sheets of paper in half, there
was a short pause as they drank coffee. And then Jimmy said,
'OK, fish face. Hand it over.'

'Simultaneously,' Oliver said and held out his sheet of paper
invitingly. After a moment, Jimmy laughed and did the same,
and with a solemn nod of each head they swopped papers.

The silence that followed was a short one, and it was Jimmy
who broke it first.

'Ah, shit,' he said disgustedly. 'I might have known it. You've
done a bloody sight better out of this than I have. Are we at the
fucking crossroads? Christ, can't you do better than that? They
used to use that one on the *People* back in the fifties, as I recall.'

'Long memory you've got,' Oliver said. 'Considering your
age – ' But the badinage was mechanical. He was staring down
with a frown at the piece of paper Jimmy had scribbled.

'Useful though . . . Listen, there has to be more to your story
than bloody cuts. That's been done to death. Even the *Guard-
ian*'s stopped beating that drum – in features at any rate.'

'No, it was that. To start with.' Oliver lifted his head. 'I got a

190

letter from a patient too. The chap I listed there as an interviewee had his operation cancelled for the fifth time, and he said this time it was to give his bed to a sex-change case. I wasn't going to bother you with that – '

'Bother me?' Jimmy howled. 'You bastard! Very tender-hearted you are, wanting to protect an old mate! That's the only interesting part of the story and you bloody know it. You just didn't want to let it go – '

Oliver shook his head. 'It wasn't like that, Jimmy,' he said and he looked up at the other with his face very straight, no hint of amusement anywhere. 'I'm not like that and you know it. I make a deal and I keep it. We go back too far for me to pull a dirty one on you, anyway. It's something personal – '

'What, leaving out the plums from the plum pudding? That's *personal*?'

'Yes,' Oliver shouted, and the woman at the urn looked across disapprovingly, and he lowered his voice. 'Yes,' he said again. 'Strictly personal. But I have to tell you, since you've got it anyway.'

'Have I ever got it,' Jimmy said in high satisfaction. 'Picked up one of the nurses, didn't I? Took her out for a drink and blowout at the local Chinese – Christ, can't these girls eat! – and I've got more than you'd believe. The name of the surgeon, all the details about what was done, the lot. Verifies the patient's word for it. She'll be worth the money.'

'You're buying the story?'

'She needs the cash,' Jimmy said after a moment. 'No, don't look at me like that. It's very easy to be high-minded when you're in the sweet backwaters of radio. Not so easy when you're paddling in the crappy sewers down what's left of Fleet Street. So we're buying – '

'This nurse told you who the surgeon was?'

'Did she ever – and there's another lollipop. A woman, no less, and a doll. I saw her. Sian – the nurse – pointed her out to me in the car park. A lady surgeon with looks no woman'd be ashamed of – '

'You don't have to tell me that,' Oliver said savagely. 'I know that perfectly well – '

'And you were holding that out on me too? Honestly, Merrall,

191

I thought better of you. It was never your style to try to steal from under a mate's nose. Not when you use him for cheap research when it suits you.'

'I wasn't trying to cheat you,' Oliver said wearily. 'I was trying to protect myself. Listen, Jimmy, can I get you to lay off on this? It's bad enough I've got to deal with it – if I'd known before I started I'd never have got so deep in. But – well, the fact of the matter is, the surgeon, Kate Sayers – '

'Well?' Jimmy squinted at him over the smoke of his cigarette, because Oliver had stopped. 'Spit it out. If you ever want to get anything else from me, that is. Not another bloody word do I ever let you see from our morgue unless you blubber your bibful. Right now.'

'I live with her,' Oliver said. 'She's my – after my marriage died, I lived on my own a good while. And then I met Kate and about fifteen months ago I moved into her flat. You see what I mean? I'm in the crap up to my elbows and I'm doing all I can to try to keep my head above water. And now you've got hold of it – '

'Oh, shit,' Jimmy said softly. 'Oh, shit! You poor old bugger.'

Chapter Twenty

Joe Allen's was fairly quiet when they got there, pushing their way through the Covent Garden crowds, and Oliver was grateful for that. Usually they chose this particular restaurant for the fun of people-watching: the regular clientele of actors, singers and dancers were as good as a sideshow as they leapt from table to table with loud cries of welcome and much hugging; but tonight he needed time to talk and the sideshow would have been a distraction. He'd almost said as much to Kate when she had chosen the restaurant after he'd suggested dinner out on this, one of the rare evenings when she wasn't on call; but had chickened out at the last minute. Bad enough he had to say what he would have to say; at least let her choose where they'd go. And anyway, saying nothing about his need to talk helped to put it all off for as long as possible.

But now, sitting in the corner table at the back of the restaurant, well away from the area of greatest traffic and waiting for the bottle of house white they were allowing themselves, he found his determination slipping ever further away. Chickening out, he thought again as he watched Kate study the menu; it was one of the newer terms that he liked, and it certainly described the way he felt at present. Small and scrawny and feathery, that was Oliver Merrall tonight, he told himself, and reddened a little as he realised that Kate was staring at him with her brows raised in interrogation, apparently waiting for an answer of some kind.

'I'm sorry,' he said. 'Did you say something?'

'I asked you whether you were going to be adventurous tonight and have something different, or was it to be potato skins and barbecued ribs as usual?'

'I don't know,' he said and bent his head to look at his own menu. 'What is there?'

'Most of the usual and a couple of new things – look, Oliver,

193

what is it? You've been anywhere but with me tonight. Would you rather abandon ship and just go home now?'

'Of course not. I'll have the skins but I'll try the – oh, dammit, no I won't. The ribs'll do fine.'

'The way they always do,' she said and pushed the menu away. 'And I'll have the gravadlax and the spinach salad and what else is new? Nice to be creatures of habit, I dare say. Makes you feel secure.'

'Yes,' he said and then leaned back gratefully as the wine arrived and there was an agreeable flurry of opening and pouring to occupy them. He gave their order then and, as the waiter went away, managed to smile at her.

'It's been far too long since we did this,' he said. 'Behaved like normal people.'

'Far too long,' she agreed. 'So now try and do it.'

'I am!' he protested. 'Aren't I? Put on a sweater instead of a suit – very normal casual person, that's me.'

She looked dispassionately at the sweater. 'Well, yes. E for effort at least. But it's hardly the sort of sweater that would make most people think of normalcy.'

He looked at the pattern of tumbling white squares that covered the black front of the sweater. 'It was a Christmas present – ' he began and then stopped, suddenly aware of the pit he had dug for his own feet. But it was too late.

'Oh,' was all she said, but it was enough. Sonia had come into their evening as surely as if she had walked in and sat down at the table with them. Oliver could have bitten his tongue off at his own stupidity. She had given him this sweater two Christmases ago, the last they had spent together, and now he couldn't imagine why he had put it on tonight. He hadn't actually thought about it at the time; just been aware that the weather had changed and it was chilly after dark and so had taken the top garment in the drawer. He hadn't, for once, thought at all about Sonia; he was far more anxious about his dilemma regarding Kate. But she didn't know that and wouldn't believe him if he said it; as far as she was concerned he'd done it again. But he didn't say anything; instead he tried to pretend nothing had happened.

Their food arrived and they began to eat, both of them clearly grateful for the distraction, and as he chewed his way through his barbecued ribs and made superficial small talk about the other people around them and the items they had read in the papers that day, Oliver let the thoughts scurry around beneath the surface of his attention, trying to work out what to say to her and precisely how to say it.

And she, apparently as relaxed and conversational as he was, felt exactly the same. She knew he was abstracted and paying her only half his attention, and she knew with all the certainty she had in her that it was his ex-wife who had supplanted her. Again. And as she swallowed her food, tasting none of it, she thought over and over again – It's not worth it. I love him, but it's not worth it. We'll have to stop all this. It isn't me he wants; it's her, and I can't take it any more. I'll have to tell him so, find the words to explain it –

'Kate,' he said as at last the waiter went away with their plates, and at the same moment she leaned forwards and said, 'Oliver – ' and then they both laughed, and for one glorious moment there was accord between them as fragile as a soap bubble.

And like a soap bubble it burst as soon as it had formed and she leaned back and said coolly, 'Yes?'

'No.' He sounded almost eager. 'You first.'

'It wasn't important.'

'I'm sure it was.'

'No.'

Again there was a little silence and then he took a deep breath and began. And because he was so anxious to get it right, to explain it all to her clearly and simply so there could be no confusion, he forgot the need to explain fully, and went in head-first. And knew at once he'd got it all wrong.

'Kate, you've got a patient in your ward – a sex-change operation. And you'll have to hand him – or her, or whatever – over to someone else. It's really the only way.'

She stared at him, her face smooth with amazement. 'What did you say?'

'Believe me, Kate, I'm not trying to interfere,' he said earnestly and leaned forwards, reaching for her hands. But she kept them firmly in her lap below the level of the tablecloth. 'It's just that I have information that you don't and that's why I had to say that – '

'Then suppose you give me the information, whatever it is? And as for not interfering – you're giving a pretty damned good imitation of it.'

'Oh dammit – I knew this'd cause trouble. Look, Kate, this patient of yours – he took another man's bed. A man who's been on the waiting list for ages. He's had five false calls for admission and each time he's been told at the last minute that his operation has been cancelled. The poor devil's nearly out of his mind with it all. That's why there was that letter – he wrote to me, you see – '

'What letter? Who wrote to you? And what has it got to do with – ' She was looking totally bewildered now and he shook his head in impatience at his own crass stupidity at explaining so badly. And to her it looked very like an expression of irritation directed at her inability to understand what his garbled account was all about. And her mouth hardened as she stared at him.

'This man, Scribner, wrote me a letter,' he said with careful patience; and again it sounded to Kate like an almost studied attack on her capacity to understand. 'Well, not to me precisely. To anyone in the press who would take up his case. Only it was me he happened to give it to. It was – it was the night we went to dinner at Esther and Richard's – '

'Oh,' she said noncommittally. The night he went to Sonia's, a little voice murmured in her deeper mind. The night he went to see Sonia, even though he didn't say he had. But I knew, I knew –

'I went back to the studio to get some stuff, you remember? And he was there hanging about and he gave me this letter. I didn't look at it for a while, though – you know how it is. Shoved it in a pocket and forgot it. So when I did read it I felt so bad about the delay I suppose I put more effort into it than I might have done – anyway, I took it up rather.'

'Oh?' she said again, still noncommittal. 'You took it up. How?'

'Went to see him. Found out what it was all about – and – ' He stopped then, awkwardly. 'I didn't realise at first it had anything to do with you, Kate. If I had known, I'd have talked to you right away. As it was, I wanted to keep you out of it. So I said nothing. But I set the story up with Radlett, and we're doing a series. Four half-hour programmes – '

'About this man who wrote you – didn't write you – a letter which you put in your pocket.'

'I know I'm not explaining well. It's because I was so anxious for you to understand properly.'

'I'm not precisely stupid,' she said and now her voice was distinctly frosty. 'I usually manage to pick up most things I'm told.'

'Of course you're not stupid,' he cried and then lowered his voice as the people at the adjoining table glanced at him. 'That was why I wanted to keep you out of it. As I said, I set up these programmes and now there's no going back. Because now another chap's got hold of the story – someone from the *Globe* – and it'd take the last trump to stop him from following up. I tried to persuade him, but it's too good a story. Anyway the chap himself wants to sell his story – needs money I gather because he's lost his job – '

'Who?' Kate almost wailed it. 'The man who didn't write you a letter?'

'I'm sorry. No, Hynes. Your patient Hynes.'

Now she stiffened. 'You know this patient of mine?'

'Not yet. I mean, we haven't met. But I know all about him. Her, now I suppose I should say.' He stopped then and made a face. 'It's a nasty business, Kate, isn't it? Why on earth are you doing cases like that? You'll be better off without him, surely?'

She raised her brows at him. 'Really? You find Kim distasteful in some way?'

'Anyone would. There's something unremittingly sleazy, isn't there, about sex changes? Real *News of the Screws* stuff – cheap and tawdry – '

'You of course have a great deal of experience in such matters.' Her voice dripped ice now and he stared back at her miserably.

'Oh, shit, Kate – I've really cocked this up, haven't I?'

'Have you? Isn't that what you intended to do? First you point out that you're wearing one of Sonia's presents, just to rub my nose in the fact that what we have isn't of course important enough to you to make a commitment of it, and then you remind

197

me, oh so delicately, of the night you went and – let's say spent time with her instead of coming back to bed with me, and then you have the brass neck to tell me how to run my job. Isn't a cock-up precisely what you intended? Because it sure as hell is what you've done.'

'Of course it isn't what I intended,' he said and now anger began to bubble in him. She can't really think, can she, that I'd deliberately try to upset her? How could she think that? 'All I wanted to do was tell you, in the best way I could, that there's trouble brewing. The *Globe* have got this story as well as me, so even if I try to hush it up – and frankly I don't see how I can, seeing I've gone so far down the road and Radlett knows about it; he'll only send someone else on it if I hand in my chips – as I say, even if I tried I couldn't stop the row happening. This case is going to be all over the place. There's going to be all hell let loose when people find out that not only are NHS services being cut to the bone even more than they know, but that cases like Kim Hynes are being given preference over cases like poor old Ted Scribner, ex-soldier, lonely pensioner – it's real hearts and flowers stuff. Jimmy Rhoda'll give it all he's got and that's considerable. And I don't want you to be caught up in it. Can't you get someone else to take the case over?'

'Let's give you the benefit of the doubt,' she said after a long moment. 'Let's pretend, just for now, that you really mean what you say, and you want to protect me. Christ, Oliver, what sort of person do you take me for? What sort of *doctor*? Do you think I'd really dump a patient just because some cheap journalist wants to peddle garbage around and then chuck it at me? I'd be one hell of a surgeon if I did that! Kim Hynes is my *patient*. I operated on her and did what I did out of something that I thought once mattered to you, but now wonder about: compassion. And care for individuals' needs. And human dignity. And old-fashioned medical ethics. Not that you'd know anything about that, would you? Anyway, that was what I did, and there is no way I would ever dream of dumping her on someone else. Why the hell should I? I'm not ashamed of caring for Kim Hynes! To run away from her now would suggest I was. And anyway, what possible good would it do your other man – what do you say his name is – Scribner? Is he a patient of mine?'

Oliver shook his head. 'Mr Le Queux's.'

'I see,' she said, and her voice dripped sarcasm. 'I have to dump Kim Hynes, *my* patient, for another patient who has nothing to do with me, who isn't on my waiting list, and who has nothing whatever to do with Kim. Is that it? Why should I?'

'Because Scribner lost his bed to Hynes, of course,' Oliver said. 'Can't you see that?'

'You're a fool, Oliver,' she said shortly. 'A complete fool. You don't even know what you don't know. Scribner's bed or lack of it has nothing whatsoever to do with me or my patient. If he's on Le Queux's list of patients, then he'd have to be admitted to one of his beds. I have mine, he has his. In fact – ' She squinted then, staring inside her memory for the way the beds on GU were currently occupied. 'In fact, I can tell you who's to blame for your Scribner's situation. His name, as I recall, is Prior. He's a wino. Admitted from the wasteground in uraemic shock, been on dialysis ever since, and they're still trying to get him stabilised. So there you are. Start a campaign against a sick sad dropout, why don't you? There he lies, a piece of human garbage suffering from self-inflicted disease – after all, he's been on meths for God knows how long – and using up a bed that ought by rights to go to your old soldier. Try that one on your friend at the *Globe*. Tell him to scream and shout to have treatment refused to characters like that, and see where it gets you. Even the Great British Public – or the segment of it that reads the sort of filth that paper peddles – with a mind as wide as a streak of slime is likely to rise up against that – '

'No one's saying that people should be refused treatment – ' Oliver began, but she gave him no chance.

'Aren't you? Of course you are! Dump Kim Hynes, you were saying, to clear the way so that your friend on the *Globe*, and you too, I imagine, can start thumping your great big drums about how wicked it is to waste NHS resources on people like that, people with different sexual needs. They're not important to people like you, are they? The fact that Kim has been to hell and back with the problem she has, the fact that she's suffered more misery than you could ever imagine in your smug life doesn't matter, does it? She's a sexual weirdo so anything goes.

Well, the man who took that emergency bed is a weirdo too – he's a booze weirdo. Have a go at him instead – '

'You're being deliberately obstructive,' Oliver said. There was a thin white line round his mouth now as he tried to control his temper. 'Of course I'm not going to start a campaign like that. I wasn't even going to have a go at your damned Kim Hynes, either. I just wanted you to realise that no matter what I do or don't do, this story is out. And other people will be hateful about the sort of work you're doing. I love you Kate, you know I do. And because I care about you, I care about your reputation as well. I just don't want you pilloried as the sort of surgeon who – '

'Who what?' she flared as he stopped. 'Who looks after sexual weirdos, right? Isn't that what you mean? Oh, Oliver, listen to yourself! The great compassionate campaigner, the man who loves the underdog, the man London listens to to find its heart: how shallow does it go? Tell me how you've managed to keep it all going for so long with no one noticing it's all a sham!'

How he still sat at the table he didn't know. His mouth was dry and his face felt as stiff as if it had been chilled in iced water for hours. 'That is cruel and totally unjust,' he said in a low voice. 'You have to know that.'

There was a long silence and then she took a deep and shuddering breath. 'All right,' she said. 'I'm sorry. It was a bit over the top, I suppose. A lot, in fact. But you must see you asked for it – saying you were trying to protect me, and all the time all I could hear were judgements about Kim Hynes and her right to be cared for. Why should I be ashamed of looking after her? Can't you see what it was you were saying?'

'I suppose so,' he said. 'It wasn't meant that way, but I suppose so. But what else could I do? You live with me, for heaven's sake! How can I carry out a proper job on this story while you're so deeply enmeshed in it? If I'd realised at the start that this was going to involve you I'd never have started on it. But now I have – I have my job to do too, you know. Just as you can't pass your Kim on to someone else, neither can I stop investigating this story. You understand that?'

'I'm not sure I do.' She lifted her chin and stared at him very directly. 'I don't want to diminish the value of what you do, but how can it help people to start digging around in the private lives of patients like Kim Hynes? How can it be of any value to anyone to – '

'Don't forget she wants to sell her story. Once she does, you'll be involved, like it or not. That's what I wanted you to realise.'

'Well, that's up to her. But you don't have to be part of the buying and selling, do you?'

'I have a story to write,' he said. 'And to broadcast. It needs to be told. The NHS is being shaved down to its barest necessities, and people should know it. I'll try not to get involved in too many value judgements about which patients deserve care and which don't, but if it happens, well it happens. And as I say, it's difficult when one of the most likely candidates for publicity happens to be the girl I live with.'

Suddenly she frowned. 'What matters most? The fact that it could be embarrassing for me to be labelled as a surgeon who does sex-change operations – or the fact that I live with you, the disinterested journalist?'

He thought for a long moment, and then looked up at her. 'Both,' he said. 'I have to be honest. Both. It's very embarrassing indeed for me. If anyone apart from Jimmy finds out the connection I could have a rough time of it. But – '

'No buts,' she said and stood up, gathering her bag and her jacket from the back of her chair. 'I'll move into the residents' quarters at the hospital. It could save us all a lot of trouble.'

He tried to get to his feet too, but was slowed down by the fact that his chair was too close to the next table. She added then, with all the malice she could and with a sense of amazement that she could behave so, 'And that will give you all the time you need for your Sonia, won't it? Goodnight. And thanks for dinner.'

And she went, walking so fast she was up the stairs and out of the restaurant before he could stop her. And by the time he'd paid the bill and run after her, it was too late. Exeter Street was deserted.

Chapter Twenty-One

The theatre block was working flat out by eight-thirty a.m. Sister Bridie Whelan had been harrying her nurses and orderlies like an excited sheepdog, her short stumpy legs in their childish white socks and plimsolls flashing from anaesthetic room to operating theatre and back via the set-up area so fast that she looked, as one of the irreverent third-year nurses said, like a toy on wheels.

'You know the kind,' she murmured in her friend's ear as they stood setting out sterile gowns and towels and gloves ready for the scrub team. 'They've got three feet and you push 'em along on a stick and it looks as though they're running like lunatics.'

'Get on with it, get on with it!' cried Sister, leaping into the set-up area and glaring at them over her mask with an experienced glitter, for no one knew better than she how to look daggers, 'And a lot less chatter! There's no sense in masking up if you cluck like demented hens and make your masks wet. That way you spray the air and the patient with organisms. I'm sick of telling you. And move, will you! I've got three huge lists and no time for any of your nonsense.' And she was gone before either of them could say anything. Not that they wanted to. The Whelan in this mood was not to be argued with.

Kate was early for her list. She liked to be early as a general rule, liked to be able to get herself changed and comfortable before any of the other surgeons came in. They made such a fuss, some of the men, about the fact that she was a female, withdrawing with elaborate care to the men's lavatory to change their trousers as though she'd never seen a man in his underpants before, and ostentatiously turning their backs if she showed a flash of bra as she got into her theatre dress. It was worth arriving half an hour before anyone else just to get the space she needed.

And today she needed to be early to clear her mind. She had slept surprisingly well, considering how bitter she had felt when she had slid between the sheets of the spare-room bed on the residents' floor, the one that was usually occupied by the house surgeon on call for the night. She had had to wander around the hospital to scrounge a new toothbrush and washing gear and then had had to wash her tights and underwear and leave them to dry overnight in the linen cupboard since she had no intention of returning to the flat to pack a bag with clean clothes until she was sure Oliver wouldn't be there. By the time she had switched off the battered bedside light it had been almost one o'clock and she had resigned herself to a night of tossing and turning as she rehearsed all the awful things they had said to each other.

And yet she had fallen almost immediately into a deep and heavy sleep and only woke when the phone beside the bed pinged with the early call she had requested from the switchboard.

But she didn't feel now as she ought to feel after a good night's sleep and when faced with a complicated list; two trans-urethrals and a repair of a messy suprapubic incision to deal with before she got to Slattery, and it had been some time since she had done any gut surgery. She ought to feel more relaxed to be sure of doing his hernia well, and she stood there in the surgeons' room in just her bra and pants before putting on her skimpy theatre dress, taking a few deep breaths, consciously relaxing. Her patients were entitled to a better surgeon than she was at the moment and she had to work hard to make sure she was in good shape. And slowly her technique took over and she felt her shoulders soften and relax and was able to finish changing her clothes in a tranquil enough mood.

She spent the next half-hour poring over the patients' notes, making sure she had each one clearly in her mind, reminding herself of her original examinations of them and planning in her head the operations each would have. If she was lucky, she'd have that sensible third year to scrub for her: Cassie Brandon. She had a real gift for theatre work, always anticipating every surgical want with swift intelligence. Doing a list with her was always a pleasure, especially as Kate often did not work with an assistant surgeon, preferring the help of just her scrub nurse. It was only when she had medical students assigned to her that she used another pair of hands, so the quality of her scrub nurse was particularly important. So, today, would it be worth ask-ing Sister Whelan to make sure she had Cassie? She thought about that for a moment and then decided against it. She had seen Bridie bustling about in one of her paddies at the far end as she had come in through the big double doors and knew she was at her least approachable when she got like that. The mere fact of being asked for a particular scrub nurse could make her bristle at what she would regard as interference. It really wouldn't be worth the risk. As long as I don't get that half-witted chap – what was his name? Cantor, Trevor Cantor. The last time she'd had him he'd been so ham-handed she'd almost lost her temper, for he seemed to be at least three beats behind her all the time, whatever she wanted. She'd made no complaint then, but had promised herself she'd object if she ever got him again. And she bent her head to her notes once more, pushing away her niggling thoughts about who would scrub for her; still unrelaxed, that was the problem – mustn't get obsessive, mustn't create troubles before they existed.

The other surgeons arrived with the coffee and she looked up gratefully as Fay Buckland came bursting in in her usual rush, spraying her possessions around so that in a matter of moments the small surgeons' room looked cluttered and rather shabby, and Kate liked that. It made her feel more at home and she grinned widely at Fay and said, 'Good morning.'

'I hope so, ducky, I hope so!' Fay said and began to strip off her top clothes, paying no attention at all to Agnew Byford who had come into the room behind her, an expression of distaste on his face as he saw her. 'Hello, Agnew – my God, but I must be mad! I put these lists together when I'm feeling hopeful and strong and then when I get here and look at them I could die before I start. I've put in two hysterectomies, a Fothergill's repair and a positive string of damned Ds and Cs. And now they tell me there's a Caesar cooking up over on Maternity – I'll be here till the cows come home. Pour me some coffee, Kate, there's a lamb.'

Kate obeyed. 'You too, Agnew?'

'No thank you,' he said austerely and disappeared with some ostentation into the lavatory carrying his theatre suit on a neat wooden hanger, and Fay grimaced at his departing back.

'Miserable bugger,' she murmured and bent to lace up her plimsolls. 'Why he doesn't come clean and do all his work over on the Private Wing and be done with it, I don't know. He clearly despises everything we stand for over here.'

'He'd never get his gong on private work,' Kate said with a little spurt of malice and Fay giggled, and then gulped coffee, fast.

'I suppose not. Though why anyone would want such a thing I can't imagine – you'd have to have all your stationery reprinted. It'd cost a bomb.'

Kate gave a little shout of laughter. 'Only you could think that a good reason for not having an honour!' she said and Fay snorted.

'There's another. If he gets a knighthood that boring fart of a wife of his gets to be Lady Byford. If I got a Damehood, there's no way my old man'd ever become Sir Teddy, is there? No justice. So, they can stuff their bloody honours. Ah, well, this won't get me anywhere. Time to get going. I hope I've got Cassie to do my list – '

'I want her!' Kate protested as she followed her into the theatre concourse, now alive with trolleys and patients as the first three arrived with their escorts of ward nurses and anaesthetists. 'And I didn't ask on purpose – '

'Are you kidding? And stir Bridie up? Never think it. I didn't say I'd *ask* – I just said I was hoping . . . Good morning Sister! Where am I?'

'You're in Two, Miss Buckland,' Sister said, busily inspecting the typed lists on her clipboard, even though everyone knew she had it all in her head already. 'I've got you in Three, Miss Sayers. I do hope you don't mind. I've had to put Mr Byford in One. His hearts, you see – '

' – are no more important than Kate's bladders,' Fay cut in. 'Or my uteruses. You mustn't let him push you around, Sister!'

Sister bridled and Kate's heart sank. Everyone knew Fay, with her sharp tongue and her total refusal – or was it inability? – to think about the effects of her words before she spoke them, and generally everyone, Kate included, loved her dearly. But Kate could have smacked her for this.

'Well, I'm sure I don't know what you're talking about, Miss Buckland! I treat all the patients who come to *my* theatres with

205

equal care – ' and Sister put considerable emphasis on the 'my'. 'And I'd be most disturbed if I thought – '

'It's all right, Sister,' Kate said quickly. 'You mustn't let Miss Buckland tease you. She's rather fond of doing that – you ought to know by now. Right, Fay?'

'Hmm?' Fay had been trying on her mask and fiddling with her cotton helmet, trying to get her unruly hair to stay inside its confines. 'Oh, yes, I suppose so. All right then. Which anaesthetic room is it?'

'Two,' Sister said icily. 'I would never risk confusing them. Each theatre has its own anaesthetic room, and always has. I won't risk getting patients mixed up. I never have so I really don't think there's any need for you to – '

'No one was saying otherwise, Sister,' Kate said soothingly and escaped gratefully, pushing Fay ahead of her and parting from her only as she disappeared into the scrub area to be gloved and gowned. 'I'll see you over some lunch, perhaps, Fay. Pace yourself!' And Fay threw a cheerful but abstracted glance over her shoulder, clearly already so deep in contemplation of her first case she had forgotten every word that had gone before, and Kate followed her, shaking her head in amused irritation. One of these days Fay would get herself into real trouble with her abrupt directness, but meanwhile thank God for her. She made a necessary and welcome antidote to the sleekness of Agnew Byford, who had now emerged from the surgeons' room in his immaculately pressed operating suit and was being fussed over by a slightly flushed Sister Whelan. He, it seemed, had the easiest list of the day, just two catheterisations and a ballooning to do, and Kate hovered at the entrance to the scrub area, fiddling with her own mask as she listened. She didn't really care what Byford did, but it was always interesting to know what else was going on while she did her own lists. And anyway, the knowledge helped to keep her personal anxieties in some sort of perspective.

'Even here he'll have to have his security people with him, Sister,' Byford was saying in that rather pompous voice that sounded as though it came from deep inside a stuffed owl. 'I've told them they must keep well out of the way, but they will have to be gowned and so forth, of course. And I suppose they might as well get an education while they're about it.'

Stupid man! Kate thought, malice returning. He just wants to be watched. He's not a surgeon, he's just a showman. But she shook her head at herself again then and went to start her scrub; he was a bloody marvellous surgeon, deft and quick and always getting excellent results. The only trouble was that he was much too aware of his own gifts and much too fond of being admired. But his patients did well enough, and that was really all that mattered.

And she went to the big sink and pushed on the long taps with her elbows and started the laborious ten minutes of hard scrubbing of hands and arms up to the elbows that were mandatory before the first case on a list. At least while she scoured her slowly reddening skin and stared at the shapes made by the suds she had time to think about what she would do, and she settled down into the routine of an operating day with a small sigh and only the most fleeting of thoughts about last night. Oliver was a million miles away, now. Not at all important.

Or not very.

By ten o'clock she was beginning to get into the stride of her day's work. The first TUR had been smooth and easy, with hardly any blood loss and a clean operating site throughout and she had seen him on his way to the recovery suite contentedly. Even though she had indeed been lumbered with the slow Trevor Cantor and had known she could not complain to Sister in her Fay-flurried state, it was going well enough; she'd have time for a cup of coffee while they got the theatre ready for the next case and got him under, and then with a little luck she might be clear of the suprapubic repair and able to start Gerald Slattery before Bridie Whelan began twittering on about her nurses' need to go for their lunch breaks. Why they couldn't work straight through as Kate herself did, and grab a sandwich afterwards, Kate couldn't understand, but she knew better than ever to say so. Nurses' health had to be protected while the surgeons' didn't and that was the end of it. Boring though.

She stood in the concourse for a moment, thinking. Fay's second hysterectomy had gone in; she could see into the recovery suite across the way where they fussed over her first patient, as well as over her TUR man, and she could see into Theatre Two where they were already at work again, and she grinned as she noticed that Fay didn't have the much coveted Cassie with her either; a new and unfamiliar face peered over the mask that Kate could see through the glass window of the door to Theatre Two. That meant that Byford had snaffled the peach of the theatre staff and she grinned sourly into the folds of her own mask as she thought of that. It was, of course, inevitable, just as it was inevitable that Sister Whelan herself would be running for him. Honestly, it was enough to make you sick –

She moved over towards the door of Theatre One to peer in to see how Byford was getting on and almost jumped as a burly figure appeared from the anaesthetic room on that side to bar her way.

'If you don't mind, madam, may I ask what you want here?' it said and she looked up, startled.

'What did you say?'

'I said, may I ask what you want here,' the man repeated.

She looked down at herself. 'I've come to sunbathe and have a nice swim,' she said acidly. 'What the hell do you think I want? I'm a surgeon, dammit. I have every right to be here.'

'But not in this theatre, I think, madam,' the large shape said and stared at her with wide bovine eyes, much enhanced by the line of green mask that was beneath them. He had absurdly long lashes, she noticed, and wanted to giggle.

'No, not in this theatre,' she allowed. 'I'm a bladder surgeon, and I'd be glad to whip out your prostate for you while you're waiting. I have no intention of doing any such thing to your charge, however, who is a heart patient, right? I take it it's the ineffable Saffron in there?'

The man seemed unruffled. 'Mr Saffron, madam, yes.'

'Hmpph. Well, I have no special interest in Mr Saffron, I can assure you. I was actually much more interested in catching Sister Whelan's eye. I need to talk to her about my next case. *If* you don't mind.' And firmly and with due force she pushed the man aside and went to the door to set her face against the glass and peer in.

As always, Sister Whelan, who seemed to have eyes in every part of her anatomy and always looked at the door the moment anyone appeared to occlude the window, saw her and came purposefully across to slip out, just as the burly watcher moved closer to Kate and set a hand on her arm.

'Sister,' Kate said wrathfully, 'do I have to put up with this sort of harassment?' And she shook her arm sharply to make the man let go, which he did as Sister stood there and glared at him. 'I need to discuss my last case with you. With this man's permission, of course – '

'He has to be here,' Sister said shortly. 'I don't like it any more than you do, Miss Sayers, but it's Mr Saffron and who am I to argue? Now, what do you want with me?'

'In the office please, Sister,' Kate said and marched away, more ruffled than she cared to admit by the silly little altercation. The theatres were a special place, a private place where only the true acolytes should be; it was not a matter to which she had ever given any direct thought but that she felt so was undoubted. Only surgeons and their attendants belonged in the theatres, and patients when they were suitably cowed by drugs and anaesthetics. A sort of holy of holies – and now the thought had come into her mind she was amused and a little ashamed and in consequence was more affable to Sister than she had intended to be. Which immediately put Bridie Whelan on the defensive; the only time surgeons were as friendly as this was when they wanted something out of the ordinary.

'Sister, I was just wondering,' Kate began. 'If I could ask some particular help from you – '

Bridie Whelan looked back at her stolidly and said nothing.

'It's my last case, you see, Sister. The one who's due in after this. He's a special one I'm doing – repair of an inguinal hernia, remember? The thing is I want to use totally no-touch technique and I don't have to tell you how tricky that is. Well, I was just wondering – by the time I get to him I imagine Mr Byford'll be finished. He doesn't take that long on his people, does he? And I was just hoping that perhaps – I mean, Trevor's a pleasant enough chap and tries hard in his own way, but he isn't Cassie, is he? I'd be most grateful if I could have her for that case – '

Almost too late she saw the frown start to creep across Bridie Whelan's forehead and added hastily, 'Unless, of course, I could have you? Now that would make all the difference – '

The frown retreated but all the same Bridie Whelan still just stood and stared at her. And then said, 'Why?'

'Hmm?'

'Why? Why do you want – '

'Well, as I said,' Kate broke in swiftly, needing to repair any damage she had done to the woman's self-esteem, 'I need someone very experienced and good and Trevor's all right, I suppose, but not as experienced as you. Or Cassie – '

'No,' Sister Whelan said with all the insulting patience she would use to a particularly stupid child. 'Why do you want to use a no-touch technique? For a hernia? It's not like a bone job, is it? Just a gut – '

There was a little silence as Kate contemplated the dreadful hole she had so carefully dug so very deeply for herself. To tell Sister Whelan why would mean explaining about the possible risk of cross infection, and to someone who was as fiercely protective of her staff as was Sister Whelan, that could be disaster. Even as she stood and stared at the slit of face and eyes that was all that was visible of the doughy face in front of her she could see the whole scenario as it flickered on its inevitable progress: Sister Whelan horrified to hear one of the patients coming to her precious theatres might be carrying HIV; Sister Whelan realising the fact that this case must belong to another surgeon by rights, since it was outside Kate's own usual speciality; Sister Whelan either refusing to allow Gerald Slattery over her portals or sweeping all her staff out – oh, damn and blast it all to hell, Kate cursed silently. What had she done in speaking to her? She should have managed with the egregious Trevor, useless ham-handed ass though he was. She would simply have to thread all her own needles and prepare all her own gut sutures and just manage – If Whelan hadn't already realised there was more here than she knew, and persisted, it could be – Oh, damn, damn, damn –

'No special reason,' she said quickly then, after what seemed an eternity but was little more than a few moments. 'I just don't want to lose my technique, you see. It took me a long time to learn it – and – '

'Well, another day, perhaps, Miss Sayers,' Sister said sharply, obviously deeply irritated. 'I really can't be expected to cope with such a – with things like that when we're so very busy. Next week possibly. If Nurse Brandon is on duty, of course.' And she swept away, her little feet twinkling busily and seeming to slap out their message on the terrazzo floor, 'And off duty she'll be, you can depend on it. Off duty she'll be – ' And Kate once more cursed under her breath and went to get her coffee before starting on her next case. At least she'd managed to stop the damage in time, she told herself. Be grateful for that.

Chapter Twenty-Two

The second TUR went a little less well. The man bled a good deal and that obscured her vision and as she became a little more tetchy, so did Trevor Cantor become a little less capable. She knew at some deep level that if she handled the boy right, he'd be fine; he was one of those who slowed down under pressure. Only when he felt really secure in what he was doing could he cope with the speed that was necessary, and if she had had enough patience for him she could have brought him along nicely. But as her operating field blurred over and over again with blood she became very irritable and snapped and that made the anaesthetist, a cheerful Maltese, become ever more flippant, for that was his way of dealing with stress.

'Thank you, Dr Azzopardi,' she said at length, when once again he had distracted Trevor's attention with one of his sallies. 'I'd be grateful if you could let this man concentrate. He's not showing a great deal of it at the moment.' At which comment the runner – Sister Whelan's second in command, who was shaping up nicely to be as despotic as Bridie herself – showed distinct signs of annoyance and Kate sighed and doggedly worked on, biting her lip beneath her mask, determined not to say another word.

When at last the case was finished and she could dispatch him on his way, they ran into more trouble. Byford's case, which had clearly taken longer than anyone had expected, was just finished and her own patient emerged into the concourse just as Saffron's trolley was pushed out of Theatre One, fluttering with drips and mobile monitors, and well escorted by no fewer than two nurses and two porters as well as the security man, as burly and imperturbable as ever. Kate stood at the door as her own runner tried to get their trolley past all the confusion, and as she saw that no one was in the least interested in anything but Byford, Byford's patient and Byford's needs, her irritation boiled over and she pushed herself forwards determinedly past the other trolley and with one hand on her runner's back propelled her firmly onward.

'This patient needs to be in the recovery suite *now*,' she said loudly and crisply and looked pointedly at Byford, who ignored her with lofty disdain. 'So if you *don't* mind – ' and then went back into the theatre to push the nurses there to work faster at getting ready for her next case, the suprapubic repair. It was already past eleven-thirty and time was running tight; there would be new lists this afternoon to be dealt with, and Sister Whelan was as edgy as a cat as she tried to get rid of Kate so that she could bustle about on her own account. But Kate was now far too irritable to be sensible and instead of retiring out of the way to leave Bridie Whelan to calm down, she stayed stubbornly put, watching them get ready with a stare of grim determination on what could be seen of her face, and feeling more and more tense as the time ticked on.

Outside there was more hubbub as the next case was brought in for Byford, and she listened, sneering a little inside her head as Byford's plump tones filled the air with his importance.

'I want a five-minute BP – yes, every five minutes. Just keep a very close watch. If necessary I'll have him back in here but I hope it won't be required. Azzopardi, are you anaesthetising this one for me? No? Then keep out of the way, will you? I really can't cope with all this hubbub – ' And he went striding into his own theatre with a great deal of hubbub, leaving Kate seething and even Azzopardi looking put out.

The next case came in then and Kate looked down at the area, once it had been sheeted and the skin prepared, and said over her shoulder to the runner, 'Staff Nurse, get my next patient up now, will you? This won't take me long at all, and I really do want to get on – '

She didn't really know why she was fussing so; there was no panic after all. If she wasn't finished before the nurses' lunches became a matter of paramount importance, too bad. They'd just have to wait and there was an end to it. Sister Whelan herself might fuss and flurry but she wouldn't jeopardise a case for such a reason, surely, and Kate knew that she'd get her list finished without undue difficulty. And yet she was now so edgy she almost felt as though she had to increase the pressure she was under, had to get Slattery up soon, get him into the anaesthetic room, hurry, hurry, hurry – and she started to clean the edges of the messy wound that lay before her in the bright eye of the great theatre lamp, very aware of the sweat that was trickling down between her breasts.

The stitching took much longer than she had hoped. The wound had been big to start with, the remains of an operation performed by another rather elderly surgeon at another hospital two years earlier, and his technique had been a very old-fashioned one. Kate had agreed to try to help the poor man who ever since he'd had it done had leaked urine from his perforated bladder on to the surface of his belly; a miserable existence. And Kate had been sure she could relieve it very easily.

And easy it was in a sense, but laborious and slow. By the time the last stitches were in, fine silk and close-set nylon, and the special impermeable dressings set in place, the clock was shouting one o'clock at her and Sister was glaring.

'I have to do the next case now, Sister,' Kate said loudly, anticipating her complaints and demands for rescheduling. 'Mr Slattery's up here and he's premedded. I'm not putting him through a delay. So, I'm sorry about lunch – '

'I'll stay, Sister,' Trevor Cantor volunteered at once. 'I'll grab a quick sandwich while someone else sets up, but I don't mind not going up to the dining room, really I don't. I'll be glad to help out.'

Kate at once felt wretched, for she had been snapping at the boy mercilessly and he was now wet with sweat and pallid with anxiety; but she had to give him his due. He was a stayer. And she flicked a glance at him and managed a smile. 'It really isn't all that – '

'There's no one else to do it,' Sister Whelan said sharply. 'So thank you, Trevor. The others have already gone to lunch except Cassie Brandon. She has to stay here for Mr Byford. He has got to get Mr Saffron in again – he's not too well and the ballooning didn't – Well, no need for fuss. But he's coming back. So get cleared up here as fast as you can.' She flicked a glare at her runner and the two juniors with her. 'And then go to lunch. 'I'll be back by one-thirty and I can run next door, while you take over here if I'm not finished. It's only a hernia so I hope we won't waste too much time in here, and I can get back to Theatre One – ' And once more she glared at Kate and went padding away to eat her own lunch.

'I'm sorry,' Kate said drearily to the three nurses now cleaning up at a great rate, hurling towels and swabs into skips and sweeping soiled instruments away to be scrubbed and resterilised. 'That last one was trickier than I thought – '

But none of them said anything and she went dispiritedly away to the surgeons' room to find a few curled sandwiches which were all that Byford had left after his own coffee break, and some half-cold coffee. And was marginally comforted to find that Fay was still beavering away in her own small theatre, the least convenient to work in, yet showing no signs of any fatigue or bad temper. Good for Fay, she thought, and stretched her shoulders. Good for Fay. I'm bushed. And she sat down and put her head back on the wall and let herself doze as she waited for the theatre staff to tell her they were ready for her, and prayed behind her closed eyes that Trevor Cantor would sweat less and move faster during the hernia repair. Because she'd need all the support she could get, she now realised. It was all getting to be a much less comfortable list than she'd expected.

By a quarter to two, as Byford went on and on with his efforts over his last case in Theatre One, and Fay was still wheeling her Ds and Cs in and out of Three, Sister Whelan was in a white-hot rage. She had spent only fifteen minutes over her lunch and then come back to realise she would have to warn Orthopaedics, ENT and Paediatrics that they couldn't operate until after four at the earliest, rather than from three o'clock. The theatres had no hope of being ready till then, the way the morning lists were going, and she marched around Theatre Two as Kate set to work on Slattery, bristling with annoyance and clearly furious with Kate for insisting, as she was, on using her no-touch technique. It could add as much as fifteen minutes or more to the total operating time, and, as far as Sister Whelan was concerned, that was a personal affront and deliberate malice on Kate's part.

Inevitably Trevor picked up his senior's mood and became slower still, and by the time Kate had cut down through the skin and fat and reached the fascia, laboriously diathermying each tiny bleeding point – somewhat to Azzopardi's surprise, for who worried that much about little bleeders? – the whole theatre was buzzing with tension. And Azzopardi didn't help when he craned forwards over the head of the table and said conversationally, 'I never saw such a lily-white job! What's the matter, Kate? This one a private patient who'd have to pay for a unit of blood? You're saving every teaspoonful – '

'I prefer to operate in a clean area,' Kate said sharply and didn't take her eyes away from the wound, looking for every little bead of blood so that she could occlude even the smallest of veins. She would have closed off capillary oozing too if she could.

'I hardly think it's all that vital for a simple inguinal,' Sister said, stopping to look over Trevor's shoulder. 'Hold that clamp more upright, Cantor, for heaven's sake! You've been shown that often enough!'

'Yes, Sister,' Trevor said and immediately tipped the clamp so acutely that it slid out of position and grimly Kate seized it and put it back.

'We're managing fine, Sister,' she said. 'I'd prefer a little quietness here if you don't mind.' It was the nearest she could dare come to telling Sister to shut up, and Sister was well aware of it and made a sharp little sound behind her teeth and began to collect used swabs with ostentatious efficiency.

Outside, beyond the thick door, the sounds of the theatre block came muffled to her ears and as Kate went doggedly on freeing the loop of gut, mobilising it, looking for adhesions and checking for the position and state of the testicle on that side, she listened as much to relax her tension as because of any interest. The rattle of wheels again: Fay's last case, could it be? Kate hoped not – it would be agreeable to be able to speak to Fay when she finished in here. It would help bring her back into a pleasant frame of mind. Fay was always in a good mood, no matter what happened. But the wheels sounded again and she heard the door of her own theatre shift and sigh as the next-door theatre opened yet again to admit another patient. Ah, that would be Fay's last one. So maybe they could meet up after all –

She had managed to push the loop of gut back safely into position now. It hadn't been nearly as oedematous as she had

216

feared it would be, after being held so long in the ring of muscle that had tethered it into the wrong place. Now all she had to do was repair the weakened wall to make sure there was no recurrence of the hernia and sew up the layers of the abdomen, and she would be able to send Slattery back to his bed safe and sound with the minimum of blood loss. Whether he was HIV positive or not really didn't matter; no one had touched his blood so far and there was no reason to suppose anyone would.

She became aware again of sound from outside, and lifted her head briefly to listen, for it was so unexpected. Raised voices, someone shouting and then someone else speaking loudly and firmly and Sister Whelan heard too and went hurrying self-importantly over to the door to push it open.

Kate went on working even as she listened, not taking her eyes from her working hands. They moved there in front of her in the pool of clean shadowless light thrown by the great lamp over her head, smooth and brown and featureless, crawling over the pinkish-grey membranes and rich yellow fat globules like busy snakes. A pleasing image, she thought, and felt as she sometimes did when she reached this stage of a long list, a little separated from her physical self, as though she were just an operating machine, while the real Kate stood to one side and watched, amused and remote and considering.

Facing her, Trevor Cantor became aware of the noise outside too, and that made him even jerkier than usual and the finely pointed scissors he had been holding ready to snip off the ends of the sutures she was tying moved convulsively in his hand.

The separate Kate watched, aghast, seeing what was coming and unable to do anything about it. The points of the scissors jerked forwards and went into the other side of the wound where Kate's brown hands were moving, and buried themselves in the tissue. And Kate stood and stared, her hands no longer moving, for a fraction of a second that felt like a year, and saw the blood begin to ooze round the glinting chrome.

Trevor was still holding the scissors by their loops and again the watching Kate realised what he was going to do and was horrified, and again the brown hands that were Kate's could not move fast enough to stop him.

Trevor gasped, and jerked his hand back, pulling the scissors

217

out, and at once the blood stopped oozing but began to pulse, bright red and glistening, into little rhythmic bubbles which became heavier and richer, and even as Kate grabbed for a swab stopped being bubbles and became a spurting series of high jets.

By the time she had managed to get a swab over the punctured artery her own gown was streaked with blood and so was Trevor's. His glasses had been affected too, and he stared at her over his blood-streaked mask, peered through the little rivulets trickling down the lenses and muttered dully, 'Ooh, Miss Sayers – ever so sorry, Miss Sayers – '

'Panic you not,' Azzopardi said comfortably. 'Our Kate'll get that dealt with in a flash, eh Kate? So much for your nice lily-white operating field though, eh Kate? Oh, well, no harm done – '

'Oh, Christ,' Kate said and pushed harder against the wall of the wound with her swab, which was rapidly becoming a sodden crimson rag. 'Give me another swab fast – '

Trevor reached awkwardly behind him for his instrument trolley, as he stood with his head turned sideways to allow the junior nurse gingerly to remove his glasses to clean them and Kate saw in a brief glance that the girl had managed to get blood all over her hand while she was doing it, and felt sicker than ever. Now two of them affected; and although Slattery had said it had been seventeen years since he'd had any partner other than his own, and although she was reasonably confident he wasn't HIV positive, still and all, maybe – and she realised she was breathing hard and fast as she scrabbled in the wound with her bloody hands and pushed with her artery forceps, snapping eagerly in a search for the source of the danger.

She found it of course. The operating Kate was too experienced and well trained to fail, and the watching Kate made a conscious effort to calm down, to breathe less rapidly and to sweat less hard as at last the bleeding stopped.

Gingerly the brown hands moved again, swabbing out the wound, and slowly the tissue reappeared underneath the folds of stained fabric: the greyish-pink fascia, the deep crimson muscle and the yellow fat, and she took the swab away and set it carefully in the bowl at her side.

'No one is to touch that,' she said sharply as the junior came

218

trotting round the table to take it all away in the usual manner. 'Do you hear me? I want nothing touched here. I'll deal with it – Now, Trevor, go away. I'll manage on my own now.'

The boy stared at her, his face wet over his mask and his weak eyes blinking without his glasses.

'I can manage, Miss Sayers, honestly I can. I'm ever so sorry I let my hand slip, but it was all that shouting – '

And indeed the shouting was still going on as Sister Whelan's voice joined in. The whole episode had lasted less than minutes, Kate suddenly realised and she took a deep breath, deliberate and slow, and managed to crinkle her eyes reassuringly at the boy now looking at her so miserably.

'I know. I'm not having a go at you. It's just that – look, I want you to do as I tell you. Take off your gloves and your gown very carefully. Don't get any blood on your hands, you hear me? Then drop them in this bowl. This one where the swabs are. I'll take the responsibility for dealing with them. Then I want you to go and wash carefully, especially your face and forehead. Watch you don't get any of the blood in your eyes. I don't think you were the target of too much of it – it's good that you wear such big glasses. But be careful – '

All the time she spoke her hands went on working, reaching for the needles, setting sutures, tying, snipping ends, making a workmanlike job of the rest of the operation. She kept her head down, but was very aware of the way all of them exchanged puzzled glances.

'For heaven's sake, Kate,' Azzopardi said goood-humouredly. 'What a fuss! The boy made a bit of a mess, I know, but what's a little blood between friends, after all?'

'I – I'll discuss it later,' Kate said and let her glance flick upwards for a moment to see them all staring at her. 'Oh, dammit, I'll talk to you afterwards. Just let me get this finished, will you? I'm nearly there – '

Doggedly she went on, setting in the skin sutures at last, making each knot as tidy as she always did, checking that the deeper sutures were firm and finally washing the area down with the wet swabs of antiseptic lotion that were standing ready at the side of the instrument trolley. And then dried the skin carefully and stood back.

219

'Nurse, you can take off the dressing towels and put on the dressing. Avoid touching the blood. Put the towels in the same bowl as the swabs and Trevor's gown. Have you any blood on you? Oh, you have. Well, get your mask off and your gown and do the same. Don't touch the blood and drop them in the bowl. You hear me?'

'Yes, Miss Sayers,' the girl said, clearly mystified, but she did as she was told and Kate stepped swiftly back to give her room as at last the dressing was put on.

Behind her she felt the door of the theatre open as the porter came in to bring the trolley and get Slattery across to the recovery room. And Kate watched as he was taken away and then slowly took off her own gown and gloves and added them to the pile of bloodstained things waiting to be dealt with. The bowl, big as it was, was piled high and the gowns drooped over the side to envelop the legs of the stand it was on and Kate thought – I'll have to clean that too, dammit, and stretched her tired back.

The door to the concourse was still open and she looked over her shoulder to see what was going on out there, as the last trolley appeared from the next-door theatre with Fay's last case. On the far side of the big area Kate could see Sister Whelan talking at a great rate with a tall man who was looking a little hunted, and Kate frowned suddenly as she realised he was not gowned and was wearing street shoes. How on earth had someone got this far into the theatres in such unsuitable garb? This security for Saffron was getting to be perfectly ridiculous, she thought; what was Sister thinking of not to push him right out of the area? And she realised then that that was precisely what Sister was trying to do, while the man was stubbornly resisting.

Fay emerged from her theatre then at the same time as once more the trolley bearing Byford's case came out of the door of Theatre One into the now very busy concourse, and Kate moved towards the door, drawn to it by the peculiar nature of the situation. There was something very important happening out there and the atmosphere was tense as the nurses and the orderlies moved around on their jobs looking both scared and avid, covertly watching Sister and the man she was berating, and

Kate stopped at the door of her own theatre as Fay, pulling off her mask, reached hers.

'Hello, Kate,' she began. 'What a bitch of a morning! I thought I'd be here till midnight and here's me with an antenatal clinic full of vast burgeoning women waiting for me since two o'clock, God help us all — '

The big man who had been talking to Sister Whelan moved suddenly, sidestepped Sister and came towards the two of them as Byford went pushing past him with his hand on his patient's wrist. He was lying on his trolley with a face as white and flaccid as the sheet that framed it.

'Miss Buckland?' the big man said. 'Could I have a word please?'

'Eh?' Fay peered up at him a little blearily. 'What do you want? Who are you? Listen, I'm nothing to do with that Saffron man — it's Byford you want. Hey, Sister, what's this man doing here in street clothes, anyway? Don't we have enough of an infection problem without — '

Sister Whelan lifted her hands in a gesture of impotent rage as the man said, 'Not Sister's fault, Miss Buckland. I tried to explain I'd be willing to wait elsewhere if she would assure me I could see you, and she wasn't able to give that assurance. So I had to wait for now.' He reached in his pocket and Kate wanted to laugh suddenly. It was all like something out of one of those late-night films she and Oliver sometimes watched on television on Saturday nights, all stereotypes and comfortable reassuring clichés.

'I'm Inspector Hyman, Miss Buckland, and I would like to have a word with you, if you don't mind. About a patient of yours, a Mrs Walton.'

Chapter Twenty-Three

'Did you see it?' Alice threw herself into the seat next to Sian so hard that she slopped some of the tomato sauce from her fish on to the table, and Sian leaned forwards and mopped it up with ostentatious care.

'You're a real pig, you know that?' she said in a conversational tone. 'Not fit to sit and eat with decent people.'

Alice ignored her, looking eagerly across the table at David who had been talking to Peter over Suba's head. She was sitting staring down at her salad and making no attempt to eat it. 'David, Peter – did you two see it?'

'See what?' David squinted at her, his face clearly unfriendly. Alice was shaping up nicely to being the most disliked member of the first year, and everyone but she seemed to know it.

'Oh, Christ, you really are dummers, aren't you? The bloody news, that's what. In the South East. Comes on after the proper news.'

'Oh, that,' David said. 'Yes. I saw it. The demonstrators and all that – '

'Oh, you fool!' Alice almost howled it. 'That was at lunchtime. I mean the one that's just gone out, the six o'clock. Did you see that?'

'Some of us have to work,' Peter said. 'We can't sit around watching telly,' and he turned his shoulder at her to exclude her from his conversation with Peter and went on talking to him in a quiet voice as Suba still sat silently between them, her head down as she stared at her untouched plate.

'Well, if you don't know you don't. You don't have to be ashamed of it,' Alice said, hugely pleased with herself. 'They've gone and arrested Miss Buckland.'

There was a sharp little silence, shocked enough to please even Alice who sat there and looked round at them all with her face glowing with excitement. 'Did you hear what I said?' she repeated. 'They've arrested Miss Buckland.'

'No they haven't,' Sian said. 'You're a bloody fool and a liar too.'

'Well, near enough! It said on the news – there was a photo of her and everything. Helping police with enquiries into the treatment of a patient here at Old East in the last month and pictures of these people from the group – you know the one I mean. The lot that Shirley Farmer's always on about. Your mate, Suba – '

She stopped then and stared at Suba and then leaned forwards and pulled roughly on her arm. 'Hey, you're on Gynae! Tell us all about it, for God's sake. What happened? Did she kill someone? This baby? That was what the woman who was on the news said. From that group. That Miss Buckland killed a baby that could have lived and that it wasn't just an illegal abortion, it was murder – is it true?'

'I don't know,' Suba said after a long moment, with a sharp scared little glance up at Alice and then a shifting of her gaze back to her plate.

'Oh, come off it, ducks, of course you know! I always know what's going on in Paediatric Outpatients, so you ought to know what's happening on a little ward like Gynae, for God's sake! We get hundreds of patients every day and you only have your thirty or so, so you ought to know. Who did she kill? What was the operation? And – '

Suba still didn't look at her, and now the others were staring at her too, and David gave her a little nudge with his elbow. It was a friendly enough gesture and he meant no harm but Suba suddenly leapt to her feet and stood almost visibly shaking as she rubbed her arm where David's elbow had touched her.

'Leave me alone! Just leave me alone! If you don't I'll – I won't let you keep on at me. Leave me alone – ' And she turned and ran out of the dining room as the others stared after her, mystified.

'She didn't take her dirty plate back,' Alice remarked after a minute. 'These Pakis, think everyone's here to wait on 'em – lazy cow – '

'Shut up,' Sian said but it was mechanical and she still sat and stared after Suba, her brows slightly twisted.

'Do you think she does know what it's all about?' David said and began to wipe the gravy from his plate with a piece of bread. 'I heard it was nothing much – just the usual anti-abortion lot. Here, I'm still starving. Want a second helping, Peter? I'll get this one if you get the puddings.'

'Get your own,' Peter said. 'I don't know. Still waters and all that. She's a funny little thing. Listen, Sian, what time are you off?'

'Usual,' Sian said. 'Middle shift. Why?'

'Meet you for a drink after? Over the road?'

'I'm broke,' Sian said. 'Stand me a couple and I'll owe you.'

'Fair enough. Oh, go on, David, get your bloody second helping! Sitting there looking all huffy at me. I'll buy you a drink too, don't worry. I'm flush.' He smirked a little. 'Would you believe a grateful patient? Went out this afternoon and tipped me a fiver, no less!'

'Unethical, that is,' Alice Abingdon said, looking up from the plate she had systematically emptied at great speed. 'You ought to be ashamed. Still, if you're sharing it, where'll we meet?'

'Who's asking you? You're not wanted. Not now or ever. Come on, David, for Christ's sake. I'll go up with you if you're that shy.' And the two boys took their plates away to the counter leaving Alice staring sulkily after them.

'Miserable buggers,' she said. 'I'll come anyway – '

'If you do, don't talk to me.' Sian got to her feet too. 'Your absence is much preferred to your company, and the sooner you know it and leave us in peace the better for everyone.' And then she too went, leaving Alice alone at the streaked and messy table, staring furiously after her.

By the time Sian got back to her ward the whole hospital seemed to be buzzing with gossip. There had been some talk earlier that afternoon as the news filtered slowly and in garbled form out of the theatres and spread around the hospital gradually and glutinously, like car oil on a cold morning, but the television news had speeded up the whole process. Now there were little knots of people with their heads together in the corridors and in the lifts, and standing around the nurses' stations. And it wasn't only Miss Buckland's troubles with the police that were causing most of the talk either.

It was the rest of the gossip that was worrying Sian the most, and she got back to the GU and looked around for Sister. If anyone would tell her what was going on, she decided, it would be Esther. After all, it was as much in her interests as in everyone else's; and if she didn't realise that then that would make it even more clear what had to be done. But Sian had to talk to her first.

But Esther wasn't there. 'Gone to supper,' the staff nurse said. 'Now, listen to me, young lady. I told you before you went down for your own meal to get that bed ready in the far cubicle, didn't I? What the hell were you doing that you left it?'

'Kim Hynes,' Sian said succinctly. 'Got an attack of the vapours.'

'Bloody creature,' Staff Nurse said disgustedly. 'Listen, you don't have to sit there and hold her bloody hand every time she gets the miseries. She does it all the time. You've got work to do and – '

'Sister said I was to try to help her,' Sian said virtuously. 'Not to let her get all worked up. She's got to go back to theatre to get her wound tidied up and she'd got the horrors over it, Sister said, and – '

'I know what Sister said,' the staff nurse snapped. 'Right now, madam, you go and make that damned bed, and let me have no more of your chat. I've got work to do and so have you. So get on with it.'

Sian made a face at her departing back and then went slowly down the ward towards the far cubicle where the beds were waiting to be made up after patients had been discharged. It wouldn't take that long to sort that out, she thought, and maybe I'll have a chance to grab Sister as soon as she gets back. I've a right to know after all. Don't I work on this ward too?

But know what? a little voice inside her asked. It's not as though you've got any facts. Just a lot of talk. And she wished again that she knew some of the people who worked in the theatres so that she could discover the truth of it. But they were such an elite lot, and never talked to anyone but each other, though she'd have risked marching up and asking if any of them had been in the dining room. But they had been conspicuous by their absence, and that too had made her edgy and suspicious. It had to be a matter for the Union surely? How could it not be?

And she pulled the bed out to make it and kicked at the phone trolley which someone had left sitting there instead of putting it back in the corridor where it belonged.

And then stopped and stared at it and laughed aloud and fished in her pocket for a ten-penny piece. Of course that would be the way to do it. And it would be fun to see him again anyway. He was a nice chap, really, and maybe he'd take her to the Chinese again. That really had been a lousy supper.

Audrey sat beside Joe's bed, and thought about the possibility of going and having a proper supper downstairs instead of the usual sandwiches they gave her. It was nice of them to give her that much really; after all, she wasn't the patient. Joe was, and there was no reason why they should put themselves out the way they did. And it was mean of her to be bothered really, with Joe so ill. She oughtn't to be eating at all, just wasting away the way people did when they were unhappy. But that had always been her trouble. When things were bad they always seemed a bit better when she had something solid inside her. And she looked at the plate of sandwiches on the tray beside her, their edges curled up to show the pallid cheddar cheese inside and knew they wouldn't help at all.

She looked then at Joe, asleep as usual on his pile of pillows and felt again the little surge of anger. How could he waste what little time they had left with all this sleeping? Why didn't he sit there with his eyes open and hold her hand so that they would be together, really together? As it was, it was like he was already – it was like he wasn't bothered whether she stayed or went, really. And she put out her hand and slid it into Joe's where it lay on the sheet, yellow with illness and marked with spots of liverish colour and the bronze tinge on the nails and the thumb and forefinger from all the years of smoking his stinking cigarettes; and the length of the nails made her think – I really ought to cut them for him. Or should I just leave him in peace? He won't care either way, and anyway what's the point? It won't be for much longer –

She shook herself out of that literally, getting to her feet and pulling her hand away from Joe's so sharply that he stirred a little in his sleep and she stood very still, holding her breath, ashamed to have disturbed him, and him so ill. Beyond her the evening sounds of the ward came thinly in through the curtains, so familiar now it was as though she'd been hearing them all her life instead of just over the past three weeks; the clatter of supper dishes as the last ones were collected and the clink of spoons in saucers as the evening teas and cocoas were taken round and the eternal murmur of the telly set in the distant day room, while beyond that the rattle of the lifts in the corridor outside the ward and the ringing of telephones and voices and chatter and laughter; and suddenly she wished Joe was already dead, dead and buried and she left in peace to go home to Dagenham and get the cats fed and the garden tidied up, so she could settle down to a quiet evening by the telly. She hadn't seen a decent film for ages, hadn't had a decent night's sleep since God knew when –

Softly she moved away from the side of the bed, for Joe had not woken, but seemed to be sleeping even more deeply, his noisy breaths escaping his crusted lips in little gusts. He'd be like that for hours yet, she knew. Until the pain woke him again. He'd had his injection less than an hour ago. She could go and get herself a decent supper downstairs somewhere. He'd never know –

Sister was sitting at the nurses' station as she went by and she stopped to tell her she was going for some supper. Sister grunted back at her in an abstracted sort of way, not lifting her head from her writing and Audrey hovered for a moment wanting her to look up, needing her to say the way she sometimes did, 'Want to talk?' Ever since that first time when she'd been so cheeky and gone and bearded that Mr Saffron where he sat they'd been on ever such close terms, her and Sister. Audrey took some pride in that. She had no illusions about herself at all: ordinary woman, ordinary family, ordinary background, no education at all really, but she and Sister had got really close. That said a lot to Audrey about herself, that did, so she would say to the darkness in the long nights when she tried to sleep without thinking about Joe. Sister thinks I'm all right to talk to so I can't be that bad –

But tonight Sister was too busy, clearly, so Audrey sighed softly and went on her way, taking the lift down to the ground floor where the little knot of special services for patients and visitors were, the flower shop and the paper shop and the little chemist's and hoped they'd still have something decent in the café the Friends ran in the far corner. She could go to the hospital's own canteen, she knew. Sister had told her that; but she didn't like to really. It was so big and there were so many nurses and doctors and all there and one day one of them'd ask who she was and what right she had to be there, and that'd be awful. The café'd do and anyway she liked to pay her way. It wasn't too expensive and it made her feel better to pay her own way.

There wasn't a lot left on the menu. Only cheese on toast or beans on toast and she had a brainwave and asked if she could have both – the cheese cooked on the toast and then beans on top. And the woman behind the counter looked flustered and worried and she said she wouldn't know what to charge, really. So Audrey settled for beans on their own and a piece of rather tired-looking chocolate cake and took them over to the corner table she favoured where she could watch people without feeling as though everyone could see her doing it. Not a bad supper, really, but the prices these days! Over a pound for just these bits of nothing. When she and Joe had married, her whole week's housekeeping hadn't been as much as four quid and she'd cared for them both and the house and later on the first couple of kids on that. Over a pound for these few bits . . . And she pondered that as she ate her meal and then sat back to take her time over her cup of tea.

That was when she saw them sitting there and she frowned. She knew that woman sitting with her back to her, she was sure she did. The way she was leaning over and chattering at the man in the wheelchair beside her was very familiar and then Audrey remembered and shrank back into her corner. That was Mrs Holliday, the one who talked so much. That was who it was. The way she was feeling right now, the last person she wanted to get involved with was her.

But it was too late. The mere fact that she had looked at the woman seemed to have alerted her to her presence for she glanced over her shoulder and her painted little face split into a great eager grin.

'Well, there you are, Reg, who'd have thought it, here's someone from the ward that you know, now isn't that nice, she'll tell you it's all right, I'm sure she will, now do come over here and sit with us, Mrs – don't be shy now – I wish I could remember your name but I was always like that, never could remember names, aren't I a silly? But it's lovely to see you, so do drink up and come over here and I'll go and get us all some more tea – '

Audrey was swept up in a tide of chatter and was deposited, breathless, on the shores of their table and sat between Mrs Holliday and her silent husband while Mrs Holliday went on pouring out words as she searched in her bag for her purse and then went up to the counter to engage the flustered woman in conversation as she laboriously prepared their cups of tea. Audrey thought about telling her she'd pay for her own, not wanting to be beholden, but knew it would be no use. She'd just run over her in her verbal juggernaut and she'd still get the tea. Might as well save her breath.

She looked at Mr Holliday then, and found him staring at her with his rather watery pale eyes. He had a ring of milkiness around the faded blue of the iris and she remembered her own old dad suddenly. He'd had eyes like that and the memory made her smile.

'How are you, Mr Holliday? You're looking quite bobbish, I must say. Did your operation help, then?'

He stared back at her and for a moment she thought he was about to weep, for the eyes suddenly seemed much more glistening. But he blinked and the moment passed and she said again encouragingly, 'Well, you certainly look well. Your wife must take very good care of you.' And she looked over her shoulder to where Mrs Holliday was leaning on the counter chattering busily as the three cups of tea cooled in front of her and the flustered woman listened with an expression of slight panic on her face.

'She's lovely,' Mr Holliday said unexpectedly. His voice was thin and low but Audrey could hear him easily enough in spite of the sound of his wife's voice behind them. 'Ever so good to me. But she's not someone I can talk to, you know?'

Audrey smiled. 'I know. I've got a sister-in-law like your missus. Heart of gold she's got. Do anything for anyone.'

'That's right,' Mr Holliday said. Still Mrs Holliday went on

229

with her chatter and Audrey looked at Mr Holliday now sitting staring down at his hands clasped over his blanketed knees and tried again.

'Just dropping in for old times' sake, are you?' she said brightly. 'It's a nice little café this. Useful – '

'Yes,' Mr Holliday said. 'And it's a nice walk. We live only a bit away and we take this walk in the evening, my exercise she calls it, and we come here for a little bit of a cuppa and then walk back. It's an outing, see.'

'Yes,' Audrey said and smiled again. 'An outing.' There seemed little else she could say.

Still Mrs Holliday chattered on at the counter and now the flustered woman was leaning forward and listening, clearly entranced. It would be some time before she got her tea, Audrey thought, and wished she hadn't gulped down the first one so quickly at Mrs Holliday's insistence.

'Did you – ' Mr Holliday swallowed. His speech had been blurred before, but that hadn't worried Audrey. Her dad had been like that, couldn't speak clearly at all, and she had long since got used to it. Now though, Mr Holliday sounded more blurred than ever, the way her dad would get when he had to say something that worried him and Audrey leaned forwards and said encouragingly, 'Yes?' as the rusty voice stopped.

'See the news?' Mr Holliday managed and stared at her. His face showed little expression but all the same Audrey felt the anxiety in him.

'On the telly?' she said. 'I wasn't really listening, I mean, it was on in the day room but that's right the other end of the ward, you see, so – Was it something bad? Another bombing in Ireland and that?'

'No,' he said. 'No bombs.'

'Well, that's small mercy these days,' Audrey said heartily and smiled at him again. Maybe if she went to help Mrs Holliday with the teas that would make her stop her chattering to the woman at the counter?

'It said, doctor here and the police,' Mr Holliday said, and now his voice was almost incomprehensible. 'I saw it. Said the police – '

'A doctor here?' Audrey frowned and tilted her head at him. 'A doctor here in trouble? I never heard that.'

'It said on the news – Dr Buckland – do you know?'

Audrey shook her head regretfully. 'I don't, I'm sorry. It's not a thing I'd – I mean, I've been busy with my Joe, you see. And really I must get back up to him, I've been down here ever such a long time already – ' And she got to her feet.

It was that that drew Mrs Holliday's attention at last and with much exclaiming and clucking she came rushing over to the table bearing two cups of tea and then rushed back for the other.

'Imagine me, gassing on and not fetching it, well there it is, I'm a terror once I get going, you ask my Reg, he'll tell you, isn't he looking well now, Mrs – er – isn't he? I keep telling him he's better every day, gets tired you know if he talks a lot, but getting better all the time.' And she beamed fondly at her husband and with swift and birdy little movements of her small hands set the tea in front of him, fixed a handkerchief over his chest to catch any drops and put the cup in his hand. 'Can manage nicely himself now he can, after his operation, a real miracle I call it, wonderful it was, a real miracle, and I tell him he shouldn't be worrying himself over it, and him doing so well, they don't do these operations if they don't know what they're doing, even if they have a new sort and so I keep on saying it but there, he's a deep man is my Reg, thinks a lot you know, very deep, and he will go on about it especially tonight after the news about this awful business here. But like I said she wasn't nothing to do with him, a baby doctor and all!' And she laughed merrily and began to drink her own tea. 'I mean a doctor who looks after maternity wouldn't hardly be on his case would she, so I tell him not to worry. But there, he's deep, is Reg, and I tell him he'd worry about the sun getting up in the East if there wasn't anything else he could fret over! Oh, are you going then? Well, lovely to see you, give the other patients our regards won't you, and to Sister, lovely to us Sister was, Reg'll be up to see her soon, got to have a check-up he has, next week, Mr Bulpitt said so, I hope to see you too, and I do hope your good husband gets on well soon Mrs – er – '

Audrey escaped, smiling vaguely at Mr Holliday who stared hopelessly back at her, and went back up to the ward. It hadn't been much of a break she'd had really. But it had been different. At least there wouldn't be Mrs Holliday chattering at her up there, whatever else there was. And she'd watch the news later, just to see what it was Mrs Holliday was on about.

If she remembered.

Chapter Twenty-Four

The programme had been a pig. He couldn't remember when he'd last had such a lousy collection of callers or when the debate had been so lacklustre, and he said as much to his engineer as he came out of the studio and found the man dispiritedly rewinding the tape.

'Well, we all have our off days,' the engineer said, not looking at him, and Oliver was out of the control room and halfway upstairs into the newsroom before he realised the chap had thought he was apologising for his own input rather than complaining about the outside factors, and nearly went back to explain to him, needing to exculpate himself. But he didn't, of course, and went on to his desk in the far corner of the big clattering newsroom, where he had the privilege of a screen of tired plants in elderly pots to mark out his territory, in a sour mood.

'They were a bunch of wankers this morning, weren't they?' Ronnie Carter said as he passed his desk, and Oliver stopped gratefully. Usually he and this man – who called himself showbiz editor and who it seemed to Oliver did nothing more than swan around at boozy receptions and thereafter broadcast limp PR handouts – were on distant terms, but this morning he needed the reassurance of another broadcaster that it hadn't been his fault his programme had been so bad.

'Weren't they just?' he said. 'That lunatic from – where was it? – Bromley. I could have cut his throat, the damned fascist that he is – '

'Oh, I don't know,' Ronnie said with a fine judicious air. 'I thought *he* was one of the more interesting ones. You could have made a bit more of that woman from Ealing or wherever it was, mind you – the one who went on about the EEC. She had some good points to make, though you did cut her off rather – '

'Yes, well, not everybody has the wit to string together half a dozen intelligent words,' Oliver said with sudden savagery. 'It's

233

a rare gift after all,' and he slammed away to his desk feeling worse than ever. If even Ronnie Carter could pick holes in his handling of his show he really was in a mess. He'd have to see her today, get the whole damned thing sorted out somehow. He couldn't go on like this, torn into shreds first by Sonia, now by Kate; he'd end up with even worse than no home life – he'd have no career either. And he could have wept at his situation, and threw himself into his chair, needing to make some sort of physical statement of the way he felt. The chair rocked and he almost toppled and that helped a little. By the time he'd rescued his balance and settled himself, he was a little calmer.

His desk was piled high with letters, mostly banal invitations, but a good many from irate listeners who hated his style and even more from those who adored it and wanted him to open fêtes, become patron of their charities, or read their novels with a view to advising them on publication., Usually he found some mild pleasure in the inanities of the postbag, but this morning it was the last thing he needed, and he pushed it all aside and reached for the big scribble pad on which he was planning *The Unkindest Cuts*, part three. He still needed material for part two of course but he had to think ahead and block out where he was going, or he'd find himself painted into a helluva corner. And he felt another surge of anger as the words slid into his head: Christ, if he was even thinking in such dismal old clichés, what sort of stuff was he broadcasting? Maybe they were right, the engineer and Ronnie, maybe he was finished, useless, dreary –

He dropped the scribble pad and reached for the phone. Talk to her right away, apologise, explain he had meant no harm, wanted only to protect her. Until he did there was no hope of doing any decent work, and he punched the nine and began to key in Old East's number.

Radlett appeared from behind the plants and stared at him gloomily. 'What are you doing here? Why haven't you gone over to the hospital? With all that's going on there this morning, you'll have enough to finish your whole bloody series, if you ask me. Or have you done it already?'

Oliver jumped a little at the suddenness of his appearance, miskeyed and swore and hung up.

234

'What are you on about?' he said. 'I'm going over there later this afternoon. There's – '

'Thought as much. Didn't listen to the news, did you, before you went on air? So you don't know – '

'Know what?' Once more Oliver was on the defensive. Usually he listened to every news bulletin religiously, making notes, needing to be ready for whatever the punters threw at him, but this morning he'd been too abstracted, too wrapped up in his own doings to be bothered; and even in the middle of the programme when they'd gone over to ITN for the half-hour bulletin he'd pulled off his cans and stopped listening, preferring to sit there and think of last night and the things they'd both said.

'The demo there. It's getting nasty. They've seen today's *Globe* – it really got up their noses, it seems. There are a lot more people there than there were and there've been some scuffles. Trying to rush the barriers the hospital's put up. And the security people looking after Saffron got stroppy too – you'd really better get over there. And – er – ' Radlett reached over and flicked his forefinger and thumb at the pile of virgin newspapers on the corner of Oliver's desk. 'Better take a look at the *Globe* on the way. It's relevant stuff, if a bit on the unnecessary side for my taste. Still, they know their readers, I suppose. Scum, that's what they are – By the way, the show was a bit under par this morning, wasn't it? We'll have to get some better controls on the callers you're getting – see you – ' And he went padding away to leave Oliver staring after him in a state of barely suppressed fury. And it didn't help that there was no one at all he could blame but himself.

He read the paper in the taxi, propping it up against the Uher on his knees and had to admit that Jimmy had done a good job, according to his lights. It wasn't what Oliver would have done, but then Oliver wouldn't have worked for that sort of tabloid. It wasn't as bad as some of the scandal sheets that masqueraded these days as newspapers, even if it was a long way from the broadsheets, and he settled to read carefully as the taxi bucketed its way down Fleet Street and on towards the City, with a scowl on his face.

'The Magic Wand Waved at Old East', read one of the cross heads, and under it gushed a torrent of inflated prose about the tragic life of Kim Hynes, the brave honest patient in the kidney ward who had submitted to such painful surgery which was to change a life that had been hitherto such a burden – and on and on. The only notable thing about the writing was the way Jimmy had managed to avoid using personal pronouns: not a he or she, him or her, appeared anywhere and Oliver had to grin a little at that. So Jimmy hadn't been able to persuade his subs to regard Kim Hynes as a woman? Interesting, that. How would the readers of the *Globe* regard her? Would they be able to say she? Or would they think of her as a mutilated he, or possibly, worse still, as an it?

He lifted his head and stared blindly out of the window of the taxi as it pushed its way through the heavy midday traffic. How did he regard Kim himself, come to that? Somewhere deep inside he had to admit that Kate had made a sharp dig when she had said what she had about his attitude. He did find it difficult to contemplate the inner life of the sort of person who would submit to having his genitals removed as part of an attempt to be something he was never born to be. And he felt an actual frisson of sensation through his groin as the image of the operation rose in his mind and his Uher rocked on his lap as his thigh muscles tensed.

He got out of the taxi at Old East and, as he was paying the driver, the man said conversationally, 'Nasty business here, mate, eh? You press, then?'

'Radio,' Oliver said briefly, and dug in his pocket for change.

'Yeah, thought so. You're that Merrall, aren't you? Saw your picture in the colour supps once – "A Room of My Own" or something. I got a memory for faces.'

'Yes,' Oliver reddened. He still found it embarrassing to be cast as any sort of celebrity, however minor; he agreed to the sort of interviews that led to this kind of recognition, flattered and amused at the time, and then hated himself afterwards for the effects publication had. Every time he did it he swore he never would again, and every time he said yes. It would really have to stop.

He was about to go and then stopped. After all, taxi drivers, famous for having opinions on everything, useful *vox pop* insert if he had anything worthwhile to say. 'What do you think of this then?' he said and lifted his copy of the *Globe*. 'Read it?'

'What, the fellow what had the sex change? Sooner him than me,' the driver said, and made a face. 'Must be barmy.'

'You think it's right for him to have an operation like that on the NHS?'

'If that's what the stupid bugger wants and what some crazy doctor wants to do to him, what's it to do with me?' the driver said and put the cab into gear. 'No skin off my nose. I belong to Private Patients' Insurance, anyway. Wouldn't get me into a place like this and no error. It's all a lot of socialist rubbish anyway, all this NHS stuff − ' And he nodded affably and drove off and Oliver stared after him and thought − Why do I bother? Why do any of us bother? Who gives a damn anyway?

A lot of people, he realised then as he turned round to look at the Medical School entrance of the hospital. The little knot of demonstrators who had been there every day he had come had now thickened considerably. There were at least a hundred of them, he assessed, looking at the mob with an expert's eye, and a great many more bystanders were just watching and waiting to see what would happen. They had been herded behind roped-off areas by the police who were heavily in evidence, and several of them seemed settled in for a good day. There were old women and several very young ones with children in prams who bawled a good deal, and not a few youths who had clearly drifted over from the Job Centre on the next corner.

Most of the crowd seemed in accord with the demonstrators, who were carrying the usual motley collection of placards such events spawned. 'Hands Off Our Old East' was a common theme and there were others that read, 'Don't Bleed Our NHS to Death'. But there were others now that he hadn't seen on previous visits and he noticed one of them in particular, carried by a tall and rather aesthetic-looking old man in a tattered raincoat but an expensive bowler hat. It read in uneven letters, 'Prostates Not Perverts', and he carried it above his head with great aplomb, not at all put out by the jeers of some of the boys from the Job Centre.

But there were some in the crowd who were not at all in sympathy with the demonstrators it seemed: several dispirited-looking people were clustered together under a banner which read, 'Gay and Lesbian Pride Group' and another little knot of even more miserable men were standing behind a poster which read, 'Persecution of Minorities is a Fascist Plot. Transvestites Say No to Victimisation'. The boys from the Job Centre were jeering at them as well as at the old man, and now and again spat in their general direction. But they paid no attention, just standing there doggedly as the marchers, who were about half of the people in the placarded group, made their repetitive circle from the front to the back of the building, through the archway that led to the courtyard beyond.

Oliver hitched his Uher higher on his shoulder, shortening the strap, and fitted the microphone in place to check sound levels. He'd pick up what he could while he was out here; why not? And then go and see Kate. Maybe they could get some lunch together, if she hadn't already had some. He realised suddenly that he was more than a little empty. It had been a long time since they had sat at Joe Allen's and he had chewed his way through barbecued ribs, and he'd not bothered with breakfast this morning.

He moved in among the crowd, collecting background sound to start with, and at the sight of him some of the more experienced demonstrators started a chant of, 'Cut out NHS Cuts, Cut out NHS Cuts!' and he nodded at them and held his microphone up to show them he was recording them, and nodded at the tall angular woman who was leading it. She had been the one he'd interviewed before about it all – a clever woman with a lot of sense in her. But he couldn't talk to her again. It would have to be someone else. He had just about chosen his target, a tall man in a rather neater suit than that of most of the other people there, who looked as though he might be useful, and was starting to make his way towards him when one of the policemen set a hand on his arm.

'Excuse me sir, but can I ask you who you are? And what you want here?'

'Mm?' Oliver squinted at him in the dusty sunshine. 'Oh. Merrall. City Radio. Picking up some quotes, that's all. Why? Any reason why I shouldn't?'

'Not at all, sir,' the man said with rather pugnacious courtesy. 'Just checking. We don't want to get this out of hand here, you see, and we have instructions to be very careful about who – you know how it is.'

'No,' Oliver said. 'I don't. You tell me.'

'Well sir, you being Press – and perhaps you'd show me your Press card if you don't mind – should understand. We have a security problem here, Minister of the Crown and all that. Can't be too careful. Anyone we see carrying packages that might hide a bomb you know – can't be too careful – '

Oliver looked down at his Uher. 'This a bomb? Hardly likely.'

'Anything's likely these days, sir. So if you don't mind, your Press card and then we'll have a look inside that there box.'

'And if I won't allow it?' Oliver said. 'Press are supposed to be – '

'Security, sir,' said the policeman woodenly and moved a little closer and Oliver saw that now there were two others flanking him and a couple of fairly obvious plainclothes men a few yards further back. 'Got to have proper security. We don't want another Brighton, do we? They was lax on security there and now we're at a hospital. Can't be too careful.'

Oliver stared at him and then reached in his breast pocket for his wallet, and flicked it open to show his NUJ card with its blank staring photograph of himself and said, 'Will that do?'

'Very nicely, thank you sir. And now if you don't mind, this machine of yours – ' and he reached forwards and with a practised hand flicked it open and looked at it.

'Perhaps you'd just take that tape out, sir, so we can look further. I wouldn't like to damage nothing, you see – '

His teeth gritted to prevent himself from saying what he shouldn't, Oliver complied and at last the policeman nodded heavily and said, 'That'll be fine, sir. Thank you. You can go ahead with your interviews now.'

'Thank you, but I don't think I'll bother,' Oliver said, his voice tight with anger. 'I haven't the time now – I've got to see someone in the hospital. Thank you so much for making my job so difficult for me.'

'In there, sir?' The policeman seemed unperturbed. 'You mean to go inside, sir?'

'I do. Any objection?'

'Not if you have an appointment, sir. Or any other evidence of your right to be on the premises.'

'Right to be on the – what are you talking about? This is a hospital! A public place.'

'Not entirely, sir. Private property, in point of law. Well, DHSS property. You have an appointment with someone there sir?'

'No, dammit. I mean, in a way – '

'Can't be both, sir.'

'I want to go and see my – my friend, all right? She works there.' Oliver was standing very straight and had his head up. His temper had been fraying steadily all day and it would take very little now for the controls to snap.

'Oh, yes, sir? Where?'

'It's no damn business of yours,' roared Oliver. 'If you think – Look, let me talk to whoever's in charge here. I've had enough of this rubbish – '

'By all means, sir. Joe, tell the Inspector, will you? This gentleman wants a word – '

'Right,' one of the other policemen said. 'Right away.' And made no move.

'*Now*, if you please,' Oliver said and his lips felt hard and tight. 'I have a lot to do and no time to waste.'

'I thought you were just going to visit your girlfriend, sir? Why should that put you in such a rush?'

'That is none of your business! Where's that Inspector? I demand the right to see him. Now!' Oliver's voice was rising and people around them were becoming aware of what was happening, and coming closer to stare and listen, and Oliver's tension tightened as the screw of anger inside his head turned another couple of twists.

'Well, so you shall, sir, when he's got time. He's a very busy man, you understand, and seeing you just want to get in to see your girlfriend – '

'I said my friend!' Oliver shouted. Why it should anger him so to hear Kate labelled his girlfriend he wasn't sure. But then he knew he was; it was as though she were some little piece of nonsense and he no more than one of the boys from the Job Centre. They were the sort who talked mawkishly about

240

boyfriends and girlfriends, and his gorge rose as he heard the snobbish sneering thought go marching through his head; and that was the last and most ruinous turn of the screw. He almost heard his control snap, felt it physically as a sensation deep in his abdomen, and with all the power he had in him, pushed on by the frustration of the morning, he pulled back his arm and hit out with a great sweep of his fist. He felt it connect with the policeman's face and revelled in the luxurious sense of joy that filled him. He'd let go; the tension was gone and he felt marvellous.

But then he didn't. He felt sick as suddenly three large policemen landed on him at once, knocking the breath out of him and throwing him to the ground so violently that it seemed to come up and hit him. And the impact was so hard and so sudden that he couldn't breathe.

He lay there for what seemed for ever, trying to catch his breath, but his throat had gone into some sort of spasm and had locked and as he struggled, feeling his ribs cave inwards with his efforts, the light in front of his eyes broke up and dazzled and then shattered into scraps of black and white jigsaw patterns. And then someone hauled him up and he was being half dragged, half pushed, across the road and his head was hurting quite abominably. But at least he was gasping and filling his lungs again. And crying too, he discovered, for his face was wet with tears.

Chapter Twenty-Five

'Does he have to know?' Kate asked and lifted her chin to stretch the back of her neck which was aching abominably.

'I don't see how we can stop him knowing,' Levy said. 'Do you?'

'I don't see why not. Oh, I mean, he can know I operated. It's the drama I'd like to keep under wraps. I'm not usually so damned hamfisted but – '

'I gather you had a less than capable scrub nurse,' Levy said. 'It wasn't your technique that failed but his.'

She reddened. 'Who said that? I didn't – Look, I don't want to make life any more difficult for that boy than it need be. And it was my case and my responsibility.'

'And his cock-up,' Levy said. 'But I take your point. Better not to try to share blame around. Especially if we want their cooperation. The nurses, that is. I imagine that's what you're hoping for? That the nurses will say nothing about the blood loss in theatre and that will be that?'

She got up and began to prowl around the room, finding the inactivity of his armchair more than she could tolerate.

'Yes, precisely that. Look, let me tell you how it was. In the middle of all that hubbub over Fay I thought – There's nothing much I can do to help, just standing here and listening. I'll get rid of that blood. So I went back into the theatre, collected the bowl in which we'd put all the stuff that had been soiled when Slattery bled and took it out to the sluice. I ran the linen under the cold tap for ages – long after the blood-staining was out. It comes out quite easily when it's fresh, you know – '

'I may be a physician,' Levy murmured, 'but I do remember about blood.'

She laughed then, her face lifting from its tired lines. 'Sorry. Well, anyway, I cleaned up and by the time the nurses came through to start their own clear-up, I'd just about finished. They were so agog over what happened to Fay that they seemed to have forgotten about our case. I realise, of course, that I shouldn't have made such a fuss over it. There was probably no need. The more I think about it now the more convinced I am that I was right the first time. Slattery isn't a risk – I just overreacted. It's been a tough morning – you know how it is. But, as I say, by the time the theatre staff tore themselves away from gawping at Fay and her policeman and listening to Byford kicking up his rumpus over Saffron's security, the cleaning up was done and that was that. I just went away and said no more about it. And with a bit of luck and a following wind no one else will. And then Lemon needn't know what happened. Just that I did his case and it's all over and forgotten – '

Levy shook his head. 'I wish I could be so sanguine,' he said. 'If you'll forgive the obvious pun. My dear Kate, you've been around hospitals long enough, surely, to know that there is no such thing as anything being forgotten. The nurses will have gossiped about what happened with that case. They'll have told heaven knows how many people that there was a bleed and that you were so upset about it you wanted to clean up the mess yourself. And then someone will talk to Slattery and notice how he behaves and put two and two together. And never think Lemon himself won't be talking, saying he refused to do the case and why and then you did – no, my dear, we really do have to take hold of this situation and handle it. No use shutting your eyes and hoping it will all go away. You have my personal guarantee that it won't.'

She leaned against the window and looked at him miserably. 'Then what do we do?'

'Nothing in a hurry,' he said. 'That much I am sure of. Now, tell me, how is the patient?'

'Slattery? Oh, he's fine. Perfectly clean wound, no problems at all. Surprisingly. The way that case went I'd have expected him to start spiking a temperature and chucking pus at us. But he's got a clean sweet wound and seems as merry as a grig.'

'I like the image,' Levy said. 'When can he be discharged?'

'As soon as you like,' Kate said. 'The sooner the better in fact. I need a bed in the ward anyway, and Esther's – Sister's – fussing. She's getting pressure from Le Queux for extra beds and if he discovers I've got a non-renal case in there he's likely to make life even harder for her. As I say, you know how it is.'

'Indeed I do,' Levy said with some feeling. 'I've had him on at me about beds already today. Wants another ward, no less.'

'Wants me out altogether?' Kate said and lifted an eyebrow. 'I wouldn't be surprised.'

'Don't take it personally. He's an empire builder, always was. Look, talk to this chap's GP and see if you can discharge him home, will you? He can come back for removal of sutures, to make sure there are no problems, and that way we can hope to have the man well and truly out of sight before the storm really breaks.'

She frowned. 'What storm?'

'Dear Kate, I'm sure you're an excellent surgeon but you have the most tenuous grasp of politics, haven't you? And hospital politics are the most inflammable around. Look down there. Behind you.'

'The demonstration?' she said, turning to stare out of his window. 'But what of it? That's being going on for ages. They don't want the beds closed, that's all. That's got nothing to do with Slattery − '

He sighed again and held out his hand to summon her back to the chair beside his desk. 'My dear Kate, I know you've been rather busy about your own affairs but clearly you haven't seen this morning's *Globe*, and nor have you really looked at the demonstrators and their placards. Look first, will you, at this?'

He handed the paper over his desk to her and she sat there and read it, her head bent so that her hair slid forwards to cover her face a little. A pretty enough girl, Levy thought as he watched her, and then got up to fetch a cup of coffee for her. I hadn't really noticed, but she's a pretty girl. I can't blame that Merrall chap. And he frowned at that thought. Poor Kate. She was in for a tough time with that one, unless he badly missed his guess.

'Damn,' she said then explosively and pushed the paper back on his desk. 'Oh, damn and damn and damn − '

'There's only one way they could have got it. From the patient,' Levy said. 'That reads to me like a personal story, hmm? And the pictures they've got they must have got with cooperation. One of them seems to have been taken actually in the ward. I imagine Sister didn't realise what they were up to, or she'd at least have stopped that, but there – it wouldn't have made a lot of difference, would it? They'd have got their pictures some way.'

'I don't believe it,' Kate said and then bit her tongue. She couldn't tell Levy she'd been worried about this possibility, that Oliver had told her it would happen. How could she? He'd be fully entitled to be furious with her for leaving him unaware and so unprepared for the onslaught of publicity. Better to be a little devious. Not dishonest, precisely, but less than fully open. 'I thought I knew that patient. Well, as much as one ever can. There was real distress there, real pain, and none of this mumbo jumbo they've got here. I can't imagine her actually *wanting* to parade herself in this fashion. They must have persuaded her into it. She couldn't have realised what it would be like and what it would mean – '

Levy laughed. 'You're a very agreeable and clever girl, Kate, but I have to tell you you're dreadfully naïve in some ways. Kim Hynes told them this story and it's the Taj Mahal to a Shadwell council house she's been well paid for it. Money opens a lot of mouths. She's still in the ward, I take it – '

'Mm? Oh, yes. I was going to take her back to theatre to do some plastic work on the wound. She's eager for further surgery later and – well, it's a neat enough wound but I could improve it. Why? Shouldn't she be there?'

'Not for me to say. You're the surgeon. But I'd suggest you go and talk to her. You'd better know the strength of what she's done. This won't be the end of it, you see.' And he flicked the copy of the *Globe* with a contemptuous forefinger.

'What more can there be?' Kate said. 'They've got enough detail there to satisfy the most prurient, I would have thought. Surely this will be the end of it.'

'Never you believe it. They'll keep this going for ages yet. I've seen this sort of thing before. Remember the fuss over the first in-vitro baby? This is just today's *Globe*. There'll be the evening papers, tomorrow's dailies and the weekly magazines and the Sundays to think of, as well as television and radio. I remember some years ago a writer – I forget his name, but he was quite well known at the time – he was a trans-sexual and decided to do it

245

publicly. Wrote a book about it, quite a good one as I recall. And for months there wasn't a day that passed without some publicity somewhere. This'll be the same, you'll see. Once they get a really cooperative subject there's no holding 'em.'

'I suppose not,' Kate said and moved towards the door. 'I'll get over to the ward, then – '

'Kate – ' Levy said then. 'Before you go – ' She stopped and looked at him miserably. All she could think of was the hateful things she'd said to Oliver at the restaurant; and all he'd been trying to do was warn her. Oh, damn her own prickly idiocy. She could have listened, even though his suggested remedy had been so crass. Why hadn't she listened? She'd had to dissemble to her Dean because she'd been so stupid and she still had somehow to patch up things with Oliver. As well as deal with Kim and Slattery – what a ghastly mess it all was.

'Come back here and sit down again for a moment. You can sort out the ward later. I want to ask you – dammit, I don't like having to do this, but I can't help myself. Your private life is of course your own, but when it impinges on the hospital, then I have to get involved. The thing is, I'm a little concerned about your friend, Mr Merrall.'

She felt herself stiffen. She had come to sit down again as he had bade her and now she sat on the very edge of the chair staring at him with a stony face. It was so shaming to have been found out in deviousness; clearly he had known all along that Oliver had warned her, she thought, and now he was going to tell her he knew. And she was mortified.

'He came to see me some time ago about a programme he was making. All about NHS cuts. He hadn't realised then that the area in which he was more interested happened also to be the area in which you work. I pointed this out to him – actually warned him that Kim Hynes was your patient. Now, I don't know if the programme he is preparing will in any way deal with the same areas as this rag here' – and again he flicked his finger at the *Globe* – 'but if it does – well, you'll need to be aware of the problems, won't you? As I say I don't like to meddle but I thought I should just mention it – '

She was so grateful that he had not realised her own duplicity that she smiled at him widely, which took him aback rather.

'Oh, don't worry about that, Professor,' she said and got to her feet. 'I can deal with that problem. But – ' and she sobered then. 'Look, I don't have to – I mean I have the right to choose my friends where I will with no reference to the hospital, but I do want to tell you I'm – er, sorry that a friend of mine should be – well – '

'There's no need for that!' Levy said strongly. 'None at all. Never think I have any objection to the fact that your Mr Merrall is a journalist. Not only would I have no right to object – I actually admire him. I've listened to his programme sometimes when I've had to drive at that time of the morning. An interesting man with a very – um – definite style. No waffle and a good deal of plain and very refreshing horse sense. No need for you to apologise at all!' His own face split into a grin. 'Just be careful, that's all.'

'I will,' she said and got to her feet and went, feeling surprisingly better than she had. Nothing was different of course: Oliver had still behaved badly and she had behaved worse; there was still the problem of what to do about Kim and how Goodman Lemon would react when he heard what had happened over Slattery; but all the same, she felt better. It was comforting to have Professor Levy's approval, that was the thing, and she felt a moment of embarrassment as she realised how much she needed someone like him to lean on. She was supposed to be a grown-up person, a professional person. Did she really need a daddy to protect her and to give her the balm of his respect? Yes, murmured her secret policeman, yes you do. But embarrassing though it was, it made her feel better to have him there.

She hurried across the courtyard towards the main ward block, making a wide circle to avoid the demonstrators. There was some sort of fuss going on in the street outside: she could hear shouts and a good deal of confused noise coming from behind the archway and many of the demonstrators had broken the curve of their determined circular march and had crowded into the archway to see what was happening.

For a very brief moment she felt herself drawn towards the centre of the excitement; her curiosity was as well developed as anyone else's, and it was irritating not to know what was

247

happening here in her own hospital. But she pushed the impulse away. She had work to do and the fact that the demonstrators' attention was distracted meant she could get away and across the courtyard without impediment and that was no bad thing. So, she widened the circle of her pathway even more and went purposefully into the main building, her white coat flapping behind her with the speed of her movements.

The ward when she got there was in its usual state of barely controlled chaos. All the dialysis beds were full, and there were two people waiting in the day room until they could take their places at the machines, as well as the usual gaggle of waiting relations who were there to be taught how to use the machines, ready for the day when their patients could be given machines of their own at home. The Friends of Old East had been running their Jumble Sales and Bring-and-Buys to considerable point this year and there was every hope that soon some of the pressure could be eased on the inpatient dialysis unit by the provision of a home machine for a lucky few. Teaching them and their families how to make use of such a windfall took a lot of nursing time, but it was well worth the investment in the long run. But today was one of the days, clearly, when the pressure was screwed down tightly and everyone was showing its effects in their behaviour, becoming edgy and sometimes snappy.

Except, to Kate's huge relief, Esther. She was wrapped in a large plastic apron and was working over one of the machines to which William Prior was attached and, as Kate came into the ward, she looked up at her and lifted her brows cheerfully.

'Hello! Haven't seen you today! What a lot of drama going on, hmm? What do you think of that Hynes madam? I've told her what *I* think of her and no mistake – you'll no doubt find her in floods because I was so nasty. But honestly – letting that damned man photograph her here! I've had the whole bloody Admin office on my back over it. You'd think I'd taken the wretched picture myself, they fussed so. But what the hell. Look at our Bill here!'

And she looked down at the man in the bed with an affectionate grin and cocked her head sideways as she stared at the face against the pillows.

The man lying there looked very different from the way he had since his admission. He was conscious now, his eyes open and showing a degree of alert awareness that was totally new in him. He was shaven and washed and looked remarkably presentable.

'Isn't this something, hmm?' Esther said and looked again at Kate, grinning. 'All this time on the machine and I thought we were getting nowhere. And now look at him. Very bobbish, aren't we, hmm, Billy? Oh, you really are the best – ' And she leaned forward and pinched his cheek gently and the man grinned back at her, revealing regrettably broken teeth; but his eyes were smiling and he looked pleased with himself.

'I ought to bring Richard in to see this,' Esther said then, as she finished disconnecting the machine. 'Then maybe he'd see why I'd rather be here than making bloody sandwiches in Gants Hill or wherever. Nurse! You can move Mr Prior's bed into the far cubicle on the other side. Then get this machine cleaned up, will you, and we can start Mary Josephson on her stint. With a bit of luck, we can get her out by suppertime and young Gary in before the end of the day. Now, Kate – your man Slattery – '

'Mm?' Kate said and slid one hand into Esther's elbow as they made their way up the ward towards the end where Slattery and Kim were. 'Listen, Esther, sorry I was so ratty last time I was in and – '

'Forget it,' Esther said sunnily. 'I have. Oh, and I'm sorry I was a bit off too. We all get days like that. I've decided life's too short to spend it in a rage – told Richard that this morning – '

Kate stopped and then peered at her. 'You two quarrelling again?'

Esther laughed. 'In spades, ducky! Or at least he is. I've told you. I've decided I'm not going to let any of it get to me any more. It's not worth the ulcers.'

'That's this week,' Kate said shrewdly. 'How long can you keep it up?'

Esther looked at her and now Kate could see that behind the cheerful insouciance there was a hint of panic. 'I'll worry about next week when it comes,' she said. 'Honestly, there's a limit to how much one person can take. I reached it this morning with Richard going on about – well, anyway, I got here and there was old Prior, bright as a button and demanding breakfast. And I thought – sod the lot of 'em, Richard included. When I've got people like old Bill to deal with, who am I to get my knickers into the proverbial twist, hmm? Listen, Kate, your man Slattery – '

The bleep in Kate's pocket began its intermittent yelling and Kate made a face.

'Hang on, I'd better see what that is – though I can't imagine – I mean I've got no one in ICU and I'm here. Has one of the nurses from here sent a message?'

'I'll check,' Esther said and went bustling over to the desk to talk to her staff nurse there. But she shook her head and Kate made a face, and picked up the phone.

Switchboard took an age to answer, but she didn't mind, whistling softly between her teeth. Esther was right; she'd have to take a leaf out of her book, as her old English teacher used to say with a bob of her tightly marcelled head, and Kate remembered her so vividly suddenly it was as though she were a child again. But she'd been right, and Esther was right. It just wasn't worth getting into a state over anything. Getting upset only tightened the pressure, and made you less able to cope with it. Accepting things as they happened and dealing with them logically, that was the way to keep your sanity. And your health.

Switchboard responded at last and when she had identified herself put her through to Accident and Emergency who had been bleeping her. And when they too at last answered Kate stood with her brows lifted in puzzlement.

'Miss Sayers?' the little voice clacked tinnily at her in the earpiece. 'There's someone down here who says he knows you. Got some nasty contusions, he has, and may be concussed and very anxious to speak to you. Could you come down, do you think? Right away, Sister says – '

'Someone who says he knows me?' Kate said, deeply puzzled. 'Who?'

'His name – er – hold on a moment – oh, here it is. Merrall. He's Oliver Merrall. You know, the chap from the radio. And he's really not feeling at all well.'

Chapter Twenty-Six

Suba couldn't remember when she had last felt so dreadful. She had thought it was hard enough going to the meeting on her own, without Shirley, but she'd managed to do that and to tell them what they asked her to. She'd thought she'd be miserable when Shirley was moved at the last routine changeover for second years from Gynae to go on night duty in the Orthopaedic ward, so that she no longer had a friend to talk to on duty and discuss things with, but she'd got used to that. This was something worse. Much worse.

It had started when they had begun making beds, she and the second year who had been sent to the ward to replace Shirley. She was Michelle Lomax, a small black girl with a cheerful grin and a stream of chatter that seemed never-ending; and she chose to talk all the time, not as everyone else was, of the story about that patient on Genito-Urinary who'd had that awful operation and who was all over the newspapers, but about Miss Buckland. And Suba had tried to change the subject but simply couldn't.

'I wish I'd been there to see it all,' Michelle said as she flipped the corner of the sheet and tucked it in with an experienced twist of her wrist. 'I mean, she must have been gobsmacked! Someone told me, she's got a friend who's working on theatres, she said it was all about abortions she'd been doing. But someone else said it was different, just about a car or something, but you can't tell me they'd come all the way into theatres to go on at someone about a car! And she a consultant too! It's not what they'd do, is it? Give us that pillow – ta – have you heard anything about it?'

'No,' Suba said wretchedly. 'Er – did you read all about that patient on GU who had the sex change? There are bits in the paper all about it – and – '

'I knew all about that,' Michelle said and shook her head in disgust. 'I said all along that was wrong. I heard about it even before it was in the paper – we all did. We were talking about it in our last block, because we'd heard, someone was over the road

251

in the pub and there was someone from the ward in there and she was saying – no, that's just disgusting really. But Miss Buckland! I mean – will she get *her* name in the papers, do you suppose?'

Suba began to feel dizzy. 'Why should she? I mean, I really don't know. Listen, do you have a lecture or anything that – '

The other rode over her as though she hadn't spoken. 'It's sure to be, isn't it, about abortions? Like that doctor over at – where was it? – I read about it somewhere, how he was doing abortions in private clinics and getting big money for it and then how he did some of his private patients in his NHS beds and still made them pay and the hospital found out and there was all sorts of trouble, do you remember?'

'No,' Suba said. 'I wanted to ask you – I've lost my medical textbook, you know, that one with the green cover and I was wondering – '

Michelle marched cheerfully to the next bed and began to strip it, flashing a smile at the occupant but still addressing all her words to Suba.

'I mean, what with all the cuts it's awful someone doing that but I don't think Miss Buckland's the sort, do you? She was ever so nice when we had our gynae lectures. I liked her a lot but I was telling my mum about it and she says you can never go by what people look like or even behave like. When it comes to money they're all devils and she could be right; but still, Miss Buckland – '

With a massive effort, Suba managed to stop listening. The words ran on at a great rate as they went from bed to bed, shaking pillows, smoothing counterpanes, pulling drawsheets through and still Michelle chattered on and still Suba tried not to think about what she'd done.

Because there could be no doubt in her mind. It was she who'd done it. How could it not be? They'd asked her to bring the details of Mrs Walton's operation and she'd done that. It had been so easy, just photocopying the sheets from the notes which were waiting to go down to the office. The photocopier was just along the corridor, in the medical secretaries' room, and she had known how to use it because Sister was often in need of extra sheets of special pages and kept running out of them. The day she'd photocopied Mrs Walton's notes she'd been sent to make some extra temperature charts because Sister had run out again, so it hadn't even been a matter of going where she shouldn't at the wrong time. Sister had *sent* her –

But no matter how she tried to wriggle around it inside her own head, Suba knew. It had been wrong to copy those notes and much more wrong to take them out of the hospital to someone else. People were always going on about confidentiality. They were so confidential, those notes, that even the patients they were all about weren't allowed to see them. And Suba had given them to outsiders – and she closed her eyes at the thought and felt sick.

'Are you all right?' Michelle's curious chattering voice broke through at last. 'You look ever so seedy. Are you having a period or something? That always makes me feel lousy. Shall I fetch Sister? Or – '

'I'm all right,' Suba managed. 'I'm fine. Look, you go and do the sluice jobs, will you? Or shall I? I don't mind but someone's got to fetch in all the flowers – '

Michelle thought for a moment. 'I'll do the flowers,' she decided. 'I'm senior to you, so you can do the sluice. And have a word with Sister and get some aspirin if your period's playing up. You look ever so green – '

It got no better as the day wore on. Wherever Suba turned, it seemed, people were talking about Miss Buckland and her brush with the police. What had she done? Why had she done it? What would happen to her? And when the first editions of the evening paper began to filter through to the wards, brought in by visitors as avid for gossip as everyone else, then the talk doubled and redoubled, for there was a report on an inside page that said Miss Buckland had been assisting police with their enquiries into an abortion performed on a patient at Old East and that she was one of the staff at the hospital already hit by unrest – and there were pictures of the demonstrators outside to illustrate the unrest, which indeed looked very lively – and also that the hospital was the crux of another scandal over the presence of a patient who had undergone a sex-change operation, when other patients were left on long waiting lists –

Suba had tried very hard to pay no attention to it all, but she hadn't been able to cut herself off from it. When one of the patients actually pushed the newspaper into her hand she felt herself forced to read it. And stood there at the side of the bed, her head down over the dreadful words, praying she wouldn't disgrace herself again the way she had that day in the operating theatre when she had fainted and Miss Buckland had been so nice to her and –

And she lifted her head and looked miserably at the patient, who peered at her and said loudly, 'Well, there you are, Alf! Didn't I tell you that Miss Buckland was a really nice lady? Of course she is, because here's Nurse all in tears over her and – oh, there, ducks, it'll be all right, I dare say! Don't you cry, dearie, now – '

Suba fled down the ward and into the best haven she knew, the linen cupboard, and stood there in its musty warm dimness, her face pressed against a pile of sheets, weeping bitterly. She'd have to give up, that was what she'd have to do. She'd have to go back home and tell Daddy he was right, and she was wrong. She didn't have what was needed to be a nurse. She couldn't cope and there was an end of it. And she didn't know what made her cry the most: the thought of Daddy's face when she told him, or the thought of having to leave the hospital behind.

Someone came in behind her and almost ran into her, and stood there blinking in the darkness.

'What on earth?' a voice said and Suba stood rigid, the tears drying in her throat.

'It's only me, Sister,' she managed, her voice quavering dreadfully. 'I was just looking for a – for a sheet – '

'Well there are enough of them there, right in front of you,' Sister said tartly. 'What do you want it for? I thought you'd finished the beds, you and Nurse – whoever is it they've sent me – Lomax?'

'Well, yes, Sister. I just wanted to check we had enough because – ' She stopped, her lies in tangles around her feet and Sister, her eyes now accustomed to the gloom, scooped up the dressing towels she had come in to fetch and then peered more closely at Suba's streaked face.

'Tears? Oh, for heaven's sake, girl! What is it now? What's upset you?'

'Nothing, Sister,' Suba managed to gulp and then to her

horror the tears began to flow again, for Sister had sounded sharp but not entirely unsympathetic, and that seemed to have pulled the stopper out of her.

'Well, we'll get nowhere steaming up in here,' Sister said in a resigned sort of way. 'Out you come, my girl, and into my office and then we'll see what all this is about — '

'It's personal, Sister,' Suba managed, clutching at the first thought that came into her head to free her from any need to tell Sister Morgan what was upsetting her. 'It's just personal — '

'Hmmph,' Sister Morgan said and shepherded her out of the linen cupboard into the comparative glare of the corridor outside. 'Well, if you say so, you say so. But you've no right to be sitting around being personal on my ward and in my time. I've all these patients to look after and no time to waste on any of your fusses! And look at you, girl! I can't let you be around the patients looking like that. Come along into my office and you can do my filing for me. That'll keep you out of trouble till you've regained a little common sense. But first wash your face and make yourself look respectable and then come along to me.' And she gave her a little push with a not unfriendly hand and, somewhat comforted, Suba obeyed.

At least she hadn't had to blurt it all out. Sister Morgan, she was quite sure, would be deeply lacking in any sympathy for what she had done. She could remember all too well what had happened that first time she had tried to explain how worried she was about Mrs Walton and taking her to theatre. And she felt the tears tighten her throat again as she remembered the way Mrs Walton had clutched at her hand in the theatres that day, when she had been sliding woozily under the anaesthetic, and how glad Suba had been that she could make her feel a bit better —

The cold water she splashed on her face helped a bit, and she was able to come back to Sister's office in a somewhat more composed state, and Sister saw her and nodded approvingly and indicated a chair in the corner and on the table in front of it a great pile of folders and an even higher pile of papers.

'All these reports are just back and have to go into the notes,' she said. 'If you make any mistakes I'll flay you alive, understand me? Make sure you staple the path reports to the path cards, and the X-ray reports to the X-ray cards — I don't want 'em mixed up. And make sure the bacteriology reports with the red stars on the corners are clipped to the *red* bacteriology cards, you understand. Not the white one. Right? In any doubt *ask* me. I'd rather be pestered now than driven mad by stupid errors later on.'

Gratefully Suba settled to her job. It was just what she needed, demanding concentration and attention to detail which would stop her thoughts running round in circles, but not so much that she'd get flustered. And after ten minutes of sorting and clipping she began to relax and feel that maybe it would be all right after all. Maybe there'd be no more fuss about Miss Buckland and the police? Maybe she'd be able to forget all about what she'd done? She could be sure of one thing: she'd never do such a thing again.

The door of the office opened and at first she didn't look up, struggling as she was at the moment with a recalcitrant stapling machine, and then she heard the voice and almost froze.

'Hello, Beverly. Have you seen the bloody evening paper? And I'm told it was even on the news on radio at three o'clock – I ask you! These *stupid* people! What am I supposed to do, ask the whole bloody country for a second opinion before I operate on any patient? Damned meddling fools – '

'Tea?' Sister Morgan said imperturbably and pushed her tray forwards as Miss Buckland almost threw herself into the other chair by her desk.

'Thanks,' Miss Buckland said and poured a cup and drank it thirstily. Suba sat and stared down at her sheets of paper, not sure what to do. Sister knew she was there, and for that matter so did Miss Buckland, for she was clearly visible. If they wanted to talk privately they'd say so, surely, and she'd be able to escape? And she coughed a little experimentally and Sister looked sharply over her shoulder and said, 'Do get on, Nurse. I want those done tonight, not next week.' And obediently Suba bent her head and began to shuffle the papers.

Miss Buckland was the first to speak. 'It's so *bloody* stupid,' she burst out suddenly. 'The trouble with most of these people is they don't really listen to me. I've turned up on a couple of TV programmes and expressed an opinion, so they decide on the basis of that to pin labels on me. Radical feminist, they're saying in the news, you know that? Me! As dedicated a non-joiner and non-labeller as anyone can be, and I get that sort of nonsense shoved at me. If they'd just read what I've written and read it properly and listen to all I've actually said and not what they choose to hear, they'd know what I'm for. I'm for choice, God damn it. Every woman has the right to choose what's right for her and her child. And to call me abortionist as though I cheerfully rip 'em out on demand – I never heard such – '

'It's no use getting so angry, Miss Buckland,' Sister Morgan said soothingly. 'Hundreds of people know it's not true. I know it's not true. If it comes to it you can always get me to stand up for you. I know what you are and how hard you work for women and babies, none better, for pity's sake! And I'll tell 'em – if I have to.'

'I might have to ask you,' Miss Buckland said gloomily. 'They reckon it'll come to court, you know. I told that bloody policeman there was no case to answer but he's got hold of some documentation in the case – don't ask me how, but he has. Several pages of Mrs Walton's notes, I gather, including the ones where there's discussion of the doubt about her dates. Do you remember? You thought she was about twenty-four weeks, and I said I didn't think so, she was just small for her dates, because she was quite adamant about her last period – '

Suba went on sorting the reports mechanically, having to read them over and over again to get any sense out of them. She knew exactly which page Miss Buckland meant: hadn't they all made a particular point of that one and got all excited over it when she'd taken the pages into the meeting?

' – and when we talked to Harry Holbeck for a second opinion he said he thought twenty-six weeks on the scan. Either way she had a rapidly growing carcinoma there with lymph node involvement and I know I was right to do what I did. And damn it, the woman *wanted* to abort anyway! Who are these bloody moralists who think they have the right to tell other people how to live their lives? Or die their deaths . . .'

'It's babies' lives they go on about, Miss Buckland,' Sister said and poured some more tea. 'Going on about what the mothers want is what gets them going. They're not interested in mothers. Only in babies – '

'I'm interested in babies too, dammit! And God help anyone who says I'm not – '

'And you're also interested in a lot of things these people disapprove of. It's no use getting mad about it, Miss Buckland, you know that! I know you're labelled as a feminist – I think you are, come to that – '

'And what's wrong with being on the side of women?' the other flared at her and Sister Morgan laughed and pushed her teacup nearer to her hand.

'Not a thing. I'm just trying to be practical. Getting annoyed isn't practical. Deciding what to do is. So what will you do? If it comes to court?'

'What can I do? Turn up there and tell 'em they're all bloody fools. What else is there?'

'That'll get you a long way,' Sister said dryly. 'I'd have thought it might be an idea to get some of the patients whose babies you've saved for 'em to turn out to support you. All those threatened abortions you do so well with. Then they'd find it harder to make the labels stick, wouldn't they?'

There was a little silence and Suba thought – Shall I tell her now? Beg her pardon? Ask how I can help? Maybe I could help, after doing all those bad things to her. Maybe I could make it a bit better –

'I suppose that might help. My own solicitor was asking about that sort of thing – character witnesses. It's just so sickening it should be necessary, for God's sake!' She seemed ready to burst with rage again. 'After all these years – and I've given them all I've got, these women and their babies – to have to dig out character witnesses? It's a bloody insult!'

'Insult or not, it could be useful,' Sister Morgan said. 'Look, let's think of some of the more recent patients we've had – what about – ' and she pulled her big ward ledger forwards and began to riffle the pages. 'Let me see: who have we had these past few months? There are those children, Tracy and – no, they won't do. You've made sure they'll be able to have babies eventually but they're really a dreadful little pair of tarts. They won't make the right impression at all . . . Ah!' And she stopped with one finger set on the page and looked up at Miss Buckland and grinned.

'Well?' Miss Buckland demanded and Suba had to hold on to the table in front of her to prevent herself from jumping up to go and look over Sister Morgan's shoulder.

'That girl Roberts – the one who went to a back-street abortionist and he perforated the Pouch of Douglas – you remember? She's still pregnant and if you hadn't been so quick and good she'd have lost the baby and herself as well probably. Bled like a – remember? She ended up having seventeen units of blood in the first couple of hours she was in. Now, if we can get her, then maybe – yes, I like it. She'd be the best possible character witness. What do you think?'

'I *don't* like it.' Miss Buckland got to her feet. 'In fact I hate it. I don't look after people in a – on any sort of conditional basis. I don't take care of 'em and then go and say, "Listen, I did this for you, now you come into court and help me out." I won't do it. It's disgusting.'

'It'd be a lot more disgusting if they win a case against you, Miss Buckland. And they could, you know. The way things are these days, people are very – ' She shrugged then. 'Intolerant. I still remember what happened to that paediatrician who was accused of killing Down's babies. They put him through hell. And then he died soon after, heart attack – these are nasty times.'

'Yes,' Miss Buckland said and stood there with her hand on the doorknob. 'I know. But I don't have to make 'em worse by behaving as they do. I'm not asking any of my patients to come to court on my behalf. It's not right, and I won't do it. Look, can we go and see the Lester woman? Have you got the histology back on her D and C?'

'I have,' Sister said. 'It's here – ' She came over to the desk where Suba still sat with her head down over the reports. 'Move over, Nurse. Let me see – now where was it – ah, here she is. Yes, I made a note to tell you. I'd have called you if you hadn't come in. She's got a CIN 3 just for openers, but there were some doubtful cells in the endometrium. They want to do a repeat. Unless you opt to do a hysterectomy anyway – '

'I'll talk to her,' Miss Buckland said. 'She might be willing. It'd certainly be safer, the speed with which some of these endometrials spread. It's getting really virulent lately – or have I just been unlucky with some of my patients?'

She sighed then and opened the door. 'Do you remember the story about the little Dutch boy who was walking on the dyke one day and saw a little hole in it? Knew if it wasn't dealt with the dyke'd break down and the whole of Holland'd be flooded? Well that's me. I feel as though out there are millions of women all with rampant cancers of their genitals and I'm the poor cow with her thumb in the dyke trying to hold it all back. God, I'm tired. Come on, Sister. Let's go and see who we can mutilate today, God help us – '

Suba sat for a little while after they'd gone, watching them through the glass wall of Sister's office and trying to think what to do. Miss Buckland might be a noisy person and she might swear more than Daddy would approve of and she might be rude to people sometimes, but that didn't mean she was bad. Suba had done a terrible thing, taking those papers to that hateful group of Shirley's. It was all Shirley's fault, she thought then, letting resentment fill her with a warm and comforting wash. If it hadn't been for her I'd never have done such a nasty thing. It was all her fault –

But you did it. The thought slipped out from beneath her resentment to bob about on the surface of her mind and sharply she got to her feet and went over to Sister's desk, where the ledger still lay invitingly open.

She stood there for a moment looking down the ward as casually as she could. From behind the glass wall came the usual afternoon clatter of teacups and the ever-present drone of the TV set in the day room, and there was some laughter and chatter too, for many of the women were up and about. She could see Sister's back, and beyond her on the other side of the bed they were standing beside, the rumpled head of Miss Buckland. Both seemed absorbed in what they were saying to the patient and unlikely to look over their shoulders at her, so slowly she bent her head and ran her finger down the column of names on the left-hand side of the page. And found it.

Prue Roberts. Of course. She remembered Prue Roberts very well. She'd been very friendly with the woman in the next bed who'd tried so hard to get pregnant and who had told Suba all about it. Over and over again she'd told her. Prue Roberts. Yes, she was the person to help Miss Buckland. And if Miss Buckland wouldn't ask her, then she, Suba Mahmoudi, most certainly would. Then maybe she'd feel better about the awful things she'd done to start the trouble in the first place. And then she wouldn't have to give up nursing after all.

She went back to the pile of reports waiting to be filed with the full name and address of Mrs Roberts carefully scribbled on a piece of paper and tucked into her waistband. She'd go and see her the first chance she got and see to it that she saved the day when Miss Buckland had to come to court. And it was really remarkable how much better Suba felt as she thought about it.

Chapter Twenty-Seven

There was always hubbub in the Accident and Emergency department but when Kate pushed open the great rubber doors to go in she felt the impact of the extra busyness of the place today almost as a direct physical blow. There were people everywhere; in the middle of the department a large, hairy and very noisy man in dirty jeans and tattered leather jacket was fighting with two of the young male student nurses and swearing at the top of his drunken voice; not far away a small child sat on its mother's lap with its mouth wide open and bawling loudly as she sat and stared blankly at the fighting that was going on while making no effort to soothe him, and wherever else Kate looked there were people sitting drooping in bandages or with bruises or clutching various parts of their anatomies, to display their justification for being there waiting to be seen, as doctors and nurses bustled in and out of the curtained-off cubicles, clearly busy about even more damaged patients than the waiting crowd.

She looked round hopefully as at last the shouting man was borne away by the triumphant young nurses and the baby stopped its crying, looking for Sister; and then saw two sizeable policemen standing in front of a corner cubicle. They were murmuring to each other and she looked at them, frowning. They couldn't have anything to do with Oliver, surely? And she wondered briefly why the idea had even come into her mind. And then thought – Traffic accident? And walked even more quickly across the broad waiting room to Sister's office.

Sister was, to her relief, in there and greeted Kate with a wide smile. They had worked together many times when Kate had been senior surgical registrar, the job she had held before getting her consultancy, and they'd got on very well. It comforted Kate just for a moment to see her, and she managed a smile too. But it was a brief one.

'Oliver Merrall, Mary? He's in here? What's happened?'

'Then he isn't just confused? He kept on about wanting to see you and I thought maybe he was just – he wasn't very rational, I must say. He does know you?'

'Yes, he knows me,' Kate said, trying not to let her impatient anxiety show. 'What's happened?'

'I'm not sure. I gather he got into some sort of altercation out there on the demonstration. I've had a couple of other people in here to patch up, because a real fight got going. I'm told there were TV cameras out there, the lot. Anyway, as far as I can understand it, your friend either was hit by a copper or hit out first – there's some argument on that point – then when they jumped Merrall got more of a bashing than they meant, I suspect, because he's concussed and he's had his face – well, you'll see. The thing is he was rolling around and carrying on alarming, asking for you, and the only way I could quieten him was to promise you'd come and see him – listen! There he goes again. He's a bit of a goer, isn't he?'

Kate hurried to the office door and stared in amazement at the far cubicle, from behind the curtains of which a great roar of rage was coming. She couldn't hear any words, but that it was Oliver there could be no doubt; she knew that voice far too well; and she moved swiftly, crossing the floor so fast that she almost slithered, and reached for the curtain to the cubicle as Sister came hurrying behind her.

'Hold on,' Sister was saying. 'Let me explain something, Kate – '

But Kate paid no attention and tried to push through the curtains as Oliver kept up his shouting, and then was stopped as a large and heavy hand landed on her shoulder.

'Sister said you're not to go in there.' One of the policemen was looking at her almost reproachfully. 'Sister said – '

Mary caught up with her and said, 'Kate, take care now. He really is very concussed and in a bit of a state. Started hitting out a bit, to tell the truth, when we tried to stop him standing up. He wanted to go and look for you, you see, and of course I couldn't let him, not till he'd had his skull X-rayed and we couldn't be sure he wasn't more damaged than we could see. And – '

'Is that why the police are here?' Kate said and glared at the policeman and pulled almost violently away from his grasp.

'Hardly necessary, I'd have thought, to control just one agitated patient. Send them away, Mary, for heaven's sake – '

'I can't.' Sister was now holding the curtain aside to let Kate follow her into the cubicle. 'I told you, he's supposed to have hit a copper and I'm here to tell you that they take a very dim view of that. No way do they go away just on my say-so – Hey, Mr Merrall, stop that racket! She's here, for heaven's sake!'

Oliver was lying flat on the couch with a nurse on each side of him trying to restrain him as he struggled to sit up and seemed to want to swing his legs over to stand on the floor. They were young and flustered and one of them had lost her cap in the struggle, and even as Kate came up to the side of the couch, he managed to release one arm from the grip of the nurse on that side and swung it out and knocked off her cap too. He had his eyes tightly closed and his mouth wide open as he shouted and Kate had to lean over and set her hands on both his shoulders, to pin him down as she shouted back equally loudly, 'Oliver, for heaven's sake – it's me, Kate – Oliver – '

The shouting stopped at once and he opened his eyes and glared up at her and she looked back at him and felt her legs start to shake as her joints seemed to become jellies.

He looked dreadful. One side of his face was coated with blood and grit from cheekbone to chin, and from his ear to the side of his nose. The eye on that side was puffy and blue with an expanding bruise and his nose had bled and left streaks of mucus and blood along his other cheek and down to his ear. His hair was matted with blood too, clearly from some sort of scalp injury, and he was sweating heavily.

'Kate,' he said and closed his eyes again and now she saw tears squeeze through his lids. 'Oh, Kate, tell them, for Christ's sake, tell them – this is hell – '

'Tell them what?' she murmured and moved closer to him as the nurse fell back a little, relieved that Oliver was now no longer thrashing about. 'What is it that – Christ, what's happened to you?'

'Make 'em let me go – ' he managed. 'They're treating me as though I'm mad – I can't stand this – ' And she nodded, remembering suddenly.

He'd never made a great deal of fuss about it, trying to dismiss

264

it casually on the rare occasions it happened but he was, she knew, bothered by being in enclosed spaces. Not precisely claustrophobic, she had thought, but very close to it at times. They'd once been in a crowd leaving a theatre which had for some reason stopped moving forwards, while people behind had continued to push onwards, and they had been pinned, unable to move, between burly bodies. And she had laughed and managed to turn her head to share some silly comment about it with him and seen his eyes were wide and staring, with the pupils grossly dilated and he was sweating hard and she had thought – He's panicking. And had with a massive effort managed to elbow aside the people closest to them and create extra space for him and he'd calmed down a little. They'd moved again within seconds of course; whatever the barrier was it had been removed and they were out in the street within a minute of the episode. But he had been pale and quiet for the rest of the evening and they had gone home to bed early, instead of going out to supper as they had planned.

Now, looking at his face against the white sheet of the couch, she realised how he must be feeling, to be confined as he was, and said sharply to the nurses, 'Let him go!'

'But Sister said – ' one of them began and Sister, standing behind Kate said quickly, 'Do as Miss Sayers says, Nurse – we'll be fine. You get on and clear up the other cubicles, will you? That's it – ' And the two of them escaped gratefully and Oliver lay there and blinked up at Kate, ignoring Sister completely and said, 'Thanks,' in a low thick voice.

'What happened?' Kate said then and perched herself on the edge of the couch and reached for his wrist. His pulse was full and bounding but it was not, she thought with the professional part of her mind, the sort of pulse that would suggest he was bleeding internally. It was steady and strong, if fast, but that was clearly due to the anxiety; and she turned her head and said curtly to Sister, 'The skull X-rays?'

'They're still looking to make sure – they've asked for an opinion from Dr Cantrip – he's the consultant radiologist on call – because the registrar says he wants a second opinion, especially as it's a police case. But he said he saw no fracture – '

She was speaking in a low voice and looked briefly over her

shoulder at the curtain. 'I really can't send them away, I'm afraid. It's a serious charge, you see, assaulting a police officer – '

'A fractured skull would be a great deal more serious,' Kate snapped. 'May I see the films? Or are they still in X-ray?'

'I'll find out,' Sister said and turned to go. 'Will you be all right with him? He seems quiet enough now – ' And indeed Oliver had closed his eyes and seemed to be sleeping, though there was a rim of white to be seen under his closed lids and his mouth seemed tight and twisted in a way that was not usual on sleeping faces.

'Oh, he'll be fine now,' Kate said. 'He just can't cope with being crowded. Nor can I – nor can most people. Putting on restraint causes more problems than it solves – ' She let go of his wrist and slid her hands round his fingers and they tightened against her grip and she knew then he wasn't asleep. 'He'll be fine,' she said again. 'I can manage. Look, Sister' – and she raised her voice – 'can you tell those policemen I have to make a careful examination and discuss the symptoms this patient is having? I can't have anyone listening to that. It wouldn't be right. Take them to the other side of the waiting room where they'll be able to see the cubicle clearly in the usual way, so that I can do my job quietly and they can still do theirs. I just don't want them within a few feet of us.'

'Certainly, Miss Sayers,' Sister said equally loudly and marched out through the curtains, and Kate heard her saying firmly to the policemen, 'You can come and sit down, over there, outside my office. You'll be able to see everything that happens here and can intervene if there's the least need, but Miss Sayers, the consultant, you know, has to make her examination in peace. You can't stay here – now come along and I'll see that someone fetches you both some tea. You look as though you need it – ' And though there were some rumbles of complaint that Kate could clearly hear, they let her push them in front of her like so many children in a school crocodile and went willingly enough across the waiting area to ensconce themselves on chairs outside her office door. After a moment Kate went and peered through the space between the edge of the curtain and the wall and watched them settle, and then went back to Oliver.

He had his eyes open now and was looking at her and she

leaned over him and touched his forehead, just above the huge contusion that marked his cheek, and said softly, 'Darling, what happened? Has anyone done anything to this yet?'

He shook his head on the white sheet and then winced and screwed up his face into a tight grimace.

'Christ, that hurts – ' he murmured thickly. 'My head feels like – have I broken it?'

'I can't be sure,' Kate said. 'Sister'll get me the X-rays. But it'll be Cantrip's opinion that matters most. He's the best radiologist there is – look, I'll start on that face. This may hurt a little, but it's necessary – ' And she turned to the trolley that stood at the side of the cubicle, all set up ready to do dressings, and pulled it closer.

'I'll wash my hands and then start. And while I do it, you can tell me quietly what all this is about. And whether you did hit a policeman or not. And if you did, why – well, let's get you cleaned up first – '

She washed her hands at the basin in the corner and rubbed in the antiseptic lotion and the smell of it filled her nostrils and managed to bring her professionalism back to the top of her mind again. She had come alarmingly close to dissolving into tears at the sight of his battered face, and was still trying to recover from the great wash of fear that had filled her when she had first seen him. Now she had to behave like a doctor again and not like a woman whose lover was injured. It wasn't easy. But having something to do to help was important; it took away some of the sense of powerlessness that had filled her. And so took away the terror.

Slowly she began to swab the crusted cheek and he lay there, his eyes open, staring up at her face as she worked and she avoided his direct gaze, afraid that if she didn't she would weep, for he looked so very woebegone and so very trusting at the same time that it took all her control to continue working smoothly.

But she did, slowly cleaning away the filth and picking out of the torn skin and underlying tissue the largest pieces of grit she could retrieve, while moving with great delicacy, for it was clear he was in considerable pain. He winced occasionally, and tears of pain dripped from his eyes, but he managed to keep his head still and she was grateful for his stoicism, for it gave her some of her own. While he was so still she could get on and do the job she had been trained to do, even though it was on the face of someone she now knew that she loved far more than she had realised she did.

For that was the worst part of the situation. That he was a person who mattered to her she was well aware. She had not decided to live with him lightly, nor had it been a merely physical need she had been satisfying with him, important though that was to her. She had admired him, enjoyed him, found him to be the best companion she had ever had, but she had thought for the past fifteen months that that was as far as it went. Yes, she had been jealous of his ex-wife, yes she loved him, but after all, what did the word mean? Different things to different people –

But now she knew that what it meant to her was a deep and total involvement with this man. Seeing him in this state was agony, a much greater pain than she would have thought possible. She was angry for him, and with him too for letting it happen to him, and at the same time felt immensely, fiercely protective. Altogether she couldn't understand her own tangle of feelings at all; all she knew was that this man was the most important person who existed in the world and that if anything happened to him it happened to her as well.

'Did you hit a policeman?' she managed to say at last when his face was looking a little less dreadful and she had applied a layer of richly emollient antibiotic cream and covered it lightly with tulle gras. She started to work on his scalp, gingerly exploring the matted hair to find the site of the injury that had shed so much blood on his clothes and snipping away the locks of hair to reach it more easily once she had located it. It was easier to talk to him while she did this, for she could not see his face, standing as she now was behind him.

'I'm not sure,' he said after a moment. 'I can't really remember properly. It all started with – ' He frowned and his scalp moved under her hands. 'Dammit, I'm not sure. I wanted to record something, and – '

He stiffened suddenly. 'My Uher? Where's my Uher?' And he moved, tried to sit up and turned his head at the same time, and she had to push him back down again firmly.

'I'll ask Sister. No point in getting agitated about it now. Your broken head matters more than any damned tape recorder.'

He subsided, but was clearly agitated about the loss, and she looked at his upside-down face and saw the tears escape again from his closed eyes to creep oddly upwards, as they seemed to do from her vantage point, and again felt that great wash of protectiveness. Poor darling Oliver, weeping for his lost toy, she thought absurdly and slid her hands down on each side of his neck and bent her head to set her face against his uninjured cheek. It felt damp and hot at the same time, and he smelled disgustingly of blood and dirt and sweat and the antiseptic and it was a queasy mixture. Or was it her own mixed feelings that made her feel so dreadful?

'I think I did hit him,' he said suddenly and his voice seemed oddly loud and heavy for her ear was so close to his lips. 'Oh, God, I think I did. He was being officious. I remember now. Wouldn't let me record, was being officious, wouldn't let me come in to find you and talk to you, wouldn't fetch his Inspector and suddenly – '

His eyes flew open and she lifted her cheek from his and looked down at him and he stared back, and his eyes looked extraordinarily deep and dark, and so odd, upside down. 'Oh, Kate,' he said. 'Oh, Kate, I did. I do remember. I just couldn't stop myself. It'd been such a pig of a morning and then that bloody man – I hit a lousy policeman . . . Now what?'

'Now I feel better about you,' she said, trying to sound practical and cool and relaxed and finding it exceedingly difficult. 'If you've remembered then you have no retrograde amnesia and that means there's not been any real damage done. I doubt you're even that much concussed. You actually remember hitting him and then being hit by him?'

'Not just him,' he said and now there was more expression in his voice, a rueful self-mocking tone that was a great improvement on the miserable way he had sounded so far. 'Half the bloody police force jumped me. Christ, it was like juggernauts. They landed on me in a great rush and I hit the ground so fast it was – I couldn't breathe, you know? That was – I can't tell you. Hell. And then someone dragged me and I couldn't get my face off the road and that was when this happened.' And he lifted his hand gingerly towards his cheek, though she stopped him touching it well before he got there.

'Leave that alone,' she said. 'We're going to have enough of an infection problem as it is. I'll have to give you systemic penicillin. Can you remember anything else that happened?'

'All of it, I think,' he said. 'I can't see any gap – it's a consistent picture – the bastards – ' And his voice rose a little. 'I know I was wrong to lose my temper, but Christ Almighty, they didn't have to land on me the way they did – '

'Sister says it's a serious charge,' she said after a moment.

'Of course it is.' He sounded very tired now, and she bent her head again to the cleansing of his scalp wound. The sooner he was settled in the ward and could sleep it all off the better. 'I know that as well as anyone. They'll throw everything at me – '

She had found the cut now, a deep one, but not too ragged, and she snipped away the rest of the surrounding hair and then cleaned it. It wouldn't need stitching, she decided, but careful cleaning was a must. And she set to work on it and then reached for a dressing. He'd have to have a proper bandage put on; there was no other way to fix the dressing in place, and she touched his cheek and said softly, 'I'll have to get Sister to bandage this. It isn't one of my major skills. She'll do it better – besides, I have to talk to her. Hold still here for a moment. I won't be long – '

She ignored the policemen across the waiting hall who got to their feet as she emerged from the cubicle, and went across to one of the cubicles on the other side with its curtains drawn where Sister could be seen talking to a patient on the couch there.

'Sister,' she said as she came up to her, purposefully formal in the presence of a patient. 'I need to talk to you about Mr Merrall – '

'Merrall?' the man on the couch said thickly and stared at her malevolently. He had a split lip and was clearly in considerable discomfort. 'Is that the bastard who did this to me? I'll have him for it, you see if I don't. Don't let him con you, Doctor – the man's a rough and a – '

'I have no wish to discuss my patient with you, sir,' Kate said freezingly. 'Sister, if you will give me a moment?' And she moved outside the cubicle and well out of earshot. Sister followed her.

'Who is that?' Kate said softly.

'Sergeant Parson,' Mary said, equally quietly. 'He was the one in charge out there. It's a nasty split – it wasn't so much the violence of the blow that did it, but he's got uneven front teeth, and the lip caught on one of them – '

'Can you put that in the notes?' Kate said eagerly. 'Oliver'll need all the help he can get on this one. Only if you're sure, of course – '

'Oh, I'm sure,' Sister said grimly. 'He's a nasty one, this chap. Most of the men in the force round here are good enough chaps. We know 'em well of course. But this one's always been a bighead, fancies himself as important. I'll see it makes the notes. There's no bruising, you see, which you'd expect from a blow violent enough to make a split in the skin. It really was just bad luck, I reckon. I'll get the houseman to see it too. He'll agree with me – '

'Will he?' Kate let her doubtful anxiety show in her voice.

'Oh, he'll agree,' Sister said firmly. 'He's a good lad and he's learning fast. He knows who to listen to. How is he then, your friend?'

'Not too bad. The contusion's nasty but the scalp wound's clean and small – no stitches needed. And he's not too head injured, I think, because he has full recall now. Which is a comfort. But I want him admitted. Can we fix that? Can you get your houseman to – '

'Just watch me,' Sister said promptly. 'Anyway, it's Alan Kippen's firm which is on intake today, and he's on holiday so his wards are fairly thin. I'll see to it your chap's admitted for observation of head injury query query concussion, and if you have a word with Sister in whichever ward he gets into I dare say you can keep him there as long as you like. Want to get the lawyers going, hmm?'

'Yes,' Kate said. 'And the sooner I start the better, I reckon. This one is not going to be a nice one at all. Is it?'

And Sister, who had a lot of experience of situations like this, said regretfully, 'No, I'm afraid it isn't.'

Chapter Twenty-Eight

Audrey was sitting in the day room while they sorted Joe out. At the beginning she used to stay there while they did what they had to do, helping them, passing them things, jollying Joe along, but not any more. She couldn't bear to do it now, to see his poor body so thin that his ribs looked like a fence, and to see his skin so yellow and so lax. It wasn't as though he really knew her any more, anyway. There were times he did of course, times he opened his eyes and looked at her and said, ''Allo, ducks,' and it was just like the old days really. Well, not exactly, but a bit. And she would smile back and say, 'Well, get you, doin' nothing but sleep all day – where do get off being so lazy?' And he'd grin and drift off again and she'd hold his hand and watch him.

But not when the nurses were dealing with him. Like now. And she leaned back in her chair and closed her eyes and thought – How much longer? How much longer can we go on like this and how much longer can I stand it? Get on with it, Joe. Get on and die, leave me in peace, don't leave me, Joe, what'll I do without you, Joe, how can I manage everything and it's taking so long –

She hadn't realised she was asleep but she must have been, because she actually jumped when he pulled on her skirt and she sat up sharply and stared a little wildly at him and then smoothed her hair with both hands and said stupidly, 'Oh, hello. How are you?'

'Check-up,' he said. 'Got to have a check-up,' and stared at her.

'Oh, yes,' she said and tried to remember his name. Her brains felt scrambled, what with one thing and another, and she couldn't even remember when she'd last seen this chap. And she gave her head a little shake and then it came back to her. Mr Holliday; they'd talked in the café downstairs, and his wife – and she flicked a glance over his shoulders, looking for her. If she was here she'd have to go and help the nurses with Joe after all. Bad as it was to see what was happening to Joe, it wouldn't be as bad as having to sit with that woman jabbering at her –

'She's gone,' he said and stared at her mournfully and she looked at him again and saw the long pale face and the drooping lower lip and felt a stab of irritation.

'Well, I'm sure that makes no difference to me,' she said sharply. 'I wasn't even talking – '

'She talks a lot, but she means no harm,' he said, and then leaned a little more closely, pushing his wheelchair towards her with a pair of bony hands.

'It's nice to see a face you know,' he said. 'All the other patients I was in with, they've gone. Except you – '

'I'm not a patient,' she said, and didn't know why it should matter because in a way she was, wasn't she? 'It's my Joe what's ill and I have to get back to him – '

'They're washing him and all that,' Mr Holliday said. 'I heard as I came past. I pushed my chair all the way. It's good, isn't it? I'm at the other end of the ward and I managed all this way. Even though it's so late. It's easier in the mornings, you see, when I'm not so tired.'

'Oh,' she said and leaned back in her chair. If his chattering exhausting wife wasn't here she could stay. No harm done. And he seemed to want to talk and she might as well let him.

'I found out what it was all about,' he said at length. 'It was on the news, like I said.'

'What?' She opened her eyes, which she had allowed to close for a moment, and stared at him a little stupidly. 'What was that?'

'Last time I saw you. In the café. I asked if you knew about the doctor who was on the news.'

She made a little grimace. 'Oh, yes, I remember. This place is always in the papers these days. I can't say I like it. It's not supposed to be like that, is it, in hospitals? It's that sex change of course. Nasty, I call it. All those awful men flaunting themselves around with their earrings and then doing that! I'm surprised they do such things in a hospital like this, I really am – '

'No,' he said and stared at her even more lugubriously, and she frowned a little. Irritating man, with his big dark eyes and his miserable expression, always making her feel guilty. It wasn't as though she'd done anything to him; hardly knew him, really.

And she considered getting up and going back to Joe's bed. They must be finished by now, surely?

'It was nothing to do with that,' he said. 'I meant about the doctor they're going on about doing abortions.'

'Oh,' she said and nodded. 'Well, yes, they're always making a fuss about that sort of thing, aren't they? Just shows how ignorant they are. If they'd been around as long as I have they'd know there's nothing new under the sun.' She nodded again and turned down the corners of her lips. 'There's always been abortions and always will. Better to have doctors doing it properly than mucking around with pennyroyal and slippery elm the way they used to – not that you'd know of course,' and then she reddened a little. It just showed you how times had changed. To think she'd ever talk to a man about such things; her old mum'd have had a fit if she'd heard her.

'I know more than people think,' he said and he seemed to sit more upright in his chair, and his voice, which had begun to weaken a little, sounded stronger. 'And I think a lot about what I know.'

'I'm sure you do,' she said and sat up a little more herself, moving her bottom forwards to perch on the edge of her chair. She could see over his head down the ward, and the curtains round Joe's bed. The moment they twitched even, she'd be up and away.

He nodded. 'Oh yes. They can't fool me any more. I know what's right and what's wrong. And I'll say so when the time's right.'

'I'm sure you will,' Audrey said heartily.

'I'll tell 'em I think it's all right to do what they do as long as the mother gives her permission, see? If she doesn't – well, it's wrong then, isn't it? It's hers, not theirs to use any way they like. It's like if I have a kidney cut out, I'd want to know what they did with it. Wouldn't you?'

She looked at him with her nose slightly wrinkled with distaste. 'I'm sure I wouldn't. I've been around hospitals long enough to know when it's best to keep your mouth shut and mind your own business. If they took anything out of me I wouldn't want to know what they did with it! Why should I?'

'Because it's you,' he said. 'Isn't it? Part of you? If you had a baby and it – well suppose it died. Wouldn't you want to know what happened to it?'

She went red. 'People have funerals,' she said. 'And souls go to heaven and that's all I need or want to know, thank you very much. I really must say I don't know what you're on about, Mr Holliday. And I'm really not sure I like this sort of talk – dead babies and kidneys – morbid, I call it. Haven't we got enough to put up with here?' And she looked at him and to her horror felt her eyes fill with tears. 'I'm sitting here with my poor husband as hasn't got above a few days left, though they never actually say so, but I know, I'm not a fool, and I shouldn't have to listen to such morbid talk. I really shouldn't.' And she got to her feet in a little stumble and moved to go.

'Oh dear,' he said and then reached out with one slow hand to tug on her skirt. 'Oh dear, I am sorry. I never meant no – I wasn't thinking. It was about me I was talking, you see. This operation I had – it was about my operation and the baby – '

She stared down at him, mystified. 'What baby? You're not talking sense, you're not. I'm going to tell Sister – I don't think you're feeling right – '

'Oh, I am,' he said and nodded again in that infuriating mandarin fashion. 'It's just that – I found out, you see, what they did. I saw it in the papers after, and I'd thought it was that, but couldn't be sure – these new operations with brain transplants, you see. They did that to me. They asked my permission, I signed a form and everything and so did my wife, they said would I agree to a new operation with them transplanting bits of brain to make mine work better and get rid of the symptoms. I tremble a lot, you see, and I get ever so weak and can't talk properly and everything – ' He gave a little gasp as though to demonstrate his dilemma. 'So I said of course because I couldn't be worse off, could I? No.'

He stopped as though to catch his breath and she could have gone then, but now she stood there staring down at him. She could see the anxiety in him again, the way it had been that evening in the café when he'd talked to her, only then his wife with her fountain of chatter had been there and he'd not been able to explain properly. Now he could, and she felt somehow that she had to listen. He had a right to be listened to. And she didn't know why she thought that. It was just there, a fact that had to be considered.

'Well, it's done you some good, hasn't it? The operation? You're talking better now than you did when you came in. I remember. You couldn't talk at all, to tell the truth,' she said candidly. 'I was really set up for you when you started talking again afterwards. I thought, that one – well, he's a lucky one – '

'But where does it come from, that's the thing.' He leaned back in his chair. His voice was getting thin again and beginning to wobble, just like it had when she had talked to him before. He got tired very quickly, she thought, and sat down again. Poor fella, she told herself. Poor fella.

'Well, I don't know,' she said. 'I dare say – I mean they do a lot of things in hospitals we can't know about. All the blood they give people and the drugs – some of them come from people, I've been told. They take bits of people and then extract important drugs. I read the papers too you know – '

'Blood,' he said and seemed to dismiss it. 'That's all right. People don't die for that, do they? But babies. That's different.'

'Babies?' she said carefully.

He was sitting with his head resting back on the cushion on the wheelchair, looking rather pale now. 'Yes,' he managed. 'Babies. That doctor that did the abortion – the police came and fetched her from here. There's to be a court case because she done this abortion. It was to do my transplant, you see. That was what happened. I know now.'

She sat there silently staring at him. And then moved awkwardly and said, 'Well, you can't be sure, can you? I mean, it mightn't be – '

Now he managed to open his eyes. 'Of course it is. Where else did they get the stuff for the transplant? Anyway, they said to me it was from a miscarriage, so I thought – well that's all right. A miscarriage, no one's fault. But an abortion – and such a big baby too. There was this piece in the paper and it showed a picture of a baby. It was a baby, you know. Not just a miscarriage. A baby – '

'Well, I'm sure – ' she began and then stopped. What could anyone say to him about such things? It wasn't right to be even talking about it. Not really.

'I didn't mind. I don't mind.' He seemed to have found some new energy from somewhere for his eyes were wide open now and he was looking at her. 'But I do think I want to know if she said it was all right. The woman. I wouldn't like to think she'd done it for nothing and never knew what a good thing it was. I want to thank her, see. I want her to know what happened to her baby, and tell her she was a good woman. Only no one'll tell me who she is — '

'Well maybe she'd rather forget all about it, whoever she is,' Audrey said. 'I'm sure if I'd had such a thing done I'd think, least said soonest mended.'

'It's all over the papers now,' Mr Holliday said. 'So it's being said anyway, isn't it? I mean, people are talking about how awful it was to do this abortion but they've said nothing about how good it was to help people like me. And not just me. They've done a few more, you know, from the ward I used to be in. I keep my ears open, I know what's going on — '

'Well, yes,' Audrey said. 'I dare say you're right. Well, I must get back to my Joe now. Nice talking to you — ' And she turned to go, once again uncomfortable to be with him. He really was rather odd, one way and another.

'I'm going to watch out and I'm going to the court when it all happens and I'm going to tell them,' he said as she reached the door of the day room. 'I've told her, my wife, she's a good soul and she mightn't like it but she won't go against me. I'll go to that court and I shall tell them it's a good thing what that doctor did. It wasn't bad to do that abortion. There's me and those other people, look how much better we are. It wasn't all wasted, you see, was it?'

'No,' said Audrey and smiled vaguely at him. 'No, of course!' and escaped at last.

The curtains were still closed as she reached Joe's bed and she hesitated outside, not sure what to do. There was nothing they did to her Joe she shouldn't be part of, of course, she knew that; Sister had said to her from the start, you stay with him all you want. And she did. But the curtains stood there like a barrier higher and harder than a range of mountains and she had to take a deep breath to make herself go inside.

277

The nurses had gone and she frowned for a moment. She hadn't noticed them go, but they had taken all their stuff away with them, and left him quietly lying there, his hands on the sheet in front of him and his head propped against the high pillows, and as she stared at him a rope of fear looped itself round her throat and pulled hard so that she couldn't move. He wasn't breathing; Joe was lying there and he wasn't breathing, and they'd gone away and left him and not told her; they'd gone so he'd died all alone without her there to hold his hand or anything.

She managed somehow to move then and pushed herself across the narrow strip of parquet floor that lay between her and the side of the bed, her hand outstretched and her mouth open to shout her fury at the nurses, at Sister who let them do it, at everyone and anyone. And then stopped as she saw the lax mouth move and the narrow chest cave in in that dreadfully familiar way that showed he was still breathing, just; and she slid to her knees beside the bed and reached for his hand and held on to it. He hadn't gone yet: oh, Joe, don't go and leave me. Oh, Joe, don't keep me in this state. Oh, Joe, Joe, Joe –

Behind her the curtains moved again and it was Sister.

'I'm so sorry, Audrey,' she whispered. 'Nurse told me that he'd – that he was sinking and I came to tell you and fetch you. We wouldn't have left you not knowing, I promise. Here, my dear, let me help.' And she put her arm behind Audrey's back and lifted her and at the same time pushed the chair forwards till it touched the back of her knees, and she sat down, never once taking her eyes off Joe's face or letting go of the thin bundle of dead bones that was his hand.

'Thanks, Sister,' she said. 'Very good of you,' and was pleased with herself. She sounded quite ordinary, really, as though Sister had just told her the weather was nice or something of the sort.

'It won't be long now, Audrey,' Sister said. 'I'm sorry, my dear. He had a minor heart attack while the nurses were bathing him, you see. It does happen that way towards the end with lungs and – well, I was afraid you'd be too late and I knew you'd be upset. I'm glad you still have time to be with him. But it won't be long, dear. Just a little while – '

'Yes, Sister. I know, Sister,' Audrey said, still quiet, still calm while inside her head the words hurled and tumbled, bounced and ricocheted. Don't Joe, hurry up, Joe, Joe, Joe, Joe –

'I'll fetch you some tea,' Sister said. 'And here's the bell by your hand. Don't hesitate – '

But there seemed no sense in any of that. The tea came and stood untouched on the bedside table and the bell sat there in the fold of sheet beside her hand and she held on to Joe until her own fingers felt dead and she couldn't have moved them if she'd tried. She watched his face, waiting for each breath as it came, so rarely and so convulsively each time, and counted them and heard the sounds from the ward outside coming from a long way away. And none of it was real; none of it mattered. Only the words inside her head mattered, really.

She didn't ring the bell when he died. What was the point? Why make them come running, make them take her away and start all the disgusting things they'd do to him once they knew? She wanted everything to stay as it was for as long as it could because at last the shouting inside her head had stopped. Joe was dead. She couldn't shout at him to hurry up, couldn't shout her fury at him for leaving her, because he was dead. Inside her head was dead too. Numb and cold and dead and that was good. It felt very good, and she wanted to make the good feeling last. Being dead inside was the best thing that could happen to her now.

But Joe being dead wasn't something she could stop them from finding out. Sister came in and leaned over the bed and then leaned closer and reached for his pulse and then gently took her elbow and made her stand up and took her outside.

'I'm sorry, dear,' Sister said and looked over her head to one of the nurses and nodded at her, and Audrey knew she was telling her to go and do all the horrible things to Joe that had to be done. 'It's a happy release, really, dear. He was having a lot of pain towards the end, wasn't he? A happy release. Now come along and I'll get you a nice cup of tea.'

Audrey wanted to laugh then. That was what they kept on giving her, nice cups of tea, as though that would make Joe's dying any better. Or easier. Or slower, or anything else. And she giggled a little inside her head and then the giggle came out of her lips and Sister sighed and said to the nurse who had come hurrying across to her, 'Fetch me some diazepam, Nurse. Mrs Slater needs a little – yes, come along, dear. You can have a nice lie down in the side ward.' And led her away, still laughing, to the side ward. And Mr Holliday, who had managed to wheel his chair halfway up the ward, watched her go with the familiar lugubrious expression on his face, and Audrey would have laughed at him, too, if she could. But she was too busy laughing over Joe.

Chapter Twenty-Nine

'Oh, you've done it now, Levy,' Goodman Lemon said, and his voice dripped with satisfaction. 'You've really done it, haven't you? You won't be able to talk your way out of this one so easily.'

Professor Levy sighed. 'I really don't know why you're making such a fuss, Lemon. I was on call that evening and you were not. This man seemed to me to be in need of a genito-urinary investigation so I arranged it. I am the Dean and the Chief of Staff, you know. I do carry overall responsibility here. And you can't complain when I exercise that responsibility.'

'That's piffle and you know it,' Lemon said. 'And so will the committee, you'll see. I'm not wasting any more time arguing with you. I shall make my comments to the committee and no one else.'

'Such a comfort,' Levy murmured and smiled at Kate who was sitting silently in the armchair near the window of Levy's office. 'Kate, my dear, some more coffee?'

She smiled back at him and shook her head, and then went back to thinking about the conversation she had had that morning with Oliver's solicitor. She ought to be worried about the forthcoming inquisition from the ethical committee for which they were here, but somehow she couldn't get at all anxious over that. All the fuss over Slattery seemed to her now to be inconsequential. It was Oliver and his appalling situation that mattered.

'There are very few options open to us,' Andrew Curlew had said, his voice clacking busily into her ear. 'I've thought about it all very carefully, and as I see it, we either plead confusion – Oliver didn't realise the man was a policeman – '

'They'll never take that,' Kate had said, wanting to shout at the man for his stupidity. 'He was talking to him, demanding to see the Inspector – '

'I'm well aware of that. I was just spelling out the options. You have to do that even if you immediately jettison them. Now, that was the first and it's out. The next is to cry confusion because of all the hubbub there was. Oliver didn't realise what he was doing – and yes, I'll agree before you say a word. That's out too, because he's a highly experienced journalist and used to any sort of hubbub. And anyway the scene was comparatively peaceful up to that point. The trouble didn't start until after he hit the sergeant. In fact the hitting of the sergeant was what started it. Which leaves me, as far as I can see, with just one other possibility. Provocation.'

'It's the only one,' Kate said. 'It's what happened.'

'You were there?' the little voice said smoothly. 'You have evidence to offer?'

She reddened. 'You know I wasn't. But Oliver's told me and – '

'I'm afraid what Oliver tells you and what constitutes evidence are two very different things,' he said with what she knew was mock regret. This man is really hateful, she thought then, holding the phone to her ear so tightly that her knuckles were white. He ought to be on Oliver's side, for God's sake, not acting like some sort of prosecutor. And then she knew she was being absurd; mere partisanship wouldn't get Oliver out of this mess. He needed legal expertise and this man was the source of it.

'Well, all the same there must be some witnesses – '

'I'm working on finding them. Some of my chaps are on the picket lines today talking to these people – '

'They're not a picket line,' she said, childishly pleased to be able to put him right. 'They're demonstrators. There's no strike going on here.'

'Not much to choose between 'em, is there?' the sleek voice said. 'These rabble-rousers are all the same.'

'Hardly,' Kate said sharply. 'People with a genuine grievance aren't rabble-rousers, as you put it.'

'Well, all that is by the by.' The man sounded impatient. 'If you could get Oliver to phone me – I gather he has access to a phone there?'

'He has, of course. But he's far from well still, and I don't want him bothered more than is necessary. That's why I'm talking to you now rather than him.'

'You've been very helpful, Miss Sayers, but I do have to consult with my client directly, you know. Some things can't be done at second hand.'

'Of course.' She felt her teeth clench at his patronising tone. 'I'll see to it Oliver phones you as soon as he feels fit enough.'

'Thank you – ' He hesitated a moment and then went on in a more affable tone. 'I'm sorry to see you're having problems of your own, Miss Sayers.'

She stiffened. 'Oh?'

'All the papers today – most unpleasant for you being labelled as – well – '

'As what?' she said softly, trying for Oliver's sake not to let him know how angry she was. How far would this man go, for God's sake?

'Well, the friend of such people as this Hynes person. *Most* unpleasant.'

'Miss Hynes is my patient, Mr Curlew,' she said. 'That is all. My *patient*. And I do not discuss my patients with anyone except my patients. Do you understand that?'

'Oh, perfectly.' He still hadn't registered how angry she was, she realised, for he said then, 'But do keep it in mind that if you need any – um – legal advice I'm always here. Any friend of Oliver's, you know – '

'Yes,' she said and hung up sharply, too furious to care how unmannerly she was, and went to see Oliver to tell him what had been said.

'He's not a bad chap,' Oliver had said, uncomfortable when she'd told him how maddening she had found his tone of voice and his attempt to discuss her affairs. 'Really he isn't. Not considering he's a lawyer. I – we owe him a lot, really. Always taken very good care of us – '

She realised then that of course he was talking about Sonia and the divorce, and the matter of the access to the children, and felt her jaw tighten. No matter what happened, no matter what the issue, that bloody woman crept in somehow and she allowed herself the luxury of a moment or two of sheer hate for her. They'd never met, and probably never would, but Kate could not remember ever feeling so powerfully about anyone ever before. But wallowing in hate wouldn't help, she thought, dragging her practicality back to the top of her mind. It's getting Oliver out of this mess that matters. And if Curlew could do it, well and good, even if the bloody man was involved with the repellent Sonia.

'He wants to talk to you when you feel up to it,' she said then. 'But don't push yourself, darling. You're really far from well.' And indeed he wasn't well. Clearly he had an appalling headache, for he squinted painfully against the light and any undue sound or movement, and around the livid contusion on his face and his now very bruised eye his face was pallid and damp. But he made a small grimace at her.

'Too bad,' he said. 'I'll have to talk to him. Find out what he's doing – '

'Provocation, that's the line he's taking.'

'Fair enough. That man was bloody provocative.'

'He's sent people to the demo to talk to them. See if he can find witnesses for you.'

'I doubt he'll get far,' Oliver said. 'People don't like to get mixed up in cases involving police, cases like this. They won't come forward. I might even – ' He stopped and swallowed. 'They might send me to prison for this, you know.'

'They couldn't,' she said, and stared at him in horror. 'I thought, a court case, a lot of publicity, a fine – all that would be bad enough. But surely not – '

Oliver shrugged. 'It's a major offence, striking a police officer. They really get very steamed up about it.'

'But this is – you were just doing your job, for God's sake! And they tried to stop you – '

'I know, I know. I've been on to the Union too. This morning. They're getting in touch with Andrew too, see if they can do anything. But I'm not sanguine. Believe me, if I get out of this with no more than a fine I'll be damned grateful. Pray for me, love, because God knows I need it.'

Sitting now in the Dean's office waiting to be summoned to talk to the Ethics Committee she tried to do as he asked; to say inside her head the sort of prayers she used to make when she was a child. Please God, make it all right for Oliver. Please God don't let it happen – But there was none of the comfort she had found as a child in the silly words. That was all they were, silly words.

The phone on Levy's desk pinged and he picked it up.

'Yes,' he said after a moment and hung up. 'Mr Lemon, perhaps you'd care to go in? They're ready for you.'

'Splendid,' Lemon said and marched over to the door. 'Now we'll see – '

There was a little silence after he'd gone and then Levy said gently, 'How are you standing up to it all, Kate?'

'Mm? Oh, well enough – '

'I was dreadfully sorry to hear about your friend Merrall. Such a nasty business.'

'Yes. He's got a severe facial contusion and a black eye. No skull damage fortunately. But some concussion.'

'I was thinking more of the – um – repercussions,' Levy said almost apologetically. 'To get involved with police in that way – very unfortunate.'

'Unfortunate is one word for it,' she said grimly. 'He could go to prison, you know?'

'Yes, I know. If there's anything I can do to help – '

'If you're willing to go to court and say you think he was justified, that might be useful,' Kate said wearily. 'But you know you can't and I know you can't. But thanks all the same.'

'No I can't do that. But anything else, just let me know. I wish I'd seen it all. Then I could have been a witness.'

'I wish I had. Then I could have hit the damned policeman too,' Kate said with a sudden spurt of rage, and Levy grinned sympathetically. 'Well, yes, that would have been satisfying. Useless but satisfying.'

'As it is, I'm just – ' She rubbed her face with both hands. 'To tell the truth, I'm so tired I can hardly think straight.'

'Try not to let that show too much when you deal with this committee,' Levy said. 'They're a pretty reasonable bunch, but we mustn't let them get the idea that you're – not on top form, you know?'

'I know. I'll be careful.'

'No need to be careful. Just be honest.'

She looked at him. 'Honest? Frankly, I wasn't planning to be – shall we say – as open as I might. I'm not admitting for example that the cystoscopy was your idea – '

'But you must!' Levy said and smiled at her. 'My dear, I need

285

no protection from you, believe me. Tell them all about it as it happened. My pressure on you, all of it. That really is the best way.'

She frowned, puzzled at the insouciance he was showing. 'But Professor Levy, you know how that'll look? As though we conspired or something – '

He laughed then. 'My dear, we did! And you must say so. No, don't look like that. I know what I'm doing. Trust me. Ah – ' He cocked his head as the sound of muffled voices came from outside his door. 'I rather think Lemon's on his way. My, isn't he cross!' And they both sat in silence as they heard more shouting outside and then the thump of feet on the stairs.

'There! And I thought he'd come back and tell us what happened,' he murmured, and Kate looked at him, still deeply puzzled. Why on earth did he look so relaxed and comfortable? After all, he'd really behaved in a very devious way, and Lemon had been justified in his anger, fully entitled to do what he'd done, which was to complain to the committee. Levy should be a little more concerned than he was, surely?

The phone pinged on his desk again and once more he answered it and then smiled at Kate. 'Both of us – ' he said. 'Certainly. We'll be in at once,' and he hung up the phone and stood up and held out one hand to Kate invitingly.

'Sensible people, want me to come with you. Feel better now?'

'Oh, yes,' Kate said and stood up. 'Heavens yes! But it still feels like being on trial or something. It's like sitting outside the headmistress's office – '

'Isn't it just?' He opened the door. 'But it won't be like that, I do assure you. I do my homework, you see, Kate. You can't be Dean of a hospital like Old East without being a good politician who does his homework. And I've done mine. So stop worrying – '

The committee room was large and cluttered, with all the assorted detritus of years set on and against its walls. Portraits of long dead members of the medical staff, framed diplomas and testimonials and pictures of classes of long ago medical students jostled with cases in which elderly surgical instruments were displayed museum-style, and rather battered and ill-matched chairs. At the big central table there were six people sitting, two

of them women, and at the head of the table was Laurence
Bulpitt. He got up as they came in and grinned at Kate.

'Hello, my dear,' he said. 'Nice of you to spare the time for us.
Do you know everyone? You do, of course, Levy. Let me see
now, Mrs Cantrip – John's wife, you know? And a Deaconess of
St Matthew's in Pennington Street. And Miss Barber from the
Nursing School you may have met. And of course Neville Carr I
needn't introduce. And by no means least, Peter Impey, our tame
lawyer, and Father Jennings who has retired from his parish but
still finds time to give us. All good friends to the hospital as I'm
sure you know. And we do appreciate your coming along to help
us.'

With a little flurry of nods and smiles she was led to a chair at
the table and Professor Levy sat down facing her and smiled
encouragingly at her.

'Now, Kate, I do want you to understand that we are not in
any way – ah – attempting any criticism here. We just need to
know, as the hospital's Ethics Committee, how things – ah – are
happening here. I don't have to tell you that ethical problems are
part and parcel of every day's work. I doubt any of us can get to
lunchtime without having to wrestle with something that has a
moral element in it. After all, it's the stuff our trade is built on,
hmm?'

Laurence Bulpitt was well launched on his way and looking at
him and his comparatively young face Kate thought – He's on
the way to a knighthood too. He'll be a major force in the Royal
College one of these days, and she tried to see the man she had
first met so long ago when she too had been comparatively low
on the career ladder; he was older than she, of course, but all the
same he'd just been a bouncy registrar then, full of himself but
very agreeable. And now he sat there at the head of a committee,
sleek and rather plump and undeniably good-looking in the way
that expensive clothes and a touch of self-indulgence always
creates good looks, and she sat in front of him like a frightened
child.

She gave herself a mental shake then. She was not a frightened
child. Nor was she a junior medical student. She was a consultant in her own right, and to make a fuss over what was

happening here was demeaning. A situation had arisen that had to be sorted out, that was all –

'We have a situation here that we have to sort out, Kate,' Bulpitt said, which unnerved her somewhat. 'And I'm sure we can. Please, will you tell me – tell the committee – how it was Mr Gerald Slattery came into your care? And what you did for him?'

She let her eyes move so that she could see Levy and he smiled at her and inclined his head gently and she thought – He's right. What's the point in twisting anything out of some sort of sense of loyalty? I'd only make matters worse and I hate that sort of thing anyway –

So she told them, exactly as it had happened, what it was all about, of the conversation with Levy in the ICU, of her conversations with Slattery on the issue of whether or not he should be tested for HIV and of what happened in the theatres and how she did her best to deal with the problems of the heavy blood loss. And they listened, all of them silent, some of them taking occasional notes, and when at last her voice came to a stop they sat, still silent, and waited.

Then Bulpitt stirred. 'Well, thank you, Kate. A most useful performance that, succinct and speedy. It was a pleasure to hear you. You agree?' And he cast a sweeping glance round his committee who murmured and nodded back at him. 'It is pretty well what I thought – '

'And as I already told you before this meeting, Laurence,' Levy said and leaned forwards to prop his elbows on the table and his chin on his fists. 'It seemed to me essential that we had the man dealt with as soon as possible and with the minimum of fuss, before Lemon could turn the whole affair into a – well, you can imagine. I was very grateful to Kate for agreeing to help me and for allowing the small subterfuge of the cystoscopy.'

'I wouldn't have done it if there was any harm in it,' Kate said then, needing to defend herself. 'A man of his age – it can be a useful screening. I know it's an invasive investigation, but all the same – '

'I agree,' Bulpitt said. 'I'm a few years younger than the patient, and I'd be delighted if any medical man caring for me took the trouble to check my plumbing as a routine. I see it much as I see the provision of cervical smears for women – a practical step. No need to apologise for that. No, Kate, we owe you our gratitude. You helped defuse what could have been a very unpleasant situation for Old East.'

Kate was puzzled and looked at Levy, her brows raised.

'I'm not sure I – frankly, I felt some guilt over all this. I thought you'd rap my knuckles hard.'

'What for? Taking on a worrying patient and handling him with great skill?' Bulpitt said. 'Why be ashamed of that?'

'I could have been accused of poaching another practitioner's patient,' Kate said. 'Dammit, I did.'

'Happily, we needn't talk in those terms,' Bulpitt said. 'It's one of the few personal benefits of NHS practice, you must admit. No need to worry about each other's incomes. No, you were most helpful. It's Mr Lemon who – well, I really can't say that.'

'I can,' Levy said unexpectedly. 'And I will. You needn't minute it,' and he looked over his shoulder at the secretary in the corner who was taking busy shorthand. 'I think Lemon behaved appallingly. We can't have people going out of this hospital saying surgeons risked their lives by refusing to operate on them unless they submitted to blood tests they had every right to refuse! And refusing to let other surgeons take care of them. A stand had to be taken and I determined to take it. I was rather afraid at first that I'd created a bigger problem than we could handle, and was concerned for Kate – but in the event it's all turning out well enough. You see the situation from my point of view – '

'We had to,' Neville Carr cut in. 'It's the same as the patient's.'

'It is also the legal way,' Impey said and squinted over his glasses at Kate. 'You were worried about the – um – tradition of practice. What some people *call* medical ethics – but they are not what *we* regard as ethics, surely? The matter of poaching of patients and who refers to whom and all that – important to the practitioners, no doubt, especially in lucrative private practice, but of no value whatsoever to the patient. In fact many of these so-called medical ethics could more accurately be labelled restrictive practices, and should be – '

'Indeed, yes,' said Bulpitt, clearly breaking into what was a familiar track. 'The patient must always be regarded as the prime issue. How is he now, Kate? Recovering well?'

'Indeed. I sent him home.' She looked again at Levy but not

for encouragement this time. Just for confirmation. 'He'll have his stitches taken out by his GP to whom I've spoken, and he'll come back to see me in Outpatients. He seemed to be in excellent spirits when he left us. And very well.'

'Good,' Bulpitt said heartily. And then smiled at her. But it was different suddenly and she felt the change in atmosphere and looked sharply at him. 'This might be a good point at which to ask you about your other patient, um – Hynes, isn't it? The reassignment of gender chap – '

'What about her?' Kate's head had come up and she looked at him very directly.

'Has he – she been discharged yet?'

'No, I have some tidying of the wound to do. To prepare her for future plastic work.'

'Well, far be it for us to tell you how to care for your patient, Kate. We do of course have full confidence in you. But we are a bit worried about the publicity the hospital is getting because of – all the fuss about Fay Buckland, you see, and also about your Hynes. We could do with a respite, I think. If the time comes soon for Hynes to be discharged I think it would help us quite a lot.'

'I'm as anxious to release beds as anyone else,' Kate said. 'But I won't apologise for admitting her or for treating her. She's been under the care of Barbara Rosen for three years, you know. She's no sudden arrival here. All the talk about the waiting list – it's a travesty of justice to suggest that Kim's occupation of a bed has any bearing on the shortage of care for other patients – '

'I agree with you totally, Kate,' Bulpitt said soothingly. 'It's just that – '

'I worry about the nurses, you see, Miss Sayers.' Miss Barber leaned forwards earnestly. 'We try to teach them not to gossip to outsiders and we do stamp on such behaviour when we can, but they're very young, you know, and it is difficult for some of them to understand . . . If a patient is on the premises, you see, it's hard to make *sure* they don't gossip. Once they've been discharged, of course – well, memories are short. You know how it is with these youngsters. They'll go on to the next piece of excitement. I really think the whole fuss will die down once this patient goes.'

290

'I'll arrange it as soon as it's right for the patient,' Kate said with a note of stubbornness in her voice and Levy grinned at her. 'But I'll keep what you said in mind. May I go now?'

'Of course. And thank you once more – ' Bulpitt got to his feet. 'One word though before you go – I'm afraid Mr Lemon is far from happy with us at the moment. He left here in a – shall we say, highly emotional state. I had to tell him that as far as we could see there was no ethical case for you to answer. Only on traditional grounds, as Impey here said which we, as a committee, discount. And he took that rather badly. Blames you, I fear, rather more than he should – '

'He should be blaming me,' Levy said. 'But Kate's an easier target, I suppose.'

'I'm just saying you should take care.' Bulpitt patted her on the shoulder and led her to the door. 'I wish you could stay, my dear. We now have to deal with the matter of poor Fay Buckland and her dilemma which is rather more difficult. But I'm sure you've got other things to do. But remember what I said – Mr Lemon could be tiresome for a few days. I'd keep out of his way if I were you.'

Chapter Thirty

———————⟨∞⟩———————

Suba used her day off to deal with it. She should have gone home, of course, and she had worried a good deal about that. She had gone home on her day off every week since coming to Old East, and if she didn't this week Daddy would be very annoyed, but this was too important; it would be worth risking Daddy's rage. So she had phoned him at the shop and for the first time in her life told him a lie. And got away with it.

'I've got to study, Daddy,' she said, staring at the scribbled wall in front of her in the stuffy little phone box on the ground floor of the nurses' home. 'We should be having exams soon and I really ought to get down to it – '

And he, rushed because he had a shop full of customers – she could hear the chatter in the background – had huffed a little and complained, but he'd accepted it. And she had hung up, feeling ashamed and deeply exhilarated at the same time. It wasn't as hard as it seemed sometimes to do what you had to do. If this could all be sorted out over Miss Buckland, then maybe in the future some time – because there would be a future for her then at Old East – perhaps in the future some time she could lie again and have a whole day just for herself? It was an intoxicating thought.

She considered carefully what would be the best time to go, and decided on the morning. People went shopping and took children out, she knew that, but most people didn't do it too early. If she turned up there at about ten o'clock, that should be about right. She'd thought of phoning at first, finding Mrs Roberts' number in the phone book, but decided against that. Suppose she said not to come? What could Suba do then? No, she would just arrive on the doorstep. Then she'd have to talk to her; yes, that was the way to do it.

It was difficult finding the place. She had the address carefully written down: Flat 179, Lansbury House, Tarling Street Estate, and she knew where Tarling Street was; she would walk it – but it was a rather long walk – or take a bus up Cannon Street and then along Commercial Road and walk a little way down Sutton Street. So she did that, and that part of the journey went well. She sat on the bus in her new tweed coat and her brown boots – she had been given those as a special present when she'd started at Old East, from her aunt, and she was very proud of them – her hands folded on her neat bag as she stared out of the window at the passing street and rehearsed in her head what she would say.

Every time she tried to plan it, though, it came out differently. Mrs Roberts kept saying different things in reply to what she, Suba, said in her imagination, and that confused and worried her. And then, as she reached the end of the bus journey and jumped down she decided wisely to stop thinking about it. Just go and tell her, simply and easily, that would be enough. She'd be sure to understand and want to help.

But then it all got very difficult. Block after block of flats lifted themselves lumpishly into the dull September sky and although she had looked carefully at the map of the estate she had found at the entrance to the great sprawl of buildings, it was difficult to work out exactly which was Lansbury House. So she walked what seemed to be miles looking for it, as her boots creaked their newness and her feet ached more and more.

But she found it at last, a tall building exactly like all the others, with the same spray-paint graffiti on the concrete walls around the base and the same litter of garbage in the concrete walkways between. She stood and craned up at the building and thought – Suppose the lift doesn't work? And the prospect of climbing seventeen floors in her creaking new boots nearly made her turn and run. But then she saw someone emerge from the battered lift, and took a deep breath and went on. She was here now. She had to do it.

The lift creaked dreadfully and she was frightened for a while that it would stop between floors and trap her there and she'd never be able to get out; but at last there was the seventeenth floor and she was standing on the winndy walkway that encircled the building and staring down at the foreshortened people below and the map of Shadwell spread out before her. She looked eastwards, hoping to find the huddle of buildings that was the hospital, needing a sight of the familiar place to reassure herself,

293

but it wasn't possible to work out exactly where it was, and with her pulse now thumping unpleasantly in her ears, she walked along the rubbish-strewn walkway, peering at door numbers.

There was someone in at number 179; she could hear the sound of a child crying, but she had to ring the bell three times, loud and long, before someone came shuffling along to the door to open it.

Suba was quite shocked when she saw Mrs Roberts. She was wearing a pink dressing gown which was badly torn and her hair was rumpled yet greasy. Her face was pale and she looked half dazed as she stared at Suba, quite without any recognition in her face.

'Er, hello,' Suba said. 'How are you, Mrs Roberts?'

There was a little silence as Prue stared at her and then she said, 'Who are you?'

But before Suba could answer there was another wail, and Prue muttered and turned and let go of the door and walked back into the flat, and after a moment, Suba followed her and closed the door behind her.

The place smelled of urine and dirty nappies and stale food and Suba picked her way past the pram which took up most of the width of the hall, following Prue to the far end, where she disappeared into a bedroom. And Suba went in too.

It was a very cluttered room with a cot, and a large Moses basket on a table, as well as a chest of drawers and a wardrobe. It must have been a pleasant room once, because an effort had been made to make it pretty, with wallpaper covered in Disney characters, and matching curtains much embellished with frills, but now it was unbelievably untidy. There were dirty clothes on the floor and the half-open drawers of the chest were filled with a tangle of garments and more were hanging over the open door of the wardrobe. In the cot a child of not yet two was standing holding on to the bars and shrieking at the top of his voice. The reek of ammonia was so strong that it caught in Suba's throat and she could have retched. But she didn't. Instead she stood there as Prue lifted the child out of his cot and lay him down, still shrieking, on the top of the chest of drawers and began hunting in a desultory fashion in one of the drawers.

'Here,' Suba said, pushed by a sudden impulse. 'Let me – '

And she came to stand beside Prue just as she fished a rather grey nappy out of the drawer.

'What?' Prue stared blankly at her. 'What do you want then?'

'Let me help you with this little chap — ' Suba said, and turned to the child. 'What's his name?'

'Danny,' Prue said. 'Oh, do shut up, you little — ' as Danny shrieked ever louder.

'We'll soon get him right,' Suba said and pulled off her coat and after a moment added it to the drapery on the wardrobe. And she began to undress the child who stared up at her and stopped shouting and lay there occasionally hiccupping.

Before starting her training at Old East Suba had spent a good deal of time with small children, not only her own younger brothers and sisters, but also the ones in the nursery her school had adopted. It had been part of her social studies O level to spend some time there and she had enjoyed it, and found she was good with the small ones. Now Danny seemed to know she could be trusted and lay there, his thumb stuck in his mouth as she took off the reeking nappy that covered him and looked round for a bucket to put it in.

'It's in the bathroom,' Prue said sulkily. 'Here, give it to me — ' And she took it and went away leaving Suba to look at the raw red bottom and belly and thighs the child was displaying.

'I'll need some water, Mrs Roberts,' she called after a few moments. 'And have you some zinc and castor oil cream? He's a bit sore — '

For the next ten minutes or so, there was an agreeable enough silence in the little room as Prue came back with the cream and a wet flannel; and Suba did the best she could to make the child comfortable again, and when eventually she had pinned on the clean nappy and taken off his shirt and found a reasonably fresh one to put on so that he could be put back into his cot, she felt a great deal more relaxed.

Prue Roberts stood at the door of the room and said, 'Who are you anyway? I've seen you before. I have, haven't I?'

Suba smiled over her shoulder at her from the cot, where she was still standing murmuring down at Danny. 'Yes, you remember me. I was on the ward at Old East, when you had your operation — '

Prue went a sudden mottled red. 'I didn't have no operation — ' she said loudly and Danny let out another wail, and Suba turned back to soothe him.

'Well, when you were ill then,' she said, puzzled. Of course she'd had an operation; Suba could clearly remember her being sent up from the operating theatre with a unit of blood dripping into her arm and looking as pale and as dead as — well, some sort of shop-window dummy. But she didn't want to argue with her; she looked too ill now to be argued with and she gazed anxiously at her and said carefully, 'How are you feeling now?'

'I'm all right,' Prue said. 'What are you doing here then? Is it that I didn't go to the clinic for my appointment? I didn't want to and that's the end of it. I've got — I made — there's other arrangements.'

'Oh?' Suba said carefully, not wanting to say the wrong thing and floundering a little. 'Oh!'

'Yes, that's it. My friend — It's been arranged, you see. I'm to have this one at this other hospital, and I'm seeing the doctor there. Well, I will be doing. So I don't have to go down to Old East. Much good they were to me anyway, when I needed 'em most — ' And she looked mulishly at Suba and Suba thought — She's scared of me.

'I've got nothing to do with that,' she said. 'Listen, can we take him into the kitchen and give him something to eat? That's why he's crying, I think — ' because Danny had started bawling loudly again — 'and then I can explain it all to you, why I'm here and everything.'

Prue stared at her and then shrugged. She came into the room and leaned over the Moses basket and picked up the baby that had been sleeping in it and Suba bit her lip in embarrassment. She hadn't even noticed there was a baby in there.

'She's easy, this one,' Prue said suddenly and, moving awkwardly, lifted the baby and set her cheek to its head and the baby woke and opened its mouth and cried, a little mew of sound that made the older child now sitting on Suba's arm yell even more loudly.

The kitchen was marginally tidier than the children's bedroom and Suba put Danny in a high chair that was standing there and looked round for something to give him to stop the shouting.

Prue, appealed to, moved heavily to a corner cupboard and found a biscuit and the child grabbed it and at last was silenced.

'Is the baby breast-fed?' Suba ventured, looking at the infant who was now rolling its head towards its mother in an unmistakably hungry way. 'Don't mind me if – '

'No,' Prue said wearily. 'Not in my state. I couldn't manage and – I'll get her a bottle.' And she went to the grimy refrigerator and reached in it for a bottle. Suba saw the teat was uncovered and worried about that; she knew that such things should be kept sterile if the baby was to be protected from dangerous infection. She hadn't done her children's wards yet, but she knew that much. But she said nothing; there seemed little point anyway, looking round at the kitchen. Not precisely dirty but far from clean.

'What does he have now?' she asked, looking at Danny, as Prue ran the bottle under the hot tap to warm it. 'I'll get his for him if you like.'

'I don't see why you should,' Prue said and stared at her with suspicion now very clear on her face. 'If you're not from the clinic what do you want here? Checking up on me, are you? I'm well enough. You don't have to come checking up on me. I've got myself all sorted out, don't need you social workers hanging around.'

'But you said you remembered me!' Suba said and tried a smile. 'I'm one of the nurses at the ward you were in at Old East. And a very new one, too. I couldn't be a social worker – I'm not old enough – '

'Never you think it,' Prue said with a suddenly savage note in her voice. 'You should see some of 'em. Still got milk teeth and think they can tell me what to do. I send 'em packing, I can tell you. So why are you here? Oh, Danny, shut up! Here, he likes that rusk stuff. Mix one with some milk and he'll eat that.'

Suba took the packet Prue had pointed to on the dresser and extracted one of the rusks, a big sugary thing, and tried not to say what she thought – that these days people gave babies fibre and not so much sugar, the way she'd learned in her nutrition lectures. But she didn't. That wasn't what she was here for, after all. And she didn't want the sort of response the social workers had clearly got from Mrs Roberts.

She mixed the rusk and milk from the fridge into a sticky porridge and began to feed Danny with it, who wolfed it down.

'I came to ask your help, actually, Mrs Roberts,' she said, and her diffidence made her voice rather low. 'I thought you might be able to give me the sort of – well, support I need. Not just me, actually. Miss Buckland.'

'Miss Buckland? Who's she?'

Prue was sitting now with the baby on her lap who was sucking steadily at the bottle. Suba felt a moment of shock. Surely she couldn't have forgotten already?

'She was the surgeon who looked after you,' she said a little reprovingly. 'She saved your life, you know. And your baby's. The new one, I mean.'

Prue's shoulders came up into a defensive posture and the baby seemed to have recognised it too, for it stopped sucking and began to wail. Prue pushed the teat back into its mouth sharply and said, 'Oh. Her.'

'Yes,' Suba said. 'I wanted you to help me with her if you would.'

'What sort of help?'

'Well, it's a bit difficult – ' Danny finished the rusk and still seemed hungry and Suba fetched another biscuit for him from the packet Prue had left on the dresser.

'Well, I'm sure I don't know – ' Prue said and then shrugged. 'I mean, what can I do for her? I'm no bloody surgeon.'

'I'll have to explain from the beginning,' Suba said and came and sat facing her at the table as Danny, at last happy, sat and smeared his face with the chewed mess he made of the biscuit. 'If you can give me a minute.'

'Well, I'm not doing anything much,' Prue said ungraciously. 'I can listen, I suppose.'

'Have you seen in the papers all about the trouble at Old East? There's been a lot there. And on the TV news.'

'I don't take papers,' Prue said. 'And I've not felt up to the telly. I sleep mostly. I'm pregnant, remember? Look at me!'

And Suba looked but couldn't see much evidence. And then smiled. 'Well, I don't have to look,' she said. 'I know. That's why I'm here.'

Again Prue's shoulders tightened but this time the baby went on feeding happily enough. 'Oh,' she said. 'Is that a fact?'

'The thing is, the papers have been on about Miss Buckland doing abortions. She's got them all on at her because – '

'Abortions? There at Old East? Don't make me laugh!' Prue said and stared at her and her face now had a slight flush on it. 'That lot there are all mouths and trousers. Full of talk and no bleedin' help at all.'

'What do you mean?'

'What I say. I went to them, didn't I, when I got into this state again? Look at me – two of 'em, and this one only a few months – what do they expect me to do? But would they help me? Would they buggery! Sent me away, didn't they, the lousy pigs. That's why I'm in this state now – '

'But – ' Suba said and shook her head. 'I thought – I mean, Miss Buckland saved that baby. If she hadn't done that operation when you were bleeding so badly you'd have lost it and – '

'More's the pity I didn't,' Prue said harshly and hauled the infant up to set it against her shoulder and began to pat its back. 'It'd have sorted me out well enough, that would. But she had to go on and – oh, never mind. What can you understand? Kid like you.'

'I wanted you to help me,' Suba said and wanted to cry. 'I did so much want you to come to court and tell them how good she was to you, saved your baby, and how – '

'Did you know why I was bleeding?' Prue demanded and, as the baby burped loudly, lifted it down to her lap again and started bottle-feeding once more.

'I – no,' Suba said. 'I've only just started on that ward. I – I'm not all that up on gynae yet.'

'I tried to get rid of it,' she said. 'Paid a bloody fortune and tried to get rid of it. And what happened? The sods made a botch of it. That was why I was bleeding. They made a botch and I landed up in Old East as an emergency. And still bloody pregnant.'

'Oh!' Suba said. There seemed nothing else she could say.

'So don't you go asking me to – oh, shit!' And she lifted her head and stared over her shoulder at the kitchen door.

Suba lifted her head too and listened. Someone was coming in. There was a rattle of a key in the lock and then steps coming along the hall.

'Is that your husband?' Suba said. 'I don't want to be in the way or anything – perhaps I'd better – ' and she got to her feet.

'No,' Prue said in a dreary flat voice. 'Not my husband.'

The door to the kitchen was pushed open and Suba stared at the newcomer and the name shot into her mind unbidden. Ida Malone, the woman who had been in the next bed to Prue, and she smiled widely at the sight of her.

'Hello, Mrs Malone. How nice to see you!'

Ida stood there, her arms full of packages, and stared at her and then flicked her gaze over her head to Prue Roberts. 'What's she doing here?'

Prue shrugged. 'Ask me! Turned up on the step, didn't she? You ask her. Nothing to do with me.'

'She's not coming into that clinic, see?' Ida said pugnaciously and plopped her packages down on the kitchen table. 'And that's the end of it. She doesn't have to if she doesn't want to. She's having her baby in a private hospital. Yes. She's gone private.'

'That's nice,' Suba said after a long pause. 'Where?'

'None of your bloody business,' Ida Malone snapped and glared at her. 'What do you want here anyway? No one wants you.'

'I just wanted to ask Mrs Roberts to help me with something,' Suba said. 'That was all – '

'Well she's not helping no one with anything. So you just be off with you, all right?'

Suba frowned and looked at Prue. 'Well, really, I – '

'You'd better do what she says,' Prue said heavily and didn't look at Suba. 'It's easier really when you do. So long then.'

'You got a coat?' Ida Malone stood at the door, her hands shoved deep into her own coat pockets.

'In the bedroom,' Suba said and Ida Malone went marching off and they could hear her banging about in the next room.

'Please, Mrs Roberts,' Suba said in an urgent low voice. 'If you change your mind – it's just that – she's so good really and I know she'd help you if you needed her. If she *knew* you did. So if you can help her – '

'This it?' Ida stood at the door again, holding out Suba's coat.

'Yes.' Suba took it and put it on, looking over her shoulder at Prue.

'Well, on your way then,' Ida said and marched up the corridor to open the front door. And Suba had to follow her. But as she went Prue said suddenly, in a low voice, 'I go to the pub opposite the hospital sometimes. Evenings. Maybe I'll see you there.' And then very deliberately turned her back on her, and left her to go along the passageway and out, past the hard stare that Ida Malone fixed on her, but feeling rather less hopeless than she had expected she would.

Chapter Thirty-One

———————— ∞ ————————

'On bail,' Oliver said. 'Who'd ever have thought it?' And he laughed. But there wasn't much humour in the sound.

'Well, at least you're here at home,' Kate said. 'It would have been a great deal worse if you'd had to stay locked up until – well, until.'

'I suppose so. It's so bloody – oh, I don't know. Sleazy, I suppose. Cheap and nasty and – Out on bail – it makes it sound as though I'm a criminal. And it's not as though I'd ever been all that rebellious. When they marched and went on demos when I was at university, I stayed in hall and wrote polemics for the newspapers, for God's sake. Half my year were arrested at sit-ins, but I never reckoned that. And now look at me – '

'You'll get over it,' Kate said calmly. 'If it's only your pride that's hurt.'

'I hope that's all it is. I haven't talked to anyone at City yet. Maybe they'll prefer not to have a presenter who gets himself in trouble with the police. Perhaps they'll – '

'Darling,' Kate said and came round the lunch table to sit on the arm of his chair. 'Listen to me. You're a bit depressed. I don't mean just low – I mean clinically depressed. It's a normal response to a traumatic experience. You've every right to react this way. But please, in the middle of it all do try to hang on to your sense of proportion! The station get rid of you? Don't be silly. They – and you – can turn the whole thing to advantage if you think about it. "Our intrepid reporter, seeking the news as it happens to bring it to you, in fracas with brutal police . . ." Can't you just imagine it? Be kind to yourself, and stop digging away at it in your mind. It won't help and it'll just aggravate the depression.'

'Ah! I see. That's your considered medical advice, is it? Snap out of it? All is for the best in the best of all possible worlds? That sort of thing? Well, I hope it works for the rest of your patients. It doesn't do a great deal for me.'

She remained there beside him for a moment and then sighed softly and got to her feet and returned to her own chair and began to eat again. She'd made the best meal she could that would be full of taste but wouldn't demand a great deal of effort to eat, well aware of how painful his face was when he moved it; and it was good. But his plate sat untouched in front of him. She knew better than to urge him to eat of course, and also knew that making any response to his jibes now wouldn't help; but for all her quiet exterior she was as tense as a spring inside.

There was a long silence and then he leaned forwards and picked up his fork. 'Sorry, Kate,' he muttered and took a mouthful of the fish she had so carefully cooked and chewed it dispiritedly. 'I'm a miserable sod. You should have left me in hospital.'

'I saw no need once I found out you wouldn't have any trouble getting bail,' she said and smiled at him and he managed to make some sort of grimace back. 'And they needed the bed. Look, darling, let's spoil ourselves. I'll open a bottle of something expensive and we'll take it to bed. What say you?'

'Sex as bandage?' he said and went on eating, but with a little more interest now.

'Why not? We've tried it every other way,' she said lightly, and looked at him from under her lashes, shy suddenly. If he refused her, she suddenly realised, she'd take it very badly indeed.

'Oh, not yet,' he said and looked at her and now he grinned almost in his old way, though it made him wince a little as his scarred face moved over the bones. 'I've got masses of ideas still. This fish isn't half bad. Have you any more?'

'Masses.' She served him and then went and found the bottle of champagne someone had brought to a dinner party months ago and which they'd never got round to opening. 'I'll put this in the fridge,' she called. 'Could you manage some ice cream after that?'

'Try me.'

'Gladly.' And she brought the ice cream from the fridge and served that too, and now they ate in a companionable silence.

They shared a shower before getting into bed, and once they were there she massaged him with some of her most expensive body lotion till he complained he smelled like a brothel. But he enjoyed it and almost visibly relaxed under her touch. And then when they made love it was prolonged and satisfying for them both and they slept long into the afternoon until she was woken from a long complicated dream about aeroplanes and parachutes by the shrieking of the phone beside her bed.

She lay there blinking into the dimness of the bedroom before answering, trying to get herself together; it took a conscious effort to remember that this was late Saturday afternoon and that she was on call for the hospital. And she reached for the phone resignedly, thinking – At least they didn't ring before, when we were still –

'Yes?'

It wasn't the hospital. 'Miss Sayers? Is that Miss Kate Sayers?'

She didn't know why she was on the alert suddenly. 'Who is that?' she said guardedly as beside her Oliver turned over and reached across her body to bury his face in her back.

'Who is it?' he muttered. 'Send 'em away.'

'This is NTV – National Television. The *Probe* programme. Is Miss Sayers there, please?'

She didn't stop to think. 'Wrong number,' she muttered and slammed the phone down on its hook.

He was fully awake now as she turned back to him and he lifted his head from the pillow and peered at her in the half-light thrown from the curtained windows.

'Who was that?'

'A television company. Some programme – *Probe*, I think he said – '

'I've seen that,' he said slowly. 'Rather good – National do it I think – '

'Yes. He said it was National Television.'

'Had they got the wrong number?'

There was a long pause. Then she said, 'No.'

'I didn't think so.' He got out of bed and went padding over to draw the curtains and open the window. The room still smelled heavily of her scented body lotion, and he shivered slightly as the cool evening air hit his bare skin and came back to bed to slide under the duvet again.

'Why did you say wrong number instead of telling me they

wanted me? It's a bit over the top to protect me that much, don't you think?'

She turned her head and looked at him and managed a smile. 'Well, well, well. How's that for self-centred? It wasn't you they wanted.'

He frowned. 'It wasn't?'

'No, dear. It was Miss Kate Sayers they were after, believe it or not. The lady who lives here. The lady whose name is in the phone book at this address. In case you'd forgotten.' She got out of bed and went to the bathroom to shower again, and when she came back he was sitting up with both hands linked behind his head.

'Sorry, Kate, I deserved that. Christ, I seem to do nothing but apologise these days. Very comforting for the male ego, that is.'

'Nice for me though. I'm sorry too. I needn't have been quite so — I mean, I was startled as much as anything — '

'What did they want?'

'I didn't give them time to say,' she said and began to rub her hair with a towel because she'd washed it under the shower, needing to be cool. She always enjoyed letting her hair dry slowly, keeping her pleasantly damp while it did.

'Why didn't you ask?'

'Kim Hynes,' she said, towelling hard. 'It's sure to be about all that, isn't it? I've stopped looking at newspapers since it all started. It's the only way — but I suppose it's still going on, the fuss. That *Globe* piece you showed me said something about there being more the next day — '

'You realise that — ' he began and then the phone shrilled again and they both remained very still and stared at it. It was Oliver who leaned over and answered it.

'Yes,' he said and she shook her head violently at him, needing to remind him she didn't want to talk to anyone from television and he looked back at her, seeming not to notice and said, 'Who?'

'I'm not here — ' she hissed.

'BBC radio . . . Yes . . . Look, why do you want her?'

He listened and then lifted his brows at her. 'Me? Oh, I'm just one of the family. Quite entitled to ask why you want her. If you want me to pass on a message, you see, I'll have to know. Otherwise – '

He listened and then frowned sharply. 'I see,' he said at length. 'No, I didn't know about this. I doubt she does – Mm? . . . No, she isn't here at present. No, I really don't know. No I couldn't say. I'll let her know when she does get back though, that you called. Good evening.'

He cradled the phone and leaned back on his pillows, frowning. 'It isn't Kim Hynes,' he said. 'Though they mentioned that in passing. That was a radio news programme – they wanted you for tomorrow morning. It seems there's been a press release. All the Sundays have lead pieces, he said. Look, I'll get dressed. We'll go down to Fleet Street, see if the first editions are out yet – you can get the Sundays on Saturday night quite early – '

'Press release about what?' She followed him into the bathroom.

'Something to do with AIDS,' he shouted. He was in the shower now and it was splashing loudly. 'I didn't ask too many questions – thought it best not to. We'll get the papers, see what it's all about – '

She dressed slowly, pulling on jeans and a shirt, trying to think what sort of press release could involve her and what they might have got hold of, these Sunday papers. Had someone blurted out the tale of what had happened during Gerald Slattery's operation? Surely not. She couldn't bear the thought of that. But what else could it be?

By the time he emerged from the shower to dress she was sitting on the edge of the freshly made-up bed and waiting for him. Her hair was curling damply around her ears and he stood in the bathroom door looking at her, his body rather absurdly streaked with talcum powder and his injured cheek looking like a layer of paint against the rest of him, and managed a smile.

'You look about ten years old,' he said lightly. 'You make me feel like a child ravisher. Has anyone ever told you you're good in bed, Lolita?'

She made a face. 'Disgusting phrase,' she said lightly. 'I'm good out of it, too – '

He managed a grin. 'Not bad in cars, either. Hey, this bloody thing hurts more when it's wet. Stinging like the very devil – '

'I'll put some more cream on it,' she said. 'Get dressed and then I'll do it. You'll have it all over your collar otherwise – '

'Try not to worry, love,' he said as he stood dressed in jeans and shirt of his own so that they looked rather absurdly alike, and she applied the antibiotic cream to his cheek. 'I dare say it's all a drama out of nothing. Newspaper people – we're a rotten lot. I say we because we do it in radio too. Make a molehill out of a pimple and call it a mountain – '

'Try not to worry about being on bail,' she retorted. 'OK?'

He hugged her briefly. 'Touché,' he said. 'Come on. I'll drive.'

'You won't. You're not well enough.'

'Bollocks. I've got a scraped face, that's all. Perfectly fit to drive.'

'Like hell you are – '

Bickering amicably they went down to the car and she gave in and let him drive because it was clear he was determined. And he seemed so much happier now, so much more relaxed than he had over their lunch. And she thought – Was that the releasing effect of sex, or is it that he feels better and stronger now than I, the one with a problem, the one with something to be apprehensive about? And pushed the thought away as unjust. But it wouldn't stay pushed away and remained there hovering, as he chattered easily at her to distract all the way up to Fleet Street.

The papers were out, piled ready on a long stall at the foot of Bouverie Street, and he parked and went to get them.

'Stay here,' he said. 'No need to get out – ' And she obeyed, scared now, wanting to run away, not wanting to see what the papers had to say after all. She nearly called after him to tell him to come back, but he was already there, one hand in jeans pocket for change, collecting all the papers with his other hand. And then after he had paid for them he came loping back to the car and threw them in on her lap and got in.

'Let's go over to Joe Allen's,' he said. 'We can sit there and have a salad or something and go through them. Don't try to read them in the light in here. You'll get a headache – '

He's seen the headlines, she thought, and sat there and stared out at the swooping lights against the deep blue of the late summer sky and held the papers on her lap in both hands. And then, as the car turned and made its way along towards the

307

Aldwych, with Oliver peering out for a parking space, she let her gaze drop so that she could see them.

And the first one that screamed up at her was, 'Sex-Change Doctor in new AIDS Scandal', and a tide of cold began to rise from the pit of her belly towards her chest.

'We'll be all right here,' Oliver said and switched off the engine and made a move to get out. But she sat still, staring ahead. 'Are you coming?' he said.

'Have you seen this?' She bent her head to look again at the huge black letters.

'Yes,' he said after a moment. 'You can't really miss it, can you?'

'I don't want to go in the restaurant,' she said abruptly. 'There might be people we know – there's enough light here. Put on the inside light – '

Obediently he switched on the overhead light and put out his hand and she lifted her own so that he could help himself to the papers, and he took half of them and began to go through them. She just sat staring out of the window in front at the traffic swooping on its way to the Strand, reading the sign over the Adelphi Theatre blinking on and off at her and letting the silly tune from the show there run through her head. 'Me and my girl – meant for each other – meant for each other and liking it so – me and my girl – '

'Who is Goodman Lemon?' Oliver said at length.

'Mm? Goodman Lemon? A surgeon at Old East. General surgeon. Is this – ' She turned her head, almost feeling it creak as she did so, for she had been holding it so rigidly. 'Did he do this?'

'Yes. He says – ' He bent his head and peered at the paper. 'Shall I read it to you?'

'Please.'

' "In a statement to the Press Agency Platt, Mr Goodman Lemon said, 'A patient who was highly dangerous because of the risk of AIDS was admitted in need of a surgical procedure. I insisted naturally that he should have an AIDS test before I operated. He refused so I, of course, was forced to decline to operate. I could not put the staff of the operating theatre or his fellow patients at that sort of risk. Despite my concern and natural wish to protect the staff and patients of this hospital another of the surgeons did operate by interfering behind my back and without my consent and did so with so little skill that the man bled severely in the operating theatre and caused a major alarm. The surgeon in question was compelled to wash out the sheets and dressing towels, which were bloodsoaked, by herself, because the staff refused.' Later enquiries have proven that the surgeon is Miss Kate Sayers – " There's a picture here too. "Miss Sayers is at the heart of the sex-change operation scandal at the same hospital. She has been accused of blocking beds for essential surgery for other deserving patients with these sex-change operations that are so controversial – " '

'The bastards!' Kate said and sat there feeling the cold tide engulf not just her chest and belly, but her arms and legs as well. She was icy with fury. 'The lying – it wasn't like that! It was nothing like that! It was – Professor Levy asked me to operate because – the man was at risk, dammit! He could have strangulated. His name's Slattery, nice man, lived with a homosexual partner for seventeen years, never slept around in all that time, very low risk for HIV. But Lemon is a prejudiced bastard as well as a liar and he wouldn't operate and the man had a hernia that was threatening to strangulate. It can be a killer – So I said I'd do it – and the scrub nurse was nervous and there was that flap over Fay that day and his hand slipped and he pierced an artery with scissors. No real harm done – I found it and closed it and the man didn't even need much in the way of post-op blood. But I decided to wash the sheets and towels myself because – well, to do a belt-and-braces thing. I was damned sure the man wasn't HIV positive and I still am. But I wanted to take no chances with the staff – and they didn't even know there was a risk. I didn't tell them. Now, of course, they'll know and there'll be this crazy panic no doubt and all because of Lemon's awful – Oh, Oliver! How could they? And then saying I blocked beds with Hynes – I didn't. The waiting list has nothing to do with her case, nothing at all – '

'Hush, darling, hush,' he said and held her close and that was when she realised she was on the edge of hysteria, shouting it all at him and with tears in her eyes. And she took a deep breath and managed to control herself and said huskily, 'Are they all the same?'

'All the tabloids are, I think. Let me look at the heavies – '

He let her go, and then began to leaf through the layers of the broadsheet papers, throwing the unwanted sections over his shoulder until the back seat of the car was adrift, and found what he was looking for.

'They're a little less excited in tone,' he reported at last, but still reading. 'But the essence is the same. Clearly they published the Lemon man's statement in full, without querying it.' He frowned. 'Someone should have called you for a check, for God's sake. This is lousy journalism! It's all I expect of the cheap end of the trade, but these should have known better – '

He read on, crouched over the papers like a predatory cat over a newly caught bird and she leaned back against the headrest of her seat and took a series of deep breaths to compose herself. There was no sense in getting so angry that she became incoherent. She had to decide what to do and how to do it –

'We need a strategy here,' Oliver said, and she opened her eyes and turned her head to look at him. 'We can't let this man get away with this.'

'What can I do, then?'

He was silent for a long moment, still looking down at the papers and then said, 'You'll have to talk to them yourself. Television wants you for *Probe*, which is – when? – tomorrow night? Then you agree. And you also talk to the radio people who called tonight and – '

'But why should I play the game his way? Go crying to the press? What good will that do? Haven't I put up with enough this past few weeks over Kim? I've had to refuse to talk to all sorts of people over that business, and I still won't do it. If I go now to these TV and radio people and say I'll talk about Lemon's lies, won't they start on about Kim? And the fact is I don't want to talk about her – there's nothing I have to say about her that's relevant. Only she can talk to them because it's her affair, not mine – but what will that matter? I can't expect them to keep off Kim and let me talk only about Lemon, can I?'

'I think you have to decide how to handle that when it happens,' Oliver said firmly. 'Right now, believe me, Kate, the best answer is to agree to talk. On your own terms if possible, but if not – well, talk. I'll stay with you, advise you – ' He stopped then, suddenly rather embarrassed. 'If you want me to, that is.'

'Want you to? God, Oliver, I'm in such a state I don't know what to do! Of course I want you to help – why shouldn't I?'

'I've not been behaving all that well this past few days – ' he mumbled. 'Been a bit wrapped up in my own problems – '

She touched his damaged cheek gently, just above the line of injury. 'You're entitled. Look, don't go getting all sensitive on me now, for God's sake. I couldn't handle that. Help me please to do the best thing. You're the expert on papers and so forth. I'll do it your way – but I won't talk about Kim – '

'Well,' he said pacifically. 'We'll see about that. But right now, come on.'

'Where are we going?' For he had turned the key in the ignition and was putting the car into gear.

'City Radio,' he said briefly. 'We'll start with my own station and then get in touch with the *Probe* programme and the rest of 'em from there. Fasten your seat belt, love. One way and another you're going to need it.'

Chapter Thirty-Two

The pub was warm and smoky and very noisy, and Suba sat in a corner seat trying to look as though she liked being there. It had been a brave and alarming expedition for her, she who had always been told by her father that decent girls never ever went into pubs; just walking through the engraved-glass embellished door had been terrifying. But then having to go up to the bar to buy lemonade — because she didn't think they'd let her just sit down and wait in the corner unless she had something in a glass in front of her — and then carrying it over to her seat had been a tremendous effort; by the time she had got there her legs had been shaking. And it was silly really, because no one had paid her the least attention. The girl behind the bar had not looked at her as she sold her the lemonade and the people standing around and shouting cheerfully at each other through the fug barely moved when she had murmured, 'Excuse me,' at them as she wriggled her way through.

Now, half an hour after arriving here and with only an inch or two of lemonade left at the bottom of her glass, she no longer felt shaky, but she did feel miserable. It had all been for nothing, after all. Clearly Prue's murmured invitation to meet her here hadn't been an invitation at all. She had imagined it; had allowed her hopefulness to overcome her common sense. And really, why should Prue help her? It was as she had said — and Suba saw no reason to doubt that it was — that she hadn't wanted to keep the baby anyway; the last thing she'd want to do would be to help Miss Buckland. Suba would have to find another way to clear her conscience over what she had done, and she bent her head now and stared down into the flat lemonade and felt her eyes get hot as she tried to think of a way, and knew there wasn't one. It hadn't even been sure that Prue could have helped, even if she'd agreed to try. It was all a mess, a dreadful mess and the sooner Suba left Old East and got right away from all the trouble she'd made the better —

'Look at you,' a voice said above her head. 'Lost a quid and found a farthing, did you? You're supposed to have fun in here, not sit looking like the dead end of a wet bank holiday.'

Suba lifted her head and tried to smile, but couldn't. Sian Bevan, oh, not Sian, with her sharp face and her bitter tongue. She could cope with anyone but Sian tonight.

'Hello,' she said.

'That's right. Be glad to see me.' Sian plumped herself down beside her and shoved at her with her hard little rump to move over. 'Make me welcome. Or are you waiting for someone else?'

'Sort of. Not really,' Suba said and reddened.

'Hey, get you! Miss Muffett with a date? Whatever next?' Sian was staring at her with those hard round boot-button eyes that always made Suba feel so uncomfortable and then she grinned and didn't look so fierce. 'Don't mind me, ducky. My bark's a bloody sight worse than my bite, you know. I'll go then, in case he comes – '

'No, it's all right,' Suba said, mortified with the shame of seeming unfriendly. 'And anyway it isn't he, it's she.'

'Oh, well then!' Sian said and plumped herself down again. 'If it's a bread-and-bread date, it might as well be bread and bread and a bready filling too. At least until my chap turns up.' She grinned then. 'I'll have to see if he's got a mate for you, Suba, eh?' She glittered a little in the soft smoky light and, looking at her, Suba thought – She's quite pretty really. I never thought so before. Looks excited and well, pretty –

'No, I wouldn't like that at all,' she said earnestly. 'I really wouldn't. But it's kind of you – '

'You a dyke then?' Sian said, conversationally. 'That why you're waiting for a she and not a he?'

'A what?' Suba looked at her blankly.

Sian laughed and shook her head. 'Never mind, ducks. If you don't know, who am I to spoil your innocent young mind? Don't you like chaps?'

Suba made a little face. 'I've no time at present. And anyway, my father . . .' Her voice drifted away.

'Oh. I suppose so!' Sian peered at her interestedly. 'You people have arranged marriages, don't you?'

'Not all of us,' Suba said, pushing down the irritation that

313

such questions always created in her. 'And it isn't that at all. It's just that he says education comes first. I had enough trouble getting him to let me come here instead of college. If I start having boyfriends, that'll really upset him – I've got time.'

'Of course you have,' Sian said, suddenly kind, and it was as though she was filled with so much contentment that it bubbled over to take in Suba too. 'Don't let me tease you, ducks. Here, what's that you've got there? Have another.'

'Lemonade,' Suba said. 'And really I've had enough – I'd better go, I suppose. There's no sense in staying any longer. She's not coming – '

'Someone from the hospital?' Sian said.

Suba stared at her and for one mad moment thought of telling Sian all about it, explaining all that had happened, and about her plan with Prue, asking her to help salve her conscience over Fay Buckland and then, even as the thought came to her, pushed it away. That would be crazy; however nice Sian might be at the moment no one knew better than Suba how sharply she could change, become jeering and unkind again. She'd heard her do it to the other people in the canteen; she couldn't risk it. And yet it would be such a comfort to share the whole wretched affair with someone, to unload it all on to another pair of shoulders, if only for a little while.

'No,' she said. 'It's not important really,' and almost got to her feet. And then stopped, because Prue was there, suddenly, standing in front of her and staring down.

'So you came then,' she said and Suba continued to stare at her wordlessly.

'Well, there you are then,' Sian said cheerfully. 'Here's your friend all right and tight! You won't mind if I stay a bit longer, though, will you? There's nowhere else to sit down and my feet are killing me – ' And indeed the pub had filled up considerably now. 'I'll go as soon as my chap gets here – he won't be long. Here, I'll wriggle over – '

And she did, and Prue sat down.

There was an awkward silence and then Sian said brightly, 'Well, shall I get them in, then? Here, what do you want?'

'I'll have an orange juice,' Prue said.

'Suba?'

314

'Mm? Oh, nothing, thanks.'

'Well, you're a cheap round and no mistake. Suits me. I'll be back – keep my seat safe from these marauders, mind – ' And she was away, pushing herself loudly but amiably through the crowd towards the bar.

'Who's she?' Prue said.

'One of the other nurses from the hospital,' Suba said.

'Is she in on this as well?'

'Mm? Oh, no. She just happened to be here – waiting for her friend, you see. I couldn't just tell her to go away, could I?'

'Why not?'

'Well, you can't – ' Suba said and then stopped, a little nonplussed.

'I do,' Prue said savagely. 'If I want people to go away I tell 'em – ' She stopped then. 'If I can. You can't always though, can you?'

'No,' Suba said. 'I couldn't – '

'But you could do it for someone else?'

'What?'

'Do it for someone else.' Prue sounded impatient. 'There's no good me being here if you can't.'

'I – well, I suppose so,' Suba said and then brightened. 'I think I could always do things for patients I couldn't do for myself.'

'Well, that's all right then,' Prue said and looked across towards the bar to see if Sian was coming back. 'Does she know about it all?'

'About what?' Suba was suddenly guarded. 'You mean about you?'

'About this business you said you wanted me to do – about this Miss Buckland and her trouble.'

'Everyone does,' Suba said. 'It's been in all the papers.'

'What? That she did abortions?'

'Yes.'

'Well, there's no news in that.' Prue sounded tired, and looking at her drawn face and puffy eyes Suba thought – She's not well. Not at all well. 'Lots of people have 'em done. Only they wouldn't do me when I asked 'em.'

'I know,' Suba said. 'But it wasn't Miss Buckland, was it? The

315

doctor you saw – was it in Outpatients? Or Accident and Emergency? It wouldn't have been Miss Buckland who said no?'

'No,' Prue admitted. 'It wasn't her. I went into A and E and saw this snotty kid, thought he was bloody God Almighty, he did. Sent me off like I was some sort of begger – '

'Miss Buckland wouldn't have done that,' Suba said and leaned earnestly towards her. 'Honestly she wouldn't. She's ever so nice. She'd have helped you. She did. I mean when you were so ill, she helped you. Did she know when you came in you didn't want the baby?'

Prue shrugged. 'How do I know? I never talked to her before she done me. I was too poorly. I'd have thought she could have worked it out, though. You don't go and get into that sort of mess if you want to keep a baby, do you?' And suddenly her face crumpled and tears began to run down her cheeks.

Once again Suba was overcome with confusion and was dreadfully aware of all the other people standing around, afraid they would see Prue's tears, afraid they would think she was to blame for them, afraid just to be there, and she leaned forwards to pat Prue's hand rather helplessly, not knowing what to do.

'Oh, Gawd, leave you for a minute and what do you get up to?' Sian's voice above her filled her with a giddy sense of relief and she looked up at her eagerly.

'She's a bit upset,' she murmured as Sian wriggled back into her seat. 'I don't know what to – '

Prue was crying hard now, sitting there with her head down and making no effort to disguise her state, with the tears running down her face, her mouth drawn back into an ugly rictus, and her shoulders heaving. Sian leaned forwards and, using the scarf that Prue had round her neck, mopped at her face, and after a while she seemed to be a little less agitated and even accepted gratefully the glass of orange juice which Sian pushed into her hand, and began to sip it.

'Thank God Jimmy's late,' Sian said and then looked from one to the other of them. 'Well, you two really are the – look at you both! You'd think the bleeding cat had died. What is the matter, for Christ's sake?'

Suba had no idea why it happened, or whether she had intended it to. All she knew was that suddenly her mouth was open and words were pouring out of it. She was telling Sian all about it, about the way Shirley had taken her to the meetings, about her own worries about what was happening in the Gynae ward, about showing them the charts from Miss Buckland's patient, the lot; and Sian sat and stared at her with her round boot-button eyes and said nothing.

'And then I thought, if Prue said to them how glad she was that Miss Buckland had saved her baby, then it would help and maybe . . .' Her voice trailed away then and she looked uneasily at Prue. 'The trouble is, I'm not sure Prue is glad.'

'So I see,' Sian said dryly, and then leaned forwards again and pulled the scarf from round Prue's neck and pushed it into her other hand. 'Do mop up, love, there's a good girl. You'll get chapped if you don't.' And Prue, to Suba's amazement, managed a watery grin and did as she was told.

I'll never manage to be any good as a nurse, she thought then with sudden cold certainty. It isn't enough to be nice to them and to care about them and to mean well. You have to be a bit hard and tough and make them know that you are, and then they feel safe with you. I couldn't have made Prue laugh, not for anything. But Sian did –

But I'm not going away, for all that, another part of her mind retorted. I'm not giving up. Why should I? Maybe I can't make them smile when they're crying but I do care about them and I can make it better for them. I will. I know I will –

'Why did you come here then, Prue?' Sian said. 'I mean, if it's like Suba said and she asked you to help her and you don't want to help on account of you didn't want the pregnancy anyway – why did you come?'

And again Suba felt despair trickle into her. That was what she had wanted to know too, but she hadn't been able to ask Prue directly; yet Sian, just arrived, knowing nothing about it all, had managed to sort it all out in her mind so quickly. Oh, I wish I were like Sian, Suba thought. If only I were like Sian.

Prue sat silent for a moment and then slid her eyes sideways to look at Suba. 'You saw that woman that was there? At my place?' she said and her voice was so quiet that they both had to lean closer to hear her. But it was at Suba she was looking and

317

clearly Suba she wanted to speak to. And Suba began to feel better.

'Ida Malone? Yes, I saw her.'

'It's all her fault, the lot of it.'

'What is?'

'All of it.' Prue's mouth set in a stubborn line, but her lower lip trembled. 'She won't leave me alone. I said I'd do it, but I'm not sure – but she never bloody leaves me *alone*! Nearly caught me tonight, she did. Only I took the kids over to my friend in George Bernard Shaw House and I saw her turn up down in the yard and hid a bit and then left the kids and come out the other way. She'll be that mad tomorrow that I wasn't there, but I don't care, it's the only way I can do it – you know, get away from her for a bit, hide from her. But she'll still make me do it.'

'Do what?' Sian said bluntly. 'You'll have to explain better than that, ducks. My chap'll be here in a minute and I'll have to go. So get on with it – '

Prue took a deep breath. 'It's all that she can't have kids, see. She was in for that – '

'That's right,' Suba remembered. 'Sub-fertility. Been trying for years – they were assessing test-tube possibilities, weren't they, for her?'

'That's right. Only she's no good for that. Too old.' Prue suddenly looked better, pleased with herself. 'Dried-up old hen, that's what she is. The bitch – I hate her.'

'Then give her the push,' Sian said cheerfully. 'You don't have to see a woman you don't like, for God's sake. And what has she got to do with – '

'I'm telling you!' Prue said, sharper now, seeming rejuvenated in some way now she had put her feelings about Ida Malone into words. 'She said to me, when we was in the ward, if she paid for everything, and she'd send me private, the best of everything, and looked after me now, and bought things for the kids, she'd have the baby for me – '

'Eh?' Sian was staring at her, her eyes wide. 'What do you mean, have the – take it from you? Christ, are you talking about some mad sort of transplant? It's amazing what they can do, I know, but this really is bloody mad – '

'Don't be daft.' Prue actually managed to giggle. 'Of course not. I just mean that she'd take the baby after it was born and say it was hers, and no one'd ever know, and I'd not have to let on to Gary and – well, it'd be all right. She paid back what I owed Jerry, and all – so I said all right in the end – '

Sian waved aside these references to people she knew nothing about and went, with the same unerring certainty that had already made Suba feel so inadequate, to the core of the situation.

'She said she'd buy your baby from you?'

There was a little silence and then Prue said, 'I suppose so. I never thought of it that way, but I suppose so.'

'Well, I'm buggered,' Sian said and then was silent.

It was Suba who spoke first. 'Do you want her to do that?'

'No,' Prue said and her voice was almost a whisper. 'I don't. And I can't tell her. She's – she's funny, you know. She'd kill me, I think. She's that – she's a bit mad, I think. She'd kill me or something, I know she would. I'm scared of her.' She lifted her head then. 'That was why I said I'd come and see you. I might help you, see, do what you want, if you help me with her.'

'What do you want me to do?'

'Tell her she's got to go and leave me alone. Tell her she can't have the baby – I don't know what I'll do but I'll manage somehow. Gary'll just have to come back from his bloody Saudi Arabia, money or no money. I'll manage. Only you'll have to get rid of her – '

'I – ' Suba stopped and swallowed, remembering Ida Malone's face and the hardness of her voice. Just imagining speaking to her, telling her directly to go away and stop bothering Prue, filled her with so much fear that she felt her hands dampen with sweat. But she swallowed again and nodded her head firmly.

'Yes,' she said. 'I'll tell her.'

'Will you really?' Prue looked pathetically grateful. 'Oh, it'd make it so much better for me then. I'd feel better, I know I would. I'd stop being sick and everything. I know I would if only she stopped coming.'

'I'll tell her,' Suba said, feeling better by the moment as she basked in Prue's approval. She hadn't looked at Sian like that.

'What about the money?' Prue said then and Suba blinked.

'What money?'

'She's spent a lot on me,' Prue said simply. 'The bills like, and the food she brings. And the booking at the hospital – they made her pay in advance. A lot too. It's one of these private places where you have to pay when you book. She told me it's cost her over fifteen hundred quid already and there's still a lot to fork out for, but she doesn't mind because it's worth it to her. But she won't go now if she doesn't get her fifteen hundred back, will she? What'll you do about that?'

'Fifteen hundred quid?' Sian said, and her voice sounded strident after the low tones that Prue and Suba had been exchanging. 'Christ, she was getting a baby cheap, wasn't she? The bitch – how can anyone be so – it's beyond me. Don't you worry, Prue. She can't get away with that – '

'If she doesn't get her money back she will,' Prue said. 'You don't know her. You do, don't you?'

And she looked at Suba again, but there was none of the engaging trustfulness that had been there before and which had made Suba feel so good. Now she looked wary and angry.

'Listen, if you want me to talk up for your Miss Buckland you've got to get rid of Ida Malone, and I'll tell you right now it won't be easy unless you find the money to give her back. I've not got it and can't get it. So, there you are – '

Now it was Suba who wanted to sit with tears running down her cheeks. But she didn't. She just sat with her hands folded in her lap, staring down at them and feeling sick. Miss Buckland was going to go to prison or something and all on her account and there was nothing she could do to help her.

'Glory be, he's here,' Sian said suddenly. 'I thought he'd never make it. Listen, don't you get yourselves in such a tangle, you two. You needn't worry – my chap'll know what to do.' And her eyes were blazing with excitement as she looked at the figure pushing its way through the crowd. 'Here, Jimmy, come and say hello to these two. This is Jimmy Rhoda, my boyfriend. He's on the *Globe*, you know.'

320

Chapter Thirty-Three

This must be what patients feel like when they come into Old East for the first time, Kate thought: all this mysterious rushing round and people speaking a language that is incomprehensible – though I know they're speaking English because I recognise some of the words – and the self-absorbed excitement of the people who work here, all apparently custom-designed to make me, the outsider, feel useless and stupid and supernumerary. And then she shook herself mentally and told herself sternly – Don't be such a wimp. You don't have to feel stupid simply because you're in a strange milieu. They need you here; you're important to them and their damned programme and don't you forget it.

But it didn't really work. She still sat stiffly in the uncomfortable leather chair in the corner of the room full of chattering people and coffee cups and glasses of sour white wine and curly-edged sandwiches, as bejeaned young men with clipboards and tangle-headed girls in layers of ethnic cotton and with earphones slung importantly around their necks posed and shouted at each other for the benefit of onlookers like herself. She tried to ignore them and looked around for Oliver but he was still locked in close colloquy with a man who had pounced on him with loud cries of greeting as he had come into the hospitality room with her. They had worked together, it seemed, long ago and now appeared to be utterly absorbed in sharing memories of those days, and Kate felt a sharp bite of anger as she watched them.

Oliver was supposed to be looking after her, dammit; it had been his idea to bring her here to do this damned programme. Why wasn't he at her side making sure she was comfortable about it all? It was all right for him, radio man that he was; he was used to this sort of atmosphere. Why couldn't he realise how badly she needed him? For two pins, she thought wrathfully, I'll get up and walk out and then where would they all be?

But then the two of them came over to her and Oliver introduced her to his companion as the producer of the programme, who with crinkle-eyed charm assured her that he was immensely grateful to her for giving up her precious time to come and help with the programme and shook her hand, holding it with two of his, and Kate thought – I hate people who do that, it's so bloody phoney and American; and her moment of juvenile chauvinism made her feel illogically better. Dismiss the man as a smoothie, a practised chatter-upper and she need not take him seriously.

'I can't tell you what pleasure it is to see old Merrall here again,' the producer was saying. 'We were all lads together back in the bad old days at the Beeb, you know – they called us the three stooges, Oliver and Jimmy Rhoda and me. And we *were*, so green and wet we were amazing. I've every hope of luring him back here to make up the old team again – a duo at least if not a triumvirate as of yore – ' And now he crinkled at Oliver and Kate thought disgustedly – Surely Oliver doesn't take this idiot seriously? But Oliver was grinning at the man with what seemed to Kate to be maudlin soppiness and she threw him a sharp glance and said, 'Really? I'm sure that will be very agreeable for you both.'

'Might even take old Rhoda on too,' the man said, apparently unaware of the edge in her voice. 'He's coming tonight, you know, Oliver – a last-minute add-on to the debate – '

Kate's brows snapped down. 'What's that? I understood that the people taking part in this were Lemon and myself.'

'Indeed, when we first arranged this with you on Saturday that was the plan – it was all we had at the time. But television programmes are organic things, you know. They grow by what they're fed on. And change of course by what they lose. Lemon has refused to come on now. Called this afternoon. Says it is not necessary, would you believe – '

'Not – ' Kate opened her eyes wide. 'Then I imagine it isn't necessary for me to be here either. Oliver? You said the point of this exercise was to refute the things that Lemon said. If he isn't here to say them – '

'We have his press release,' the producer said. 'He gave an interview to the Platt Agency, remember, and that's on the record – so we're using that. We've had time to make up cap gens to show his comments one by one – and – '

322

'Cap gens?'

'I'm sorry – dreadful the way we all use jargon, isn't it? Almost as bad as you doctors. I mean, I put up the things he said as captions on the screen, and have a voiceover read them. Then you can answer them one by one. It'll suit you better, my dear, I do assure you. It means you get the last word, you see. He's the fool for refusing to come on the programme. There's every likelihood that doing it this way you'll emerge whiter than white – '

'I'm not interested in any sort of – of exculpation drama,' Kate said angrily. 'I've got nothing to be ashamed of and no need to be painted whiter than white. I'm a responsible consultant and do what I do because – '

'My dear Kate, I know that! You don't mind my calling you Kate, I hope? We're all informal here – so much pleasanter, don't you agree? – '

She didn't, but she couldn't say so without sounding childish and churlish.

' – but I do think it will help you not to have Lemon here. By refusing to take part he does rather condemn himself out of his own mouth, you know. You agree, I know, Oliver – '

'Yes,' Oliver said quickly and reached out one hand to take Kate's elbow. 'You're in safe hands, Kate, I promise you. This isn't a programme where there's any submerged hostility, believe me. I've been involved with a few of those. Everyone falls over backwards to be scrupulously fair to the protagonists but if that same everyone has taken against one of them there's no question but it makes a hell of a difference to the outcome. They're pitching here for you. This'll stop all the fuss, I do promise you, Kate. Just you wait and see.'

'Why is that man Rhoda going to be on the programme?' Kate demanded, still not mollified.

'Because of this morning's piece in the *Globe*, of course.' The producer opened his eyes wide and gazed at her limpidly. 'You saw it of course.'

'Of course I did not,' Kate snapped. 'I've better things to do with my time than read rags like that.'

'A pity,' he murmured. 'It would have been an idea to see it. I'll – er – I'll see if I can find a copy somewhere – ' And he drifted away with a last slap on Oliver's shoulder and vanished into the crowd, now thicker than ever.

'Ye gods, what a repellent man,' Kate exploded and Oliver lifted his brows.

'Not at all. He's a very decent man. If you knew as many television people as I do, you'd be on your knees praying thankfully because you'd got him doing this programme. A very good chap – and he controls J.J. very well indeed – '

'J.J.? Oh, the one who – yes, I've seen him do this programme. Seems rather a smooth type – '

'Oh he is. Bit long in the tooth now – been doing this programme for ever – but he knows what he's doing. And he can be very tough. But with this producer in the gallery you'll be in safe hands, and never you doubt it – '

'What's this about your friend Rhoda being on the programme? I didn't count on that – he's the ass who made such a drama over Kim Hynes, isn't he? Started all the hubbub in the first place – '

'Kate, you're not being entirely fair, are you? I know you dislike him, but that doesn't justify misrepresenting him. He didn't start it. Kim Hynes started it herself, as you well know. We've talked about this. She sold her story for a fat fee. It's no good getting annoyed with Jimmy over that – '

'Oh, I suppose not – ' Kate sat down again with a little thump, tired suddenly. 'Oh, hell, I wish I'd never agreed to this. Better to be dignified surely and say nothing when people attack you. *Qui s'excuse s'accuse* and all that – '

'Piffle,' Oliver said shortly. 'Goodman slandered you, dammit! You don't sit down under that. You could sue him, for God's sake. You've got justification!'

'No way!' Kate was very emphatic. 'The last thing I do is go to law. That just drags it on and on – '

'Fair enough. A reasonable decision. But the last thing you do after *that* last thing is let the man get away with it. You've got every chance of putting the record straight tonight and that will be the end of Lemon and his bile. That's why you're doing this programme and getting irritable with me is no help at all.'

'I put the record straight this morning,' Kate said sulkily, aware at a deep level that he was right, of course. 'That radio programme.'

'That reached about two million people at a time when they were concentrating more on their cornflakes and marmalade than they were on what you had to say. *Probe* reaches something like eleven million and it's an audience that is sitting on its sofas and really listening – or mostly listening. This is the one that matters, my love, and the one that'll stop all the fuss for good and all. I hope – '

'Make-up, Miss Sayers. *Would* you be so kind?' One of the ethnic cotton brigade was bobbing about in front of her and after a moment Kate got to her feet.

'I don't wear a great deal,' she said suspiciously. 'Won't I do as I am?'

'I'm sure you will,' the girl said soothingly. 'We just like to check – for the lights, you know – if you'll just come along. The other one isn't here yet – ' She looked down at her clipboard, fussing a little, and then smiled brilliantly at Kate. 'Not to worry. That means the girls will be able to concentrate on you – if you'll just follow me – '

Kate did, and said as they reached the corridor outside and began walking towards the lift, 'The other one? Which other one is that? Mr Rhoda? I gather he's taking part as well, though I don't know why – '

'I really can't say,' the girl said vaguely, peering down at her clipboard. 'There are various people due in make-up it seems – ' And she smiled brilliantly again over her shoulder and led the way into the lift apparently very casually, but Kate noticed how she now carried her clipboard firmly held against her so that there was no chance of Kate looking over her shoulder to see what was written there; and a little worm of anxiety wriggled in her belly.

Who else was to be in this wretched programme? Who else had they arranged to set against her? But once more she managed that mental shake. This was paranoid thinking. Oliver had said the people here were on her side, that there was no unspoken hostility at work; why not believe him? He may have seemed to her to be overly captivated by his encounter with his old colleague – and Kate had to admit that much of her reaction had

325

been due to her own sense of insecurity in an alien atmosphere — but there could be no doubt that he was concerned to protect and help her. And he had been quite adamant that taking part in this programme was the right thing to do, and her own common sense told her the same. The trouble is, she thought gloomily as they arrived in the large, over-bright, lavishly mirrored and scented domain that was the make-up department, the trouble is I'm terrified. It makes me think stupidly and behave worse, being so frightened. And she swallowed, feeling the lump in her throat and the cold sick dullness in her chest, and tried to think dispassionately of the adrenalin levels in her blood as the cause of such nasty sensations as well as of the damp hands and shaky knees of which she was so aware. Perhaps applying a little medical academic thought would help bring the levels down — but it didn't and she allowed the girl in the pink overall to settle her in a high chair and drape her with a matching pink cape with what insouciance she could muster.

She had to admit that she quite liked what the girl did with her eyeshadow and mascara and blushers and by the time she had finished was feeling a little better; less jellified and rather more poised. She looked good in the new dark red wool dress she had chosen to wear, and knowing that helped a good deal. And unobtrusively she tightened the belt and smoothed the fabric of the skirt over her hips. She'd show them, that she would; and there was no need to be so agitated after all: this was just an unimportant episode in her life. Tomorrow she had her usual lists to do, with a couple of prostates needing TURs and a nephrectomy as well as a couple of papillomatous bladders to tidy up; *that* was what mattered.

And then she frowned, remembering that there should have been Kim Hynes' wound toilet to do as well. She had planned to get that out of the way and Kim discharged the following day, but Esther had told her this morning that Kim had suddenly asked to be discharged on the previous afternoon and had signed herself out, promising Esther she'd be back to the clinic on Wednesday and would talk to darling Miss Sayers then about the next stage of her treatment.

'But she said she had to go and there was an end of it — had the chance to earn some money, I gather,' Esther had told her. 'And what could I say? She's been a bit happier since she arranged to get all that cash from that damned newspaper – maybe they're taking her off to earn some of it somewhere.' And she'd sniffed and sent Kate off on her day's rounds and said no more about Kim, clearly glad to have her bed released.

Now, standing in National Television's make-up department Kate's brows tightened again as she thought – Could it be? They couldn't possibly be bringing her here as well, could they? And she remembered the producer's vagueness when she had asked why Jimmy Rhoda was on the programme, and the clipboard girl's evasiveness over the 'other one' expected in make-up and suddenly she knew she had been set up. They were bringing Kim on as well as herself, and that was the last thing she wanted; and she felt her face redden angrily as she looked around for someone to complain to, someone to check with, who could sort the whole thing out.

'I've got to talk to someone about this programme,' she said abruptly to the make-up girl who smiled sweetly at her and said, 'Of course. I'll get someone to take you down to the studio. They're all there now and ready for you. You'll be able to see anyone you like there – '

'Right,' Kate said and turned on her heel to follow the messenger the make-up girl had beckoned and, ignoring the silly chatter she produced, marched behind her to the lift and then on into the big studio.

It was disconcerting at first, because the girl led her behind tall walls of canvas, over snaking cables which were surmounted in places with orange plastic bridges to form walkways, and she had to concentrate to avoid stumbling in the dimness. From behind the canvas wall, which was brightly lit on the far side, she could hear the rustle and chatter of a sizeable number of people and she thought suddenly – They do this programme in front of an audience. I'd forgotten that. And all at once a renewed adrenalin surge caught her in the middle so sharply that she gasped. Her pulses began to thump thickly in her ears and she felt a little dizzy and had to stop.

The girl looked back anxiously and hissed, 'Are you all right?'

'Yes,' Kate managed. 'It's just a bit dark here.' And after a moment managed to go on walking as though nothing had happened. But now she had stopped worrying about who else was to be on the programme with her; all she could think about was the fact that she had to walk out in front of a live audience and talk; and the idea of it dried her mouth and made her tongue feel like a piece of very thick and very unwieldy leather.

There was a sudden shout of laughter from the crowd on the other side of the canvas, in response to a blurred comment made by a heavily amplified voice, just as she reached the end of it and found her leader standing poised beside a large swathe of dark curtain.

'Look,' Kate hissed at her. 'I really do have to speak to someone about this – could you ask the producer please if I could have a word? I can't remember his name – '

'Angus McSorley,' the girl whispered. 'He's up in the gallery now – hold on a moment – Ah – now!' And she lifted the curtain just as Kate heard her name called out in that same hoarsely amplified voice, and she was pushed forwards and found herself standing in a big space staring foolishly around.

It took a moment or two to take in what she was seeing, for there was a steep series of seats built on rostra lifting high above her on her right and occupied by a large number of grinning faces; and she remembered suddenly, absurdly, the wall-of-death lecture theatre of her student days, as everyone had called it, because from the well of the room looking up at the students, the lecturers said, that was exactly what it looked like.

On the left was a sight that was both alien and familiar and she struggled with it for a moment; staring at the tall canvas walls and the desks and chairs in front of them, all in shades of rich yellows and fawns and brilliantly lit, and above them on the canvas wall below the abrupt edging of it – for it stopped short of the dark ceiling by several feet – where the word 'Probe' was written in a huge flowing script. Overhead there were banks of lights and ominous brooding unlit lamps, and in front of her, a microphone in one hand and with the other crooked into a beckoning posture towards her, was a man she had never met yet knew as well as she knew her own face in the mirror. And she walked towards him obediently, thinking – Gerrard. This is J. J. Gerrard. And then thought – perhaps I can ask him –

But it was impossible to say anything, for he smiled at her

widely, his teeth glinting enamel white in an obviously painted face, and then turned to the audience and with the microphone held close to his face bawled, 'Miss Kate Sayers, ladies and gentlemen. A splendid hard-working doctor who will, I am sure, defend her reputation here tonight. If you would just sit over there, Miss Sayers' – at which someone behind her took her elbow and began to urge her away towards the desks sitting there in their brilliant pools of light inside the canvas walls – 'we'll get ourselves together! After the break, ladies and gentlemen, we'll have another important medical story to bring you from this very same hospital – tonight, believe me, the doctors are under the microscope! Now, we have just a few seconds to go – so, settle down, studio, and all of you – be *interested*, be *involved* and don't be afraid to ask your questions and make your comments! Just watch for the girls with the roving mikes and our eleven million viewers will be out there watching for *you* and listening to *you*. Because you and only *you* are the show. You are *Probe*, ladies and gentlemen and I am J. J. Gerrard here to help you make the most of *your* programme! Over to you!' And he tossed the microphone he held to a waiting bejeaned and earphoned acolyte and ran with carefully lissom youthful energy up the steps that led to the set where Kate, unable to resist the directions of the man who had taken her elbow, sat waiting for him, sick with fright and still not knowing who else was to be on the programme with her.

Chapter Thirty-Four

At first it was as though she wasn't there at all. She knew her body was there, sitting in a singularly uncomfortable chair that hurt her back, and being bathed in light that made her face bead with sweat and sent trickles down between her breasts, but the real Kate, the person she actually knew as herself, was somewhere quite else, standing to one side and watching dispassionately what was happening. That Kate was scornful and amused as she watched the body of Kate sitting there so stiffly with her back hurting. She was jeering too, and Kate in the chair heard her and was angry.

'It's your own fault, of course,' the watching Kate whispered inside the listening Kate's head. 'You should have walked out when they pushed you into that damned chair. You should stand up now and tell them what they can do with their ridiculous TV programme. You should get up, walk out now, and leave them all looking as stupid as they're making you feel – '

And for one minute fraction of a moment the Kate in the chair felt her thigh muscles tighten and her body lean forwards ready to get to her feet and walk out, so as to stop the watching Kate's jeers; they would meet, the two of them, somewhere out of the pitiless gaze that now glittered so hatefully in her eyes and would merge and become a whole person again –

'That then, ladies and gentlemen,' J. J. Gerrard was saying, 'is the nub of the matter as it stands. We asked Miss Sayers' accuser to come on the programme and face her directly but for reasons best known to himself he refused. But we do have the statement he issued through a Press agency so we can offer his comments one by one and give Miss Sayers the chance to deal with them. Now, Miss Sayers – '

The watching Kate slid into the bright lights and moved into the sitting Kate who stared at the silly painted man as he gazed at her, a whole person again at last, a frightened person, but also an angry one. Who the hell did he think he was to set her up in this fashion and throw his questions at her? He had no jurisdiction over her, no right to pillory her in this manner. And the anger seemed to stiffen her back and take away the pain there and it dried the sweat on her body and she lifted her head and looked coolly back at him.

'Yes, Mr Gerrard?' she heard herself saying and was delighted with the steadiness of her tone.

'Let us start with the first statement Mr Lemon made to the Press agency.' He turned his head and looked above and beyond, and Kate followed the line of his gaze and saw a big screen and huge words that appeared on it. *A patient who was highly dangerous because of the risk of AIDS was admitted in need of surgical procedure.*

'I think we can take that as accurate, Miss Sayers?' Gerrard asked, and Kate flicked her eyes down to look at him again. 'This is the basis of Mr Lemon's complaint so of course we must assume that – '

'Then you assume wrongly,' Kate said crisply. 'The patient who was admitted in need of a surgical procedure and to whom Mr Lemon was referring was by no means "highly dangerous" because of the risk of AIDS.'

J. J. Gerrard opened his eyes more widely and Kate thought briefly – Is he acting? Does he know what I'm going to say? Or is he really as surprised as he seems to be?

'Oh!' he said. 'Not dangerous? But I understand that he – that his sexual lifestyle was – er – likely to give rise to anxiety – '

She leaned forwards then and grinned at him, a wide toothy grin that showed on her mouth only. There was no amusement in her eyes.

'Mr Gerrard, according to the newspapers I see, there are a great many well-known people in this country who have sexual lifestyles of such fluidity and variety that they are indeed putting themselves at risk of a range of very unpleasant infections. No one is suggesting they are highly dangerous.' There was a little titter then from the audience and a small part of her remembered suddenly that Gerrard's own marital and extra-marital exploits had had a good deal of publicity. 'It is quite unjust to suggest that this patient was at any particular risk. He has lived in a faithful relationship with one equally faithful partner for seventeen years. He is in no way a dangerous patient in any hospital.'

'Did Mr Lemon know this?' Gerrard asked, riding magnificently over the titters, and the audience stilled again to hushed attention.

'Of course he did,' Kate said scathingly. 'He was told. But he chose to make assumptions about this patient simply because he thought he was homosexual.' She sat up very straight then, and turned her head and stared at the audience, or at least to where she knew it to be; she couldn't see them but there was a dull whitish blur there and she had a need to talk to them directly. 'All because of his style, the way he talked and behaved – it's as bad as looking at a man and saying, "He's dangerous because of the colour of his skin, or the shape of his nose or the language he speaks – " Would any of you want to think that if you were ill and had to go to hospital the doctors there could legitimately decide whether or not to look after you on the basis of such – such blind stupidity?'

There was a little hush and then someone clapped at the far side and after a fraction of a moment more and more people joined in, and she sat there staring at the blur of white and thought – I'm as bad as the rest of them. I'm just as bad as the other people who work here that I was sneering at. Talking to the audience, putting on a performance – except that I'm not. I'm *not*. It's true. I mean it, and I don't think they do, these television people. Or perhaps they do? Perhaps I'm making silly judgements. And with her head whirling with the confusion of her thoughts she turned back to look at J. J. Gerrard.

He was sitting with his head on one side and looking at her, and above the paint-clogged lines of his face she saw now that his eyes were shrewd and far from as vapid as she had at first thought. And he smiled at her and said softly, 'Well done, Miss Sayers. Well done. Now let me take you on to some more of Mr Lemon's statements, if you please – '

And he turned again to the big screen upon which more words had appeared. *I insisted naturally that he should have an AIDS test before I operated. He refused so I, of course, was forced to decline to operate.*

But from now on there were no more problems. She felt as

though she had climbed a steep hill, painfully and breathlessly, had achieved the crest and was now sliding comfortably down the other side. Her answers to the questions Gerrard put to her came smoothly and easily, and indeed in many ways the questioning now seemed perfunctory. It was as though he had decided that Kate had no further call to answer, that her trial by television was safely over and that she had won. All they had to do now, his behaviour and his manner seemed to suggest, was put in the time to underline the facts that everyone already knew were fully established.

She was almost disappointed when he smiled at her and said, 'Miss Sayers, thank you. Your contribution to *Probe* tonight has been fascinating and most helpful. But now it is time to throw the question open to the floor, because never forget' – and here he swung his chair round to face the audience – 'never forget that *Probe* is *your* programme, *your* place to speak, *your* right to express your views. So, over to you – '

For a moment she braced herself again, waiting for hostility, but she need not have worried. One after the other members of that semi-invisible audience took the microphone in their hands, were briefly illuminated by a travelling spotlight and spoke in her defence. One after the other they made it clear they despised the man who had complained about her, not only for what he had said, but also for not having had the courage to come and say it to her directly; and she sat there smiling and nodding at them all, not sure how to behave. Praise was something she never handled well and they were dishing it out in great dollops. It was not a comfortable experience, and again she became aware of the sweat on her body and the ache in her back from this awful chair she occupied.

'Ladies and gentlemen!' Gerrard's voice came booming at her again, and she blinked, for she had lost interest in him once he had got to his feet to stand in front of his audience. 'After the break we'll be dealing with another medical question, and one that will touch many hearts and minds, just as Miss Sayers has already. Stay with us, and meet – '

She felt her mouth go dry and her legs start to shake. She had forgotten. How could she have forgotten her first fear? That Kim was to be brought on, that she would have to defend herself yet again and this time on a much less defensible wicket. There would be many people who would doubt the legitimacy of using scarce resources for patients such as Kim Hynes; hadn't she herself been worried about it? To have now to wrench herself back up into the sort of mood and fluency that she had already displayed and which would enable her to cope with being quizzed over Kim – she wasn't sure she could do it. In fact she was certain she couldn't.

' – and meet,' J. J. Gerrard went on, 'a most notable and most senior doctor, a lady obstetrician and gynaecologist, Miss Fay Buckland. The issue will be abortion and the rights of mothers as well as babies. Stay with *Probe*, ladies and gentlemen – *your* programme remember and no one else's – '

'I take it all back,' Kate said and giggled into her glass. It was amazing how pleasant the wine tasted, remembering how sour she had thought it when they had given her some before the programme. Now it seemed light and flowery and a perfect match for the way she was feeling. Even the sandwiches seemed worth eating now, for she was ravenous; she had eaten little all day, ever since the morning radio programme she had done which had quite destroyed her appetite. 'He really is all right, this Angus McSorley man, isn't he?'

'I told you,' Oliver said. 'I know he's a bit fulsome and it's not what you're used to. But people are in this business. It's the theatrical overtones, I suppose, affecting even sensible journalists. They're much worse on light entertainment shows – they'd drive you potty there.'

'Are you coming to work here with him then? Or was that just talk?' He looked uncomfortable for a moment but she was too relaxed now and a little too glittery with wine to pay as much attention as she might have done to the nuances of his mood.

'I thought you liked radio best of all,' she said. 'You always said so. Or was it just a case of *faute de mieux*?'

'Not at all,' he said a little sharply. 'I do like radio. Immensely. But he's offering me a remarkably interesting job. He needs a solid journalist here and I could do the job well – '

'But you wouldn't be seen, would you? This is J.J.'s programme, isn't it?' she said in a moment of shrewdness and he laughed at that, a little ruefully but a laugh nonetheless.

'You can be as sharp as the proverbial, Kate. Yes, that's the rub. I don't think I want to be deep background for anyone, even J.J. On City I do my own thing, get my own airtime – I'm pretty autonomous, too. It's a comfortable way to be. Maybe that's what's wrong with it.'

'Then stay there.'

'Money's better here.'

'Oh, blow money,' she said. 'We get on well enough on what we have – '

'Oh, yes,' he said. 'We do – ' and then reached for some more wine and as though he had actually tossed a glass full of the cold stuff over her to make her catch her breath she realised she had done it again. Opened the old sore, started the dialogue going again, reminded him of Sonia. She was always needing more money, always complaining that the children needed things, always nudging and pushing at him – and Kate swallowed the rest of her own wine recklessly and held out the glass for a refill.

'Well,' she said lightly. 'I dare say you'll do what you think is best. Oliver, did I do all right?'

He laughed then. '*Mah*vellous dahling,' he drawled. 'Too too *mah*vellous. Oh, you are funny, Kate. You people who sneer the hardest at showbiz types are really the worst. The first time you get within a sniff of an audience it's, "How was I, darling, how did I do, darling? Was I super, darling?" Well, you did well enough.'

She made a face. 'It's all right for you. You're used to this sort of thing. Me, I'm a complete tyro. All I know is that it was the most nerve-wracking thing I've ever done. I'd sooner go through my fellowship vivas again, and you can't say worse than that.'

He reached out and hugged her and laughed, but it was kinder now. 'Kate, my love, you were splendid. Dignified and honest and – well, splendid. Lemon must have realised you would be or he was tipped off. I can't see any other reason for him staying away. If he'd been here you'd have showed him up for the pompous gasbag he is – '

'Believe it or nor, I'm a bit sorry for him. Professor Levy says he's a sick man. Paranoid. Needs psychiatric care. And I must say I begin to agree with him – '

She lifted her head to look down the room to where Angus McSorley was talking to Jimmy Rhoda, their heads close together. 'And I suppose I must also say that I now know I've been less than fair to your friend Rhoda.'

'Wow! Nothing like a little time in the hot limelight to soften a woman!' Oliver said and laughed softly. 'Why, all of a sudden?'

'This other business – the one about Fay Buckland – he handled that exactly right, didn't he?'

'You mean it was all right for him to run a story about one of Fay Buckland's patients, not right for him to run one about one of yours?'

'Pig,' she said equably. 'No. I don't mean that. I mean the way that poor woman was being bullied – attempts to buy babies – there are some things that have to be exposed. That was one of them.'

'And the problems of operating on patients who may or may not be exposed to AIDS and may or may not infect others, including hospital staff, and the problems of dealing with patients who demand sex-change operations? They're different?'

'Stop being so pompous, Oliver! You know bloody well what I mean. And I wish you'd listen to what I say – though thank God it didn't come up on the programme, and I didn't have to say it to Gerrard. But I'll say it again to you – there's no such thing as sex-change operations, only gender reassignment treatment. You can't change sex – real sex. Only the *appearance* of it. So you can't call the sort of surgery Kim had more than that – '

'A rose is a rose is a rose,' Oliver said. 'Answer me. Why is it all right for Jimmy to write an exposé of a woman who is suffering from sub-fertility and who gets so desperate to have a child that she resorts to admittedly unpleasant subterfuges such as trying to buy another woman's baby, but not right for him to expose the problem of gender reassignment operations in crowded poverty-stricken hospitals where all sorts of other possibly more deserving cases are on the waiting list?'

She blinked. 'You'll have to say that again. The state I'm in I couldn't take it all in – you really should stop addressing me like a radio audience – '

He had the grace to look embarrassed. 'Well, all right, I'm sorry. But it's true, isn't it? What Jimmy did in writing about that Malone woman seems on the face of it to be highly virtuous. The noble knight carrying his lance into battle against plain evil. But that woman isn't evil any more than you maintain your Kim is evil. She's just a poor sad creature who couldn't have what every other woman takes for granted, and when she's faced with someone who tries to get rid of a baby with an abortion offers to take it on. Looked at that way, she's not so wicked, is she? Though I gather she has an unpleasant personality – but that's no crime. Yet when Jimmy wrote up Kim's story – at Kim's own request remember, and for her own profit – you regarded that as sinful in the extreme. Yet to lots of people what she had done was as close to sheer evil as you can get – flying in the face of God and Nature – '

'No!' Kate was flushed now and standing close to him, staring up into his face, prodding him with one finger to push home the emphasis of her words. 'Kim is as sick and unhappy as any old man with an enlarged prostate who wakes up umpteen times a night. Her distress may not be the sort most people can empathise with, but that doesn't make it any the less real and important, and – '

'Put that man down, Kate, you'll break him!'

Kate whirled and after a moment smiled widely and held out both hands. 'Fay, I can't tell you how glad I am to see you – and how thrilled I am you did so well. You did, you know – '

Fay, looking as rumpled and messy as ever, grinned at her complacently. 'I did, didn't I?' she said. 'I've been talking to my solicitor on the phone – I told him to watch as soon as I knew I was going to do this damned programme and he called the barrister and he watched too. And they both say the same – after this, it's very unlikely the DPP will take the matter any further. Those mischievous anti-abortionists will have to shut up and leave us in peace – '

'The day they do you're in trouble,' Oliver said dryly. 'Hello, Miss Buckland. Do you remember me? We met at one of the Old East parties last Christmas – '

'Mm? Oh, yes, you're Kate's young man, aren't you? I

remember perfectly well – What do you mean, the day they do I'm in trouble? They're the bane of my life, these people – '

'But you need them. Without them you might not stop and think about what you're doing – '

Fay rubbed her head with one hand, managing to make herself look even wilder, if that were possible, than she usually did. 'Piffle! I think carefully all the time. The difference between me and them, though, is that I think about each individual case. They just go in for their damned blanket condemnations. God, how I hate these absolute moralists! There can't be any such thing as an absolute morality – it's a philosophical impossibility. Listen, let me – ' And she was clearly about to launch herself on a long diatribe but Kate jumped in before she could get going.

'How did it happen that you were on the programme?' she asked. 'I was so worried. I'd guessed they'd got someone else to be on, and then when I heard Gerrard say it was going to be another Old East issue I thought – well, I'm not sure what I thought. I was afraid they were going to wheel Kim Hynes out. You remember, my reassignment case. It's the sort of thing she'd love and she's discharged herself from the ward so – and then when they brought you on I could have cheered – oh, damn!' She looked deeply flustered then. 'That was bloody selfish of me. I mean, I'm not glad you've got this wretched problem – but I have to admit I was damned grateful they weren't pushing on Kim's case – '

'That's all right,' Fay said cheerfully. 'I'd be the same, I dare say. It's all so silly, all this fuss, isn't it? Why can't they trust us? We do the best job we can, we always put our patients first, so why do they niggle away at us like this? I'd be much better off at home reading up on the work I'm doing tomorrow – I've got a hell of a long list – instead of wasting my time here. But there it is – '

'But why should we trust you, Miss Buckland?' Angus McSorley had joined the little group and now he stood and smiled round at them all with that same emollient grin he had worn before, and Kate looked at him a little sharply. She could see him now much more clearly: behind the urbane manner there was a mind and a will that were not to be dismissed easily as mere showbiz exuberance.

'Would you want patients to trust the Goodman Lemons of

this world?' he went on. 'He'd have turned that patient out of the hospital untreated, because of his own prejudice and ignorance. I know more about HIV, dammit, than he seems to! But he's been exposed now – partly of course through his own stupidity rather than journalists' rows, but let that be for the moment – but would you say we ought to trust the likes of him?'

'Heavens no! His sort need watching a lot. And there are one or two others at Old East I'm not too sure about!' And she slid a wicked little sideways grin at Kate and laughed. 'You too, Kate? But we've got an Ethics Committee to keep an eye on 'em – we muddle through well enough – '

'It's because muddling through isn't good enough when it comes to people's lives, Miss Buckland, that journalists like us do what we do. I know you were furious when Jimmy ran that story this morning, but you must admit that taking it all round it's done you no harm, has it?'

'I suppose not,' Fay said, and then shook her head as she caught sight of the clock. 'Oh, heavens, I've wasted enough time on all this. Is it all right if I go? I'm operating at eight o'clock tomorrow morning and I really can't sit around here getting my head in a fug – see you at Old East, Kate – 'bye all – ' And she was gone in a little flurry of shed scarves and gloves, her rumpled hair bouncing on her neck with the speed of her movements as she pushed her way out of the crowded room.

'Is she always like that?' Jimmy Rhoda said, amused. He had been standing behind Angus McSorley and now bobbed out of his shadow to grin at Kate. 'I thought we had a few nutters hanging round Fleet Street but Shadwell seems to have its share.'

In spite of her new willingness to accede to the suggestion that there was some virtue in Jimmy Rhoda, Kate could not warm to him and she said a little dampeningly, 'Miss Buckland is a very fine surgeon and a superb clinician. Her concern for her patients is beyond criticism.'

'I'm sure of that. You've only got to be with her five minutes to know that she drips with integrity – but is she always in such a tangle and a flap?'

'Most of the time,' Kate admitted and Oliver grinned.

'Old East is full of the strangest characters, Jimmy,' he said. 'If you take this investigation of yours any further you'll find out. It's a haven for nutters one way and another – '

'Investigate further?' Kate said quickly and looked from one to the other. 'For heaven's sake, haven't we had enough? What else can there be to write about? The ingrowing toenails clinic on Fridays perhaps? I've been told there's a somewhat outrageous chiropodist there – '

'Don't be so scratchy, Kate!' Oliver said. 'There's plenty there yet. I've still got my series to finish on the cuts – you've got a demo camped out there virtually permanently, and – '

'And you've got the Junior Minister for Health among the suffering multitudes as well,' Jimmy said. 'Old Saffron. Could be worth doing a bit of poking around there to find out if there's any naughtiness going on – '

'What sort of naughtiness?' Kate demanded. 'How could there be? Just because he's a Minister doesn't mean he'll be ill-treated as a patient – '

'I wasn't thinking of ill-treatment,' Jimmy said smoothly. 'I'm just wondering whether the reverse is the case. He's sitting there, has been for ages, a much-vaunted NHS patient in an NHS ward, but what special privileges does he get? Is he just in an ordinary bed or does he get a nice little side ward all to himself? Does he get the same food as everyone else? The same sort of care? Or does he get the VIP bit to make sure he gets the equivalent of private care, while the DHSS gets the good publicity about having its junior chappie being one of the great unwashed and nobly sitting it out in an NHS dump? Oh, there's plenty I could deal with there for the *Globe*, my dear Kate! And I rather think I will, you know. Too good an opportunity to miss. Especially as I've got a nice little girlfriend there with as sharp a nose for news as any Fleet Street hackette. You'll be hearing from me – ' And he tipped his hand to his forehead and slapped Angus and Oliver on the back and turned to go.

'I'll see you two villains around, no doubt. Keep in touch, Angus. One good story deserves another – you scratch my back and I'll scratch whichever bit of your anatomy you care to offer. Night all – ' And he went, leaving Kate to stare after him with her forehead a little wrinkled.

'Will he do all that, Oliver?' she asked after a moment. Oliver, who had been talking to Angus, looked over his shoulder briefly.

'Mm? Oh, I rather think so. You can't stop Jimmy when he's got a story in his nose. Your original damned bloodhound, that's what he is. Listen Angus, I do have a couple of ideas you might like to consider.'

They moved away from her, heads together, and she filled another glass of wine and stood there sipping it thoughtfully. Around her the room still hummed with activity; in the far corner she could see J. J. Gerrard surrounded by a number of people and apparently holding forth at some length. He caught her glance and lifted one hand and bowed slightly and she smiled back, albeit briefly. She hadn't liked the man at all, but she had to admire his skill. He had stage-managed the strange debate between herself and an absent Lemon with great skill, making it seem like a deliberate and well-chosen method of developing the argument, instead of what it was, a makeshift way of dealing with the matter in the absence of one of the main protagonists.

And he had indeed been on her side; he had made it crystal clear to his audience in the studio and, she imagined, the wider television audience as well, that far from behaving badly in the matter of Gerald Slattery, Kate had been brave and resourceful, doing exactly what was right for the patient, and caring for him before her own welfare. 'Whether it is right,' Gerrard had said smoothly, 'to treat possible sources of infection of this dreadful plague in ordinary hospitals among innocent people, is a question we will all have to address seriously soon, if not on this occasion. But in the meantime,' he had finished triumphantly, 'the patient in question is well and has been cured of his life-threatening condition and no one has been hurt.' And he had led the applause for, 'Miss Kate Sayers, ladies and gentlemen, a great example of the loving and superb tradition of British medicine at its best.'

And Kate, revolted by the awful emotive language he had used – 'plague', she had thought with deep distaste when he had said it, the man's a fool; and when he'd gone on about 'innocent victims' she could have shouted at him, but had bitten her tongue – but at the same time deeply grateful that Gerald Slattery's name had not been mentioned, had escaped from the studio, giddy with relief that her ordeal was over. She had sat then in the hospitality room and watched the monitor screen as Fay Buckland had spiritedly defended her own stance in the matter of the late abortion she had performed, and also had castigated the selling of babies to the infertile, and had wanted to cheer aloud. She had been so very much herself, so unstilted, so passionate, that Kate had been even more convinced that her own efforts had been puerile. But, she had told herself pragmatically, it was over now. So what did it matter? And she could not deny the programme had been helpful to her. Goodman Lemon could do her no further harm now, of this she was almost certain.

Altogether it had been a vintage piece of *Probe* programming, and now, Kate thought as she watched its anchorman preening among his admirers in his corner, now it's all over and forgotten and people will put the cat out and put the kettle on for their bedtime cuppas and forget all about it. What a silly fuss over so little. And yet over so much –

She stood there thinking for a little longer and then moved over to the side of the room where she had seen a phone. There would be no harm in calling him; he had given her his phone number and she was sure he would want to tell her how he felt she had coped with her interlocutor. It had all worked out well, of course it had. There would be no more fuss over this issue of AIDS patients in Old East at present, but still it would be nice to hear directly from his own lips that he was pleased with her. His approval mattered a good deal to her, one way and another.

He was at home and was as lavish with approval for her performance as she could have hoped. She felt as though she was being stroked as she listened to his agreeable voice on the phone and smiled to herself happily as he added in echo of her own thoughts, 'And I think that will be the end of it, my dear. Even Goodman Lemon couldn't go on batting on a wicket that has been so very thoroughly demolished. Now I hope we'll have some peace from all this wretched publicity.'

'Oh,' she said then and her face straightened. 'I'm afraid it won't, Professor Levy. I rather think it might get worse for Old East, I mean. Not for me personally. And I'm not sure how we can get over it, either.'

She heard the little sigh at the end of the phone. 'Bless you for

342

the "we", my dear. It comforts me a great deal. Perhaps you'd better explain.'

And she did, telling him all about the conversation with Jimmy and Oliver, pushing away the faint sense of disloyalty she felt in talking so. Of course she was loyal to Oliver; how could she be otherwise, loving him as she did? But she owed a loyalty to Old East as well. The place mattered a great deal more to her than even Oliver realised, and so did its patients. And as she told the Dean of what was being threatened by Jimmy, and to a lesser extent by Oliver with his radio programmes, she felt depression settle on her. And it wasn't all the effects of the wine she knew she had used rather more recklessly than she usually did.

'Well,' he said when at last she stopped. 'Thank you for telling me. I'll have to give considerable thought to this. We've managed to sort things out well enough so far – but I'm not sure how I'll handle this one. Getting Lemon to issue that ridiculous press statement of his was child's play compared to this – '

She blinked. 'What did you say?'

'Ah – perhaps I shouldn't have mentioned that – ' She could hear the glint of laughter in his voice at the other end of the phone.

'You *persuaded* him to do that? But it could have been a disaster!' She felt a wave of indignation fill her. 'When I think how awful I felt when I saw that stuff in the Sunday papers! I really could – '

'My dear Kate, I'm sorrier than I can say if I upset you – but it was a temporary upset, wasn't it? And once my good friend Mr McSorley agreed to do the programme I knew all would be well. Even after I – um – warned Lemon he might do better not to take part directly himself – And you really have acquitted yourself extremely well – and will again, I have no doubt – '

'Professor Levy!' she said. 'You really are a very slippery customer, aren't you?'

'Well, you could say so,' he said modestly, but clearly pleased with himself. 'I wasn't cut out to be a politician but once I was pushed into this chair, I had to learn to be one – *c'est la guerre*, you understand – '

'Whatever it is, you do it damned well,' Kate said and tried to sound shocked, but couldn't. The more she thought about it, the more admiration she felt for him, however much she herself had been discommoded by what had happened. He really had handled the Lemon affair with great skill. But would he be able to do the same with someone as sharp as Jimmy Rhoda, and Oliver too?

She said as much to him and he laughed softly. 'Well, Kate, I don't know whether I can. But I'll tell you this much. I'm going to try! Good night my dear. And thank you. You did superbly well. I'm proud of you.'

Chapter Thirty-Five

———————— ∞∞∞∞ ————————

Mr Holliday saw the dapper man in the dark suit come in and go down to the end of the ward where the VIP was, and thought hard about him. He looked important but that could be just because he was wearing a suit without any white coat over it. He mightn't even be a doctor, but Mr Holliday had a feeling he was. There was something about the way he'd talked to the sister when he'd come in, the way she'd been so easy with him. She wasn't at all easy with the people who usually came to visit the VIP. He had to be a doctor, Mr Holliday ended his deduction. And an important one at that. Maybe he'd be able to help.

Male Medical had been quiet for once this morning and Sister Sheward stretched gratefully. She finished the last chart and looked down the ward approvingly. The nurses had done well this morning after her spectacular if rather contrived loss of temper about tidiness. All the curtains were pulled well back from the glass dividers, and each bed was neatly made with its red blanket folded tidily over the foot rail and the lockers were well scrubbed and not too heavily laden with detritus. Leave it to the patients and they'd have nothing inside, everything out on the top, but now it looked almost as nice as the wards had used to look when she had been in training fifteen years ago. And she sighed again, this time with agreeable nostalgia. Those had been the days, before all these chits made it such a struggle to keep a ward running smoothly.

But she couldn't complain today. It was sad about Joe Slater of course; but he shouldn't have been occupying one of her beds anyway, so she'd been relieved really when he'd died at last. It was hell for him anyway, as well as for his wife, the way he'd lingered. Definitely a happy release. And really he shouldn't have been in the ward at all; she'd only kept him to please Neville Carr, and, she had to admit, to spite that damned Saffron man. When he'd intervened after Audrey Slater had bearded him in his corner there it had given Sister Sheward considerable pleasure to look down her nose at him when he'd spoken to her about it and say that Joe Slater's bed was assured and there had never been any intention of discharging him. Worth lying about really, for the way it had spiked the man's guns.

She could see Professor Levy's back now, distorted like a hunchback's through the three or four layers of glass which stood between herself and him, where he sat beside Edward Saffron's bed, and wondered what they were talking about. This was the first time he'd come up to see him, and that had seemed odd at first to Sister Sheward; after all, Levy was the Dean, and Saffron was a particularly significant patient for Old East. But he had come now and maybe that meant that the man was to be discharged? He was a lot better than he had been, she knew, not that he was under her care, but she had her ways of finding out what was happening. It would be good to be rid of him in some ways, though tiresome in others. It would be agreeable to have her ward back *in toto*, looking as it should without the beds pushed too close together in the other cubicles to accommodate Saffron's solitude in the far bay; but it would mean more battles with Agnew Byford and Neville Carr and Laurence Bulpitt; all of them fighting over the available beds. And again she sighed but this time with irritation, and got to her feet to go down the ward to harry the nurses some more. That boy David Engell, the first year, needed a good deal of chivvying: too fond by far of lingering by the beds of the better-looking younger patients and chatting to them. She had her doubts about that boy's masculinity, though she'd die rather than admit it, because it was unfashionable to say the least ever to let on you felt like that about male nurses, but there it was; she didn't like 'em and never would. Having a bit of a go at David would do the boy a lot of good and if he couldn't take it, he shouldn't be in nursing anyway. And she bustled down the ward, passing Professor Levy on his way out. But he seemed a little abstracted, and she settled for just a smile and nod as he hurried past her. He seems pleased with himself, she thought as he went by, really has got cream on his whiskers. Better have a word with Saffron's private nurses. Maybe he is on his way out. Glory be.

*

Mr Holliday pounced as the man in the black suit reached the door of the ward, pushing his wheelchair in front of him so that he had to stop.

'Er, sir,' he said. 'Sir?'

Levy stopped at once and smiled at him, the soul of courtesy.

'There was something I wanted to ask – are you a doctor, sir?'

'Yes,' Levy said, still courteous, but watchful as well now.

'I thought you was. You look like a doctor. An important one. Are you important?'

Levy smiled, very urbane, and flicked his eyes swiftly at the clock on the wall above Holliday's head. Two minutes. That was all he could manage. Just two minutes.

'All the doctors at Old East are important,' he said. 'Who is the doctor who looks after you? You know his name?'

Holliday nodded. 'Mr Bulpitt,' he said and there was a little animation in his voice now; he sounded less flat to Levy. He's a Parkinson's, he thought with a corner of his mind. One of Laurence's old Parkinson's –

'Mr Laurence Bulpitt,' Holliday repeated. 'He did my brain operation you know, though he's not a surgeon as a rule, so he told me. He's a neurologist. Yes.' He nodded slowly, pleased with himself at enunciating the word. 'Neurologist.'

'Ah,' Levy said and smiled. 'Well, I'm sure he is giving you excellent care. Now, if you'll just – '

'Oh, I'm not complaining about the care.' Holliday sounded shocked, but also tired, the moment of animation quite gone. His voice, which had seemed strong, seemed weaker now and Levy cocked a sharp eye at him and said soothingly, 'Well, I'm delighted to hear it. And now I really must – '

'It's just that I have to know, you see. I have to know about that woman. The mother, I saw the programme last night about Miss Buckland and all that, and I did agree, didn't you? I'm sure you saw it. It's all wrong, selling babies – '

'Yes,' Levy said. 'A most interesting programme. And now if you don't mind I'll – '

'But what's the difference between selling and using, you tell me that?' Holliday managed to sound triumphant, but his voice was failing rapidly now.

'It's hard for me to say,' Levy said with his customary care and smiled charmingly at the man, and leaned down and patted his shoulder. 'Now you really must let me go. I have an important meeting, I'm afraid, or I'd gladly stay and discuss the television with you. But there it is – do talk to Sister. I'm sure she'll be delighted to talk to you. Good morning!' And moving with a skill that hid his haste, he went, leaving Holliday staring dolefully after him.

'Well, I'll need more assurances than just your word, Professor Levy,' Mrs Blundell said. 'With all due respect, of course.'

'Of course,' Professor Levy said and smiled. 'I quite understand. Some more tea? You must be chilled out there in the cold so long.'

'Oh, I'm used to it,' Mrs Blundell said, managing, just, not to sound like a martyr. 'But I won't say no. Ta – '

There was a little silence and then she said suspiciously, 'Why?'

'I beg your pardon?'

'Why, all of a sudden? I mean, we've been on this demo for weeks. No one's paid us a blind bit of notice. You'd ha' thought we wasn't there most of the time. Just one radio chap gets involved – ' She laughed appreciatively. 'It did me good to see the way he popped that sergeant. He's a right Hitler he is. We've been complaining about the way he's been shoving us around all the time, laid an official complaint we have. But apart from the radio chap and a few bits in the *Globe* who gives a damn? The telly stopped covering us ages ago and it don't seem to matter a tuppenny fart to that Saffron up there whether he can see us or not. He's certainly paid us no attention, and no one's come from the DHSS to talk to us. So why all of a sudden are they giving in?'

He looked at her speculatively and then leaned forwards to prop his elbows on his desk and his chin on his fists.

'Did you see the programme *Probe* last night?'

'Me, watch telly? After a day out there freezing my arse off – if you'll excuse me, and I think you will – I need a bit more entertainment than that. I went out for a drink with my old man. Why?'

'They were investigating various Old East matters.'

She lifted her chin sharply. 'You mean they clobbered us? No one said anything to me this morning. Someone must have seen it, surely, if – '

He shook his head. 'No. It wasn't your demo. It was – various other matters that have caused some fuss here in the last few weeks.'

She grinned and nodded at him over the rim of her teacup. 'I can imagine!' she said and then laughed. 'You've really been copping it one way and another.'

'You could say that.' Professor Levy smiled back at her. 'Well, last night we won, if it can be described in that way since it wasn't precisely a battle. But the issues that came up were developed nicely and at the end of it all it was clear to most of the audience, I'm sure, that there were no sins being committed here – or none that we were accused of anyway. Even the reviewers who covered it in this morning's papers seem to accept that we at Old East do our best in difficult situations to behave – um – ethically and wisely – '

'Oh, I'm sure you do,' she said, with a hint of irony in her voice but no real malice. 'It's only when it comes to cuts that the ethics wobble a bit, isn't it?'

'Cuts in services are hardly our fault,' Professor Levy said. 'As I've told you before and you actually know perfectly well, Mrs Blundell. That is a matter for the various bodies set in judgement over us – our masters in Whitehall, ultimately – '

'I know,' she said. 'I don't mean to – but that's what worries me, you see. You call me here to tell me we can all go home, thanks very much, it's all right, they won't be closing any of Old East's wards, they won't be shoving us over to St Kitts or wherever, we'll still keep our hospital, all right and tight, but what evidence are you giving me? And like I said, *why*?'

'You're a politician, Mrs Blundell,' the Professor said. 'And if anyone will understand you will. After last night's programme, one of our doctors who took part discovered – um – became aware that rather than interest in Old East being slaked by the publicity we'd had, it had been increased. One of the journalists who has been active – the man who writes for the *Globe*? Yes, you know the one I mean – He's been sniffing around a good deal, I imagine. He says he's going to do more. And he says that he is going to investigate in particular Mr Saffron's presence here. How much of an NHS patient he actually is, d'you see – '

She was watching him with wide intelligent eyes, her long bony legs wrapped round each other, and he became aware, as he had before, of the sexuality she exuded. It was extraordinary how powerful an effect she had on him. It made the task of explaining to her much more agreeable.

'And it occurred to me, when I was told this, that Mr Saffron himself would find it deeply embarrassing to have such an investigation done and reported.'

He chuckled then, a deep rich sound in his throat. 'So I went and warned him about it this morning.'

She laughed too and for a moment there was a closeness that seemed to tie them together in a web they both wanted to be in.

'Did it work?'

'Not at first, to tell you the truth – ' He hesitated for a moment. 'He's really rather slow on the uptake, you know. For a Minister of the Crown.'

'Hmmph!' she said. 'That's why they're Ministers of the Crown. It makes 'em workable, you know. Their boss isn't the sort to fancy clever people around.'

'You could be right.' He leaned back then. 'Anyway, once I'd explained how uncomfortable things could get for him once the press really got going on him we agreed a strategy. He will be transferred home. His consultant, Mr Byford, tells me there is small risk to his health now, and he can and will make sure he has all the necessary home nursing and supervision. And Mr Saffron has agreed it would be – um – politic to keep the hands of the cost-cutters off Old East for the present.'

'For the present?' she said sharply, and the web of amiability broke into fine shreds and vanished into the dusty light from the window.

'That's the best I can offer,' he said a little apologetically. 'And I'm being as honest with you as I know how. I needn't have mentioned it, after all! But I can tell you that he's agreed to intervene personally and see to it that we here at Old East are left off the current round of economies in the present financial year. But after next April, they'll start looking again. That should give you some time to get your support going, shouldn't it? Time to involve more local people – MPs perhaps and so forth? It will certainly give me some time to bring in my own big guns.'

He smiled again then. 'I do have one or two. The odd Royal ear you know – this place has a long history of being involved with interesting people. And you must remember that though they'll leave us alone, they still need to make their economies. It'll be St Kitts that will lose beds this round of cuts, I imagine. And that may mean – indeed I'm sure it will mean – that when they come to look at the area's bedding situation next time they might find that they can't cut any of ours, because of the losses from St Kitts, you see.'

She looked a little sulky now, and far from being willing to agree to what he was asking of her. But then he said softly, 'It could be a considerable effort for you, of course, to organise a bigger and even more powerful opposition. But with extra time I suspect you could do a great deal. And I gather you have some ambitions in the political area – local government, and so forth? Maybe a tactical retreat now could pay big dividends in attacking strength later. An old military simile, you know – '

There was a long silence and then she nodded and set down her teacup and got to her feet.

'All right. You win. I'll tell them and we'll let the demo go. But I claim the right to tell the papers that we've won – '

'I don't think Mr Saffron will object,' he said. 'Nor will he change his mind. He's been ill long enough to start worrying about whether he'll lose his portfolio, I suspect. He wants nothing that will draw the wrong sort of attention. If you make it clear you – um – appreciate his willingness to listen to you, the grass roots and so forth – I don't have to tell you how he wants it, do I? – it's my guess you'll do rather well out of the whole thing.'

'Not as well,' she said, and grinned sharply, so that she looked suddenly like a rather wicked little squirrel, 'not as well as you will.'

'She wants what?' Kate said and Esther lifted her shoulders expressively and shook her head.

'I agree with you. She's outrageous. Comes on with all the delicate grace of a crack Panzer division, but there it is. She's sitting outside there now like Venus on a rock cake waiting to have a word with you about it.'

'You have to give her top marks for cheek,' Kate said.

'And the rest. Will you agree?'

'I don't know. I'll see after I talk to her. Anything else?'

There was a little silence and then Esther said, 'Um. Yes.'

Kate had her head down over her charts and didn't look up at first, but as the silence prolonged itself she felt the tension and lifted her head. Esther was staring down at her with her face rather red and Kate said lightly, 'My dear, you look suddenly as though you've been stuffed and boiled. Whatever is it?'

'I feel stuffed and boiled,' Esther said. 'The thing is, I've given in my notice.'

Kate dropped her pen and stared at her in consternation. 'No! You can't!'

'I can and I did,' Esther said shortly and turned away. 'I couldn't stand the nagging any longer.'

'Richard?' Kate said.

'Richard,' Esther repeated bitterly. 'My husband, remember? The chap I tied myself to some time back with a bunch of fancy promises. The bugger I love, God help me.'

'Do you? Or is he just a habit?'

'Do you love your Oliver or is he just good in bed?' Esther retorted and then shook her head at herself as she saw Kate's face redden. 'Shit! I'm sorry, but I couldn't help it. I'm as mad as hell at him, but he has to be right. They pay me bugger-all here to work my guts out all the hours God gives, and we've got two kids and out there there's money to be made. It's not the be-all and end-all but, Christ, it comes bloody close to it. With me to organise things properly there's no question that we can do well, and as Richard says, my first duty is to my own family, surely, rather than this lot here.'

She lifted her chin and stared down the ward stretching away each side of the nurses' station; at the humped beds, the tube-tangled machines and the clusters of visitors round each patient and sighed, a sharp little intake of breath that seemed very loud in the small space they were in.

'I mean, look at 'em, will you? They're dropouts and idiots who've ruined their own bodies with all sorts of rubbish and smoking and the rest of it and whatever we do for 'em they're back in a matter of weeks, no better off and needing patching up again. It's like that story we were told at school, do you remember? The Augean stables, wasn't it? However fast you sweep up the crap, there's twice as much there when you turn round. Well, with Richard there'll still be crap but at least there'll be some sort of reward to show from dealing with it. The sort you can show, that is. Cash. Here all I get is a good feeling and a lot of gratitude. Big bloody deal, gratitude – '

'I shall miss you,' Kate said after a moment and Esther flicked a glance at her and said roughly, 'Not as much as I'll miss you, you old bat. You and everything else about this bloody place. Poured my guts out here for years and it's all I can do to tear myself away. I really must be mad – '

'You're not mad. It's the people who don't think it's better to give you enough to make staying here more attractive than going off and selling aubergine quiche to yuppies – ' Kate said and reached out one hand to her. 'Try not to get too mad at Richard. He isn't entirely wrong.'

'Of course he isn't! If he was, do you think I'd have agreed? It's because he's so damned right that I'm going. Oh, Christ! Aubergine quiche! I suppose it's not much worse than infected piss and blocked cannulae and meths drinkers in uraemic shock. Not much worse – ' And she grinned at Kate lopsidedly and then leaned over and hugged her and they clung together for a moment or two.

'What's with you, anyhow?' Esther said then. 'That programme was bloody good, you know. I was worried that they'd start on about Kim, mind you. Bloody glad I am they didn't – but after that little parade last night I don't imagine you'll get any more fuss over that chap Slattery. Nice fella he turned out to be, didn't he? He's due next week to have his follow-up. Give him my best, won't you?'

'Are you going so soon?'

Esther nodded. 'I've got three weeks holiday due to me, and I thought I'd take it out of my notice. Hanging round once you know you're going doesn't do. Listen, you'd better go and see your bloody Kim. And Kate – when they start to collect for my present, tell 'em I want something frivolous and deeply personal.

If I get any household gear I'll wrap it round their lousy necks. A huge bottle of Joy'd be nice.'

'I'll tell them,' Kate said and went to see Kim.

'It was money,' Kim said. 'What else? I got to earn what I can when I can.'

'What sort of video, for pity's sake?' Kate said. 'What could possibly pay you enough to make you sign yourself out the day before you were due to go to theatre for your tidy-up? I've had to reorganise all the lists, upset a lot of other patients – '

'Porn, what else?' Kim said defiantly and stared at her. She had even more make-up on than usual today, and looked magnificent. Her hair was tumbling halfway down her back in a richer-than-ever cascade of curls and she was wearing a suit made of mulberry-coloured leather, the skirt so tight fitting Kate winced to look at it and the bloused top lavishly equipped with glittering steel studs.

'They gave me five hundred to show 'em – '

'Show them what?'

Kim giggled, a high-pitched little sound. 'My operation,' she said. 'What else?'

Kate stared at her. 'And now you come back here to ask me to take you in again and still do your tidy-up operation? After that?'

'Why not?' Kim said and lifted her eyes to stare at Kate. 'I've made sure not to eat or drink this morning. And you know you said it needed doing. You can fit me in anywhere you like, end of the day, anything. And – ' She stopped then and let her overintense stare drop away. 'Anyway, you want to. You're a surgeon. You like to do your job properly. I'm not finished yet, am I? If you don't take me back, then you've let yourself down, haven't you? And if you thought I was worth dealing with in the first place, thought I was worth taking on, what's changed? Are you saying I'm a person not worth bothering with because I had to make a few bob for myself in a way you don't like? Listen, Miss Sayers. It may turn out I've got to make my living in the future as a brass. How about that, then?'

She made a face at Kate's look of incomprehension. 'A rotten word, isn't it? Means a whore, a call girl, a prostitute, call it what you like. I'd be good at it. They don't all want the usual, you know. A lot of 'em'll settle for all sorts of other funny business from someone who looks like I do. And I've got good muscles. So aren't I worth bothering with if I have to make my living that way for a while? Till I've got enough for my own business again?'

There was a long silence and then Kate closed her chart and got to her feet. 'I'll fix it with Sister,' she said. 'I think there's a bed you can have. It won't be the same one, but we'll do the best we can. I'll do you at the end of the list.'

And she turned and went.

Chapter Thirty-Six

———————⟋⟍⟍⟋⟋———————

By the time Kate had finished it was past eleven o'clock, and the hospital was settling down for the night with sighs and sudden little flurries of movement, like a great animal. On the Genito-Urinary ward most of the patients were already asleep, although lights burned over the beds of those on dialysis, and she straightened her back gratefully as she closed the last of the charts and said good night to the patient, who just murmured back at her, half asleep himself. Just one last look at Kim to make sure she wasn't bleeding – that had been a more complex piece of wound toileting than she had expected, because there was some infection there – and then she'd be free to get some sleep. And she stood there in the half-light of the end cubicle listening to the soughings of the machine and the more distant sounds of breathing from the patients and thought – Shall I just slide into bed here? The overnight room in the doctors' mess should be available. A shower, a cup of tea and then I can be asleep before midnight –

But she knew suddenly that she needed to see Oliver, to feel and touch him. He might even be in bed by the time she got home; he had taken to earlier nights since his beating-up and she thought of him lying there humped beneath the duvet, his legs sprawled wide the way they always were and her skin crept with the need to be there, feeling his skin against hers. It wasn't a sexual need; that was the last thing she would have energy for tonight. It was much more basic than that, like the desire of a baby for contact with its mother's warm body. And she stared out of the back window, trying to see beyond her own reflection into the darkness outside and thought – Primitive, that's me, primitive. Wanting the warm pelt of someone reliable and safe to creep into –

Kim was sleeping heavily, and after standing looking down at her Kate decided not to disturb her, contenting herself with a look under the covers to make sure there was no obvious bleeding into the dressing. She looked different now; the curly hair was tied back in a ragged piece of gauze bandage and the face, innocent of make-up, was smooth and childlike in sleep, even though there were lines to be seen round the eyes and running a channel from mouth to nose on each side. Kate looked down at her, and tried to imagine what she might be dreaming; did she dream herself man or woman? What was it like to live inside a head as soaked in an obsession as Kim's was? What was it about her personality that made it possible for her to persuade not only Barbara Rosen in the first instance, but Kate herself that she had a real need for the sort of mutilation she had submitted to? And she couldn't find any answers and pulled the covers back gently over the slightly snoring form and went away down the ward to leave the charts on the night nurse's desk – who wasn't far off snoring herself, it seemed to Kate – and make her way home.

All the way in the car, moving easily and comfortably through the thin midnight traffic, she thought of herself sliding into bed beside Oliver. It became the one thing she most needed, that first soft contact with the smooth firmness of him and his sleepy protests as she slid her coldness against his warmest bits; and she smiled contentedly into the windscreen as the street lights overhead swooped down and then disappeared behind her as she sent the little car bucketing along. It was a pleasure to break the law at this time of night, it really was. And the fatigue that had been threatening to engulf her after what had turned out to be a hectic day stepped back a little and crouched low inside her, temporarily forgotten.

She was so eager to get to bed with Oliver that she didn't bother to open the garage and put the car away, relying on the alarm to protect it if anyone tried to break into it in the night, as had happened once before; local people knew she was a doctor and the police had warned her that hopeful drug seekers would make her a regular target, and to lock her car away safely every time. But tonight she was reckless and urgent, and she pushed her key into the lock on the front door to let herself in, feeling as excited as a girl on a first date; oh, but it was good to come home to Oliver, good to be about to crawl in beside him –

But he wasn't in bed. She stood in the hall and gazed, startled, at the wedge of light spilling out into the dimness from the living-room door, and heard the faint murmur of the voices from the TV and felt a chill plunge of disappointment. She had made the scenario of how it would be so vivid in her mind that for a moment she didn't know how to cope, and the fatigue lifted its head and growled at her. But then she shook her head in impatience at herself and dropped her bag and keys on to the chair beside the hall table and went into the living room.

He was stretched out on the sofa, his head on a pile of cushions and his bare feet propped up on the coffee table, wrapped in his old dressing gown and staring sombrely at the TV screen. There were talking heads there, but the volume was turned down so low Kate couldn't identify who they were or what they were talking about, and it was obvious Oliver couldn't either. And she frowned, puzzled, and said, 'Well. Good morning! Why did you wait up? No need!'

'Mm?' He stared at her, almost as though he was surprised to see her and then dragged himself upwards, pulling his bare feet off the table and sitting up so that he could rub both hands through his tousled hair. 'Oh, hello, love. Home so early?'

'Early?' She almost gaped at him. 'Idiot! It's gone midnight!'

He peered at the video machine below the TV set to see the digital clock there and then shook his head. 'Ye gods, so it is! I hadn't realised — listen, have you eaten? Or do you want something? There's some soup in the fridge — I opened a can and only used some of it — '

She shook her head. 'I had operating-theatre sandwiches. Disgusting enough to see me well through to tomorrow. Darling, why aren't you in bed? You look worn out!'

'Oh, I'm all right. Can't keep on going to bed immediately after *The Archers*!' And he grinned at her, trying to remind her of their silly joke about early nights, and she looked back at him and knew at once.

'What's happened?' she said quietly and came and sat down on the sofa beside him. 'And whatever it is, why didn't you call me at the hospital and tell me right away? I could have coped, you know, and I might have been useful.'

He grinned at her a little lopsidedly. 'Oh, Earth Mother Kate! Knows it all, sees it all, wants to cure it all — '

'Well, what if I do? Isn't it what I'm for? And anyway – oh, tell me love! What's happening? Have you heard? Is it likely to be as bad as you thought? Or will they be easy on you?'

He looked puzzled. 'What?'

She could have shaken him in irritation. 'Do you think it'll be – will it be a sentence or a fine?'

He stared at her for a moment and then his face cleared. 'Oh, that! No, that's all right. Andrew said they've quashed all the charges. He's got them to repay the bail, the lot. It seems there've been a good many complaints about the way this chap's been handling the demo from the start. And Andrew says that they prefer not to start any dramas. He reckons they know they couldn't get far – and it might cause internal police problems. No, you can forget all about that – '

She sat there very still, and then said quietly, 'When did you hear this?'

'This morning.'

'And you didn't think to call me and let me share the good news? You didn't think I'd been frantic over this, even more than you were, and might like to be put out of my misery?'

He looked at her and seemed to be fighting with a confusion of feelings: shame and anxiety and irritation and something else undefinable. It was the irritation that won.

'For pity's sake, Kate! I can't run to the phone every time something comes up! Getting an answer from that bloody switchboard at Old East takes a week and a half anyway. I can't be doing with it. And I'm telling you now, aren't I? It's all right. No need to fret over the thought of me eating skilly and sewing mailbags on Dartmoor. No case.'

'I'm delighted to hear it,' she said with a sardonic note in her voice. 'And delighted to see you so happy with the outcome. Turning cartwheels and leaping about in joy and so forth. It's a real heartwarmer.'

He was silent for a long time and somehow she managed to sit there and not attempt to prod him into speech. It wasn't easy.

'Well there – other things came up,' he said at length. 'It took away the – it just didn't seem to matter so much any more – the case, that is – '

'What came up?' She asked it as coolly as she could, knowing somewhere at a very deep level what it was.

He got up and went padding over to the door that led to the kitchen. 'I'll make you some Horlicks or something,' he said. 'A few tatty sandwiches aren't enough to see you through the night. You'll get that damned indigestion again.'

'Thank you,' she said and made no attempt to follow him, sitting there on the edge of the rumpled couch and listening to him crash cups and pans in the kitchen and feeling the dull sick feeling settle inside her belly, where it lay uneasily alongside the fatigue that still skulked there. But she said nothing, waiting as patiently as she could, and at length he came back with a mug full of Horlicks and a plate with digestive biscuits on it, and set them in front of her on the coffee table. She looked down at their homely ordinariness and tears pricked her lids and it needed a lot of control to make sure they were not shed. He could be so caring and thoughtful, so very comfortable and easy and yet at the same time put her through this hell over and over again —

She lifted her head then and said calmly, 'Well, you might as well get it over with. What else did Andrew have to say? About Sonia, I mean.'

His face went a dull mottled red and she sat and looked at him and made no attempt to go to him to touch him and hug him the way she always tried to do when things got painful for him. This time he'd have to manage on his own.

'Is it that obvious?'

'Oh, of course it is!' She made no attempt to disguise her impatience. 'I've lived with you long enough to know more about you than you can possibly imagine. And that particular look of misery is one that Sonia engineers. And that you allow her to — '

'Kate, let's not. Please,' he said and closed his eyes.

'I have to. You *let* her get to you and hurt you and it's that which makes me so — that I find so repellent. If she was just making life hell for you, I could sympathise totally, do all I could to help you cope, but it's worse than that. You collude in her ill-treatment of you. You let her hurt you. You roll over and expose your underbelly to her so that she can shove the knife in, over and over again — '

360

'Kate, I've asked you. Please don't.'

She took a deep breath and opened her mouth and then looked at him and saw the expression on his face and closed it again. What was the point? She'd said it all before, and to say it again would be like putting on an old and cracked gramophone record so that it could grind out its tedious maddening repetitions; who needed that? She didn't, he didn't – where was the sense in it? And she sat and looked at him and waited.

'It's different this time,' he said eventually, and his voice sounded different. Flatter and harsher.

'This time she's got a handful of trumps and she's willing to play every damned one of them. Whatever I do, whatever I say, she's the winner.'

'You'll have to explain,' she said and her own voice sounded flat too, with exhaustion, with disappointment, with every bad feeling she could think of.

'Andrew told me that she called him this morning. Him, not me.' He managed a sort of grin then, strained and more of a rictus than a smile but at least it was an attempt. 'I thought that would please you. Not to call me – it has to be a step in the right direction. At least, that was what I thought at first. Anyway, she phoned him at his home. He told me, after he told me about the case over the sergeant.' Now he even managed a short laugh. 'I didn't even have time to feel relieved, you know that? I've been worried sick for God knows how long and the way Andrew gave it to me, I didn't even have time to feel good about it. He said Sonia insisted on seeing him first thing this morning. She was waiting when he got to the office.'

'Well?' Once again he had lapsed into silence and she felt the anger rising in her and couldn't risk being patient.

'She – she saw last night's programme.'

Now it was her turn to laugh. 'Surprise, surprise! So did everyone else. I've heard of nothing but that damned programme most of the day. Not that it's done me any harm – the reverse, since you were kind enough to ask. Clearly it's made a big difference to all sorts of things. Life'll be a little easier at Old East for a while.'

'I know,' he said. 'I should have asked.' He came to sit down beside her and took her hand and began to play with her fingers,

361

smoothing each one in turn as though she was wearing crumpled gloves. 'I've been obsessed with my own problems and I know that. You needn't call me a selfish shit. I'm well aware of it.'

'Oh, you're not,' she said a little wearily. 'Not really, you poor devil,' and bent her head to watch his hands on hers.

'Thank you for that much. Well, the sooner I explain, I suppose, the sooner we'll – the thing is she says that she could go to court and apply to have all my access to the children stopped on the grounds I live with you. That you are morally unreliable because of your attitudes to such matters as homosexuals and transsexuals – and that makes you an unsuitable contact and influence on young children. And she says, and Andrew agrees with her, that finding a judge who'll agree won't be at all difficult – '

Kate caught her breath. 'She can't – '

'Oh, she can,' Oliver said grimly. 'She can do anything. Haven't you realised that yet?'

There was a long silence as she digested it all and then she said sharply, 'What was that you said? That she said she *could* go to court? Does that mean she isn't going to unless – what is it she wants? More money? It won't be easy, Oliver. We're tight-pressed enough as it is – '

He shook his head. 'No, not money. But you're quite right. There's a stick as well as a goad.' He smiled bleakly. 'She's got something else on offer, and whichever I take is going to be hell. And I don't think I have any other alternative. One of them I'm going to have to accept.'

'What's the other one?'

'She's met someone else.' He leaned back then, letting go of her hand and linking both of his behind his head. 'I thought that one day I'd have my prayers answered. That she'd fall for someone else and get off my back, and that somehow we'd sort it all out. I had this fantasy, you know? A decent sort of chap who'd make her happy enough to leave me in peace. Who'd make her see that sharing Melissa and Barney with me wouldn't hurt her, and would be good for the kids. Who'd maybe give her another child or two to think about. That was the daydream. And now she's gone and done it, but done it all wrong.'

'How wrong?' She knew she was walking on eggshells; inside

she was boiling with anger, with hurt, with the dog of fatigue that was now lifting its muzzle inside her and growling danger-ously. It would take so little to make her lose her temper with him, with the miserable way he looked, the obvious pain he was in. She ought to be all sympathy and patience, but it was impossible. There was a thin skin of such virtuous feelings stretched over her, but it bulged with pressure from the bad ones, and especially with her fury at the way he let it happen to him, time and time again.

'He's an American. From Dakota or somewhere. Well-off I gather – something to do with newspapers.' He tried to laugh. 'Old habits seem to die hard with her. Anyway, she wants to marry him and take the kids and go and live in Dakota.' And he pulled his hands from behind his head and set them over his face and sat there, hunched and hidden from her.

Oh, God, Kate thought, sitting staring at the cooling Horlicks in the beaker beside her, wrinkling under its thickening skin. Oh, God, I prayed for that. I thought of her going away, far away, thousands of miles away so that she'd leave him, leave us, in peace. And now, look what I've done – and as the sense of guilt added itself to the queasy mixture she was already filled with she had to bite her tongue to stop herself shouting at him.

'I'll hardly ever see them again,' Oliver said, and his voice was muffled behind his hands. 'They'll grow up and when I do manage to get over there, or persuade her and her chap whoever he is to let them come here for a visit, we'll be strangers. I can't bear it. It's like knowing they're going to die – '

She managed somehow to school her voice, but she knew when she spoke that it came out cold and hard and accusing.

'I see. So, what are you going to do? Look for a job in Dakota, I imagine?'

He took his hands away from his face and she looked at the red eyes and the smudges of tears and steeled herself not to feel pity. She couldn't. She was feeling too much already.

'Or are you going to assure her you'll get rid of me, as long as she stays here and lets you see the children whenever you want? Is that it?' She listened in a sort of vague surprise to her own voice, so icy and uncaring. 'You'll refuse to let her take the children away, which of course you have every right to do, but to make that possible and keep her away from the court, you'll get rid of me so that she can go on driving you crazy dancing at the end of her string. You'll stop her from marrying her Dakotan – which I strongly suspect you want to do anyway – and you'll keep her and the children and I can go to hell – '

'Kate, stop it.' He was white now, and she looked at him with a sort of contempt and he saw it and shrank into himself.

She stood up and pulled her jacket closer around her. 'I'm going back to the hospital,' she said. 'I'll sleep there. You have to make your own decisions, Oliver. I can't help and I can't sit here while you try to make your choice. I'll be back here tomorrow evening. By then I should know where I am, shouldn't I? One way or the other. Because you'll either be here. Or you won't.'

'Kate!' He was on his feet, following her into the hall as she scooped up her bag and keys from the chair. 'Kate, don't do this to me – I need you – '

'I'm sure you do,' she said, her hand on the front door. 'I need to be here. But we have to sort this out for good and all. Sonia has to be dealt with, and you're the only one who can do it. You have to choose, Oliver. The children or me. It's as simple as that. And though I'm sick with anger I'm sorry for you – it's a hell of a hole to be in – '

'Kate,' he said as she pulled the door open, and she looked back at him, standing there barefoot in his rumpled dressing gown, his hair tousled and his eyes red-rimmed. 'Kate, I love you.'

'I know,' she said wearily. 'I love you. That's why I have to go and leave you on your own with this. You know that, don't you? Good night, Oliver.'

And she went and got into the car and thought absurdly – I wonder why I didn't put it away tonight? I must have known –

Chapter Thirty-Seven

Six a.m.

It is dark and very cold in the courtyard and the light spills out of the Accident and Emergency department entrance to make the wreaths of steam coming from the breaths of the ambulance men look lurid and theatrical. They are manhandling the big trolley out of the ambulance, and puffing a good deal and fussing as they go, and a tall stooped man, thin and gangly inside his oversized coat, watches them with dull eyes and seems not to be breathing at all, for no clouds can be seen coming from his mouth, standing as he is outside the main beam of the light. He follows the trolley into the department and it is noticeable how the ambulance men avoid looking at him, they who are usually amiable and indeed cheerful souls, jollying along the sick and their accompanying relations like so many burly nannies. But there is no jollying for this relation; or for the patient, who is either dead or deeply comatose.

The senior man, the driver, explains in a low voice to the staff nurse on duty about the patient and his distaste for the gangly man in the large overcoat is made clear as the man himself stands drooping and silent in the middle of the waiting room, paying no attention to anyone.

'Tricky one 'ere, Staff. Sent for us, told us calm as you like 'e'd done 'er in and 'ad good reason. We called the police o' course, they're on their way, but we thought we'd better get 'ere fast, on account she was still breathing when we got to the flat. Not so sure now, mind you.'

She is still breathing, just, as the staff nurse finds when she uncovers the livid yet cadaverous face of the elderly woman on the stretcher. 'But she won't be much longer,' she adds and slides her hand under the blanket to find a pulse on a flaccid wrist.

'Said in the ambulance, he did, to my mate, "I'll tell you all about it", said as 'ow she was in such pain and begged 'im to 'elp 'er. Got cancer of the ovary, it seems. So 'e did. But when she was right down like this 'e couldn't stand it no more and wanted 'er brought in. So there you are. The police'll be 'ere I dare say, eventually – '

'I dare say,' says the staff nurse and peers more closely at the woman on the couch and adds, 'She's dead now, I think. I'll get the casualty officer to confirm – oh, dear, I hate these cases. Nasty – '

'Do you get a lot, Staff Nurse?' asks the first-year student nurse who has been helping her, lifting the patient on to the couch, getting a set of notes out and now standing waiting for instructions, and she looks at him and makes a little face.

'Enough,' she says. 'And half the time you can't blame 'em. If it was your old mum who was dying and in pain, what would you do? You wouldn't keep a dog alive the way some people have to be. You'd get taken to court for cruelty. But not when it's people – '

'But you can't have people killing their relations just like that – ' the first year, who is David Engell and has just started in Accident and Emergency, having finished his first three months on Male Medical, looks a little shocked and Staff Nurse looks at him and raises an eyebrow and says, 'Can't you? This one did – ' and pulls the sheet over the dead woman's face and goes to phone the casualty officer to get him out of bed.

There will be a good deal of discussion and trouble over this case she knows; she has had to deal with such before, and she does not relish this one. Her own grandmother has Alzheimer's disease and her mother is going through hell on a plate looking after her. There have been occasions when Staff Nurse, her dangerous-drugs keys in her hand, has thought undiscussable thoughts about what she would like to do and how easy it would be. She has not done it, of course, but who can tell what may not happen one day?

Six-fifteen a.m.

Audrey cannot be said to have woken up, because she hasn't really been asleep, or she doesn't think so. She goes to bed, of course she does; a person needs her sleep and Audrey knows she has to take care of herself. But it is not easy to lie in the big old double bed on her own, trying to pretend that Joe never slept there.

Sometimes she drifts away into a sort of not-quite-there state and hears Joe telling her sternly that of course he was there beside her, that he still is, if she'll just make the effort to turn over and look, but she is always paralysed when this happens and cannot move and she knows unless she does he will be disgusted with her and go away. And so he does, for she cannot move, ever, when it happens. And then she tries to cry when she knows she is awake but that is no help because crying just doesn't happen. It would be good if it did, but God, she has decided, is angry with her and will not let her cry.

Now she gets out of bed in the dark wet cold morning, glad to feel the pain in her joints and the stiffness in her back. It proves to her she is awake and that the night is over. All she has to do now is live another day. That's all.

Seven-thirty a.m.

The rain that started a while ago has settled in seriously now, and under the heavy indigo sky the courtyard is beginning to show blacker patches where the puddles are forming. Inside the wards the sound of the rain on the windows is agreeable, underlining the cosiness of being safely within doors, and the nurses bustle a little more noisily than they did when they started the day's washes and treatments an hour ago, not caring whether they wake the patients or not. After all it is Christmas Eve tomorrow, and the wards' decorations tinkle and whisper in the draught as the nurses bustle by: silvery strips of aluminium foil on all the lights on the Gynae ward and a tree decorated mainly with balloons which, Miss Buckland told Sister in her usual rough fashion, 'look for all the world like so many multicoloured boobs. Was that why you did it that way?'; red and green streamers all over Male Medical, and a display of tastefully painted fir cones in gold and silver in Sister Sheward's office, on top of the carefully padlocked cupboard where she keeps the whisky and sherry meant for tomorrow's jollifications (mainly with the doctors; she still has great hopes of getting somewhere with Neville Carr, in spite of his bloody wife); and in the children's wards, such a proliferation of paper chains, trees, balloons and streamers that the children lie and stare silently, overawed rather than excited.

Suba, happily washing the geriatric women in the Neurology ward annexe, is very cheerful. She had been disappointed when they sent her here from Gynae, having hoped to go to one of the children's wards, especially for Christmas, but the old ladies are as good as children, really, to look after. Helpless and smelly just as babies are, but less difficult, less likely to cry for their mummies. Though, she thinks with an indulgent smile as she scrubs old Mrs Renfrew's dentures, some of them do that, even though they are great-grandmothers themselves. And she pops the teeth back into the old lady's mouth and smiles at her as the old lady glares at her balefully. Only another hour to go and there will be breakfast, thinks Suba, and then I am off duty and Daddy'll be waiting for me.

And she thinks again about the possibility of not going home and setting out instead for the West End to look at the Christmas shops. But she knows she will not. She thinks a lot about doing what she wants rather than what Daddy wants, but it rarely goes further than just thinking, and that is all right, because isn't she here at Old East and doing what she wants in that way? Going home in all her off-duty time is a small price to pay for that amount of freedom.

Across the ward she sees Alice Abingdon sulkily dealing with her set of patients and feels a little less cheerful. Alice is not happy to be on this ward, and hates all the patients with a deep passion. She tells Suba over and over again that at this stage they ought to be put out of their misery, and when she does things for them is often rough and quick and even makes them cry sometimes. Suba had thought once about talking to someone about it, because she is so worried about the old ladies, but she only thought it, and then only once. Never again will Suba ever tell anyone anything about things she sees if she can help it, however much it might worry her and however wrong it might seem. It is the most important lesson she has learned since she came to Old East to train as a nurse. Do your own job and never mind what everyone else is doing.

Nine-thirty a.m.

Kate is throwing up in the small sluice at the top end of the Genito-Urinary ward and doesn't mind a bit. It has been happening now for over a week and she has said nothing to anyone, not even Oliver, but he is no fool, she tells herself as she catches her breath and lifts her head slowly and carefully, not certain that the spasm of nausea has completely passed. He must have noticed the fact that her periods are haywire, but he has said nothing; and she knows why he has not. Like me, she thinks, and washes her face and powders it to cover the shadows under her eyes, like me, he wants to be sure, wants to make the delicious uncertainty last, wants to relish every moment of it.

And she draws a deep breath and tries not to think of how Oliver will be tomorrow which is not only Christmas Eve but also Melissa's birthday. He sent her the most ridiculous pile of gifts weeks ago, and tomorrow, she knows, will slip away to the studios to phone her. He is very punctilious about never phoning Dakota on the phone at home, as though doing so would somehow pollute their life there in Finchley Road, and that worries Kate.

If he had really made up his mind completely, she thinks, had really meant what he had said that evening when she had come home and he had been sitting there waiting for her, his mind made up, he had assured her, would he be so very scrupulous about the way he uses the phone? Kate thinks not; and tries not to think about the implications of that thought. Instead she pats her belly, childishly pleased with herself that they have managed to make their plan to underline their commitment to each other so successful so soon, and goes down the ward to see her dialysis patients.

It is going to be a difficult day. There are seven patients needing dialysis, and only three machines available. Four must be sent home in the hope they will not go into irreversible uraemia. Not very agreeable at Christmas, thinks Kate, and picks up her charts ready to start her ward round with the new sister in charge, Daphne Royden. She is young and ambitious and not nearly so efficient as Esther would have been, and certainly not so much fun, but she does well enough. And Kate smiles at her and leads the way down the ward, wondering whether she will be sick again. It is very agreeable to be in the state she is in, of course, but it has its drawbacks.

Ten a.m.

Ted Scribner moves gingerly in his bed and then sighs in relief. It is dry, after all, and he feels a great rush of gratitude for that. He had fallen asleep after having his breakfast instead of going to the lavatory the way the nurses had said he must. Go regular, that was the thing, to get himself trained again, and he had meant to. But the porridge had been good and lots of it, and it was no wonder he fell asleep. He ate better here at Old East than he ever did at home, no error, and he thinks a little wistfully of how nice it would be to stay here over the next few days.

It is going to be good here for Christmas, he knows that; he has seen the tree all loaded with parcels for the patients – nice of them to do that, he thinks, real nice – and he's heard about how the turkey is carved by Mr Le Queux, making lots of jokes all the while about how much nicer it is than carving people's kidneys, and how there are drinks all round on the house.

But there it is, they said he could go home today and thought he'd be glad of the opportunity and he hadn't liked to say he'd rather stay where he was. After all, he'd waited long enough to get in here, hadn't he? And only had his operation less than a week ago? But he is doing fine they say, so he has to go and anyway, the next-doors might be fed up with the cat, so he'd better get back to her.

And he swings his scrawny legs carefully over the side of the bed and puts on his dressing gown – and he wishes he could take that home too, instead of leaving it behind as hospital property – and goes to the lavatory. It is easier now, nothing like as bad as it was, and he should be grateful. And he is grateful, really. He just wishes he could stay here in the warm with all the good food just a little bit longer. His pension doesn't go far these days and specially not at Christmas.

Ten-thirty a.m.

The meeting in the nurses' home sitting room is not very well attended and Sian sits and glowers sulkily at the few people who are there. Just the usual ones; how can they ever get anywhere if they have just the usual ones? And she says as much and the others stare at her and shrug and say nothing useful and she launches into one of what the others call her tirades. She knows they are bored but she can't help it.

'Why are they so stupid?' she cries. 'Are they waiting till a nurse dies here? It's been weeks since it happened to that enrolled chap in that mental handicap hospital. If we don't make sure they arrange for us all to be vaccinated here, then it could happen to us.'

'They've offered people here hepatitis B vaccine ever so often.' One of the night nurses who is only present because she came off duty exhausted and stopped in the sitting room to sit down by the radiator to get warm, and now can't be bothered to get to her feet and go to bed, speaks up. 'But no one took it up. Not even the ones in the path lab and they're handling blood all the time.'

'And no one here's likely to get bitten like that other fella did. We don't have any mentally handicapped here, do we?' says Peter Burnett. He is only in the sitting room to wait for David Engell because they both have a day off and are planning to go to the West End together and have a bit of fun. 'I'm buggered if I'd go on strike for anything so daft.'

'It's not daft,' retorts Sian. 'Not if you could die for want of it. And as for being buggered – you should be so lucky,' and Peter shouts back at her and for a little while it seems there will be a real fight, and the others watch, interested. It is better than watching television which is only Schools and a lot of women talking at this time of the morning.

But then David arrives and Peter goes off jeering at Sian and the meeting goes on, and when they get to the vote on the motion which is 'It is determined all the nurses at Old East should strike in sympathy with the St Kitts' demo and that all nurses should be vaccinated against hepatitis B', the vote is so small there is no hope of getting a strike going, and Sian marches out in a temper.

She works so hard to organise the nurses and they are all so wet, they don't know the price of bloody eggs and care less.

And she goes to bed, because she too is on night duty now, in the children's ward, and tomorrow will be a busy day, and sleeps badly because she is so angry. And not only with the apathetic apolitical nurses of Old East. Although she wouldn't admit it for the world, it hurts that Jimmy Rhoda never phones any more. But there, Old East stopped being in the news weeks ago, and she knows now that was the real reason he used to take her out. Thank God for politics, she thinks as she throws herself over in bed again. It may be tough to get anywhere, but at least it's more honest than bloody sex.

Eleven a.m.

Professor Levy pushes his chair back from his office desk and looks gloomily at the two men sitting on the other side of it.

'You realise,' he says, 'that this will not be done smoothly or easily? There will be considerable opposition.'

'There always is opposition to change,' one of them says. 'It is in the nature of mankind to resist it.'

'No doubt,' says Professor Levy a little dryly. 'But I was thinking less of basic philosophical concepts and more of local feeling about this hospital. There is a well-organised lobby to protect Old East, you know. The woman who leads it has a considerable flair for this sort of politicking. You'll find to your cost that any attempt to go back on the DHSS's word at this stage will cause an almighty uproar. We were assured we were safe till the next financial year. Mr Saffron said – '

'Ah yes, Mr Saffron,' the man interrupts smoothly. 'But he is no longer Minister, you see. Sad about him, wasn't it? But there you are – and the new Minister is really quite adamant. He has listened with great sympathy to the representations made to him, but he is certain that Old East, like many other similar establishments, must lose some of its fat and become one of the newer more sinewy hospitals of the nineties – Either that or we close down and sell the site.'

'Lose fat?' explodes Professor Levy. 'What fat? This place has as much spare on it as a ballet dancer with anorexia. We're

372

running on a shoestring as it is. We do miracles here on the budget you give us, do you know that? If I could persuade you to do some of the cutting we can't, at admin level, now *that* might get us somewhere. But as it is – '

'Well, there it is, Professor.' The man zips his briefcase and gets to his feet, smiling, and his silent companion copies him. 'I'm afraid there is little more we can do to help. I'm glad we were able to have this little discussion. It does clear the air, doesn't it? I see your hospital tree is up – beautifully dressed and lit, isn't it? Yes – '

Professor Levy is also on his feet and comes to join them at the window. 'It was both provided and dressed as a gift from the local Chamber of Commerce,' he said dryly. 'I can let you see the correspondence if you wish. We paid for nothing, not even the electricity for the fairy lights. It's connected to one of the shops outside the gates. You can see there, the cable is carried over the archway. There – '

'My dear chap, you really mustn't think we're Scrooges, you know!' The Ministry man smiles at him with crinkle-eyed *bonhomie*. 'I was just admiring your tree, no more! Well, goodbye, Professor. Merry Christmas!'

After they have gone Professor Levy stands staring out at the tree for a little while, and then goes to his desk to pick up the phone. He has just time to deal with this before he goes to the medical students' last lecture round before the festivities overtake them all.

'Mrs Blundell?' he says into the phone at length. 'Ah, how are you? I just thought I'd call with the greetings of the season – '

Eleven-thirty a.m.

Fay Buckland's antenatal clinic is nearly finished. There are just four more patients to see, but since between them they have eleven children the waiting room is noisy and hectic as the children roll around the floor and fight with each other and make a great deal of noise. Fay Buckland, although she can hear the noise, will not be hurried, however; the woman she is examining has a difficult breech presentation and she is seizing the opportunity to show her students how to make an attempt at manual version.

The third-year nurse running the clinic because Sister is busy elsewhere is irritated and restless because she has a great deal to do to get the big waiting area ready for the outpatient children's Christmas party this afternoon, and she can't get going with those spoiled noisy brats all over the place. So when one of the patients comes and tells her truculently that her appointment was for ten-thirty and she's damned if she's going to wait another minute, and even though the woman looks pasty and tired and has somewhat swollen ankles she does not remonstrate with her and try to make sure she stays as Sister would have done. But then the third-year nurse has not done her midder training yet, nor even worked on a midder ward, so she does not notice this and is quite happy to get the woman to go and take her two children with her, especially as one of them, a little boy, is the noisiest and bounciest of them all.

So Prue goes, pushing the baby's pram and dragging Danny along with it, miserably aware of her aching head and her dreadful tiredness. She hasn't seen the doctor for ages and she ought to have seen her today but how could she sit there any longer? They had no notion of what it was like to have two screaming kids and another on the way and no husband here to help, because he wasn't supposed to get to England till the end of January, bloody Gary; and she feels the tears, the all-too-frequent tears, slide down her nose again as she sets out on the long walk back to the messiness of Lansbury House and another long and miserable day at home with the kids. And tomorrow bloody Christmas Eve too. And she thinks about Ida Malone as she trudges on her way and wishes she hadn't moved away the way she had. She'd been horrible, but all the same, it had been someone who looked after her, hadn't it? And there wasn't anyone else around to do it.

One p.m.

Mr Holliday has been watching TV all morning. There has been nothing on, just a lot of talking people and stuff for schools, but it is better than nothing, and now the programme is changing maybe it will be better. The news. That wasn't better. But maybe, after the news? She'd be back from the shops soon and then it'd be the end of watching anything. She'd talk and jabber at him and he'd not be able to hear a word from the screen. It is funny, thinks Mr Holliday, how the best programmes are always on when there are other people around to spoil them, but there's never anything worth seeing when you are on your own and really have the chance to concentrate.

There is something then on the news that is worth concentrating on; another bit of news about brain operations. A doctor somewhere is doing them for epilepsy now, using the same sort of baby cells, and Mr Holliday listens, staring hard at the screen, slumped in the chair with his hands twitching as usual on his lap and his useless legs swathed in a rug and thinks – Did anyone listen to them when they asked about it? Were they the sort that got to know what it was all about? It must be easier to be epileptic, he thinks. At least you can make them listen to you, make them understand what worries you. They never listen to me.

Three-thirty p.m.

Kim Hynes is the last appointment on Dr Rosen's clinic list, and she is there well on time. When she walks into the consulting room she sets a cake box in front of Dr Rosen and says, 'I made it for you. Myself. It's a very good recipe – high fibre, low fat, everything just as it should be. I hope you like fruit cakes.' She giggles then. 'What a thing to say to a shrink! Fruit cakes – of course you like them. Well, how could you manage if you didn't?'

Dr Rosen smiles, and looks at the cake and says gravely, 'It looks delicious. I shall take it home and have it tonight. My daughter will help me eat it. How are you, Kim? You look well enough – '

'Really? You like the new-look Kim? Are you sure?'

She does indeed, thinks Dr Rosen, look new. The rich tumble of curls has become a sleek French pleat, pinned high on her head. The make-up, though still obvious, is less heavy and the clothes are a little less outrageous. Still very soft and frilly, but lacking the extravagances that had once been so much part of the

Hynes Effect, as Dr Rosen had described it in the notes of this most interesting case.

'I'm sure,' she says at length. 'Does it mean anything more than a look, though? Or are you new in any other way?'

Kim nods, very satisfied. 'Oh, yes. It's – I can't say how wonderful it all is. I nearly went all wrong, you know. After the operation – losing my job and all, it made me act – well, I'm really embarrassed now when I think of it.' She giggles, bright-eyed and not really ashamed at all. 'Very naughty I was there for a while. Films, a bit of tarting – the lot. But it's not for me, not even for the money. I'm a nice girl inside. You know that, don't you, Dr Rosen?'

Dr Rosen smiles and says quietly, 'Yes, Kim. I know. A very nice girl.'

'But not everyone does. So I thought – I'd better make sure I look the part, eh? It used to be I just wanted to look like a woman, so I suppose – I went a bit OTT, you know? But now, as I am a woman, aren't I? A real woman – the operation's only a bit of it – the drugs and all – anyway, now, I thought, I don't have to look like I did. Now I can be more like me. The real woman. The elegant sort – yes?'

'Yes,' says Dr Rosen. And doesn't look at the very red nail varnish and the little gold chain Kim has round one ankle, the one she has crossed over so far that most of her thigh shows under her sleek skirt.

'I'm still trying to get the business going,' Kim says. 'The bank's being – well, forget it. But I've met this lovely man, very high class, you know, a businessman and he's advising me.' She flashes her brilliant smile at Dr Rosen and then says, 'Now, do tell me. When do you think we can persuade Miss Sayers to do the next bit? It's not that I've got to have a proper you-know-what – I mean I've proved you can get away with murder and the poor devils don't know what's there and what isn't, you know what I mean? But I'd feel, you know, better. I know I'm a real woman now, but that would make all the difference – '

Five-fifteen p.m.

There are three women in labour in the maternity unit and Fay Buckland gets there just in time to deal with the most worrying of them. She is almost forty and has been under the care only of a midwife, refusing any sort of doctors or hospital intervention at all. But after being in labour for almost a day and a half the midwife has become very anxious and has insisted on transferring her to Old East. Now Fay has to see why the delay and see what she can do to help, for the baby's heartbeat is very poor and the foetal monitors show it is fading rapidly.

It is difficult to do a Caesar so far on in labour, Fay tells her students, but what else can she do? And when afterwards she and Sister stand and look down at the gasping pallid baby with the massive meningocele sprouting from its back like a great obscene piece of leftover meat, they say little to each other. They watch and hope the baby will stop breathing of its own accord. But it is a tough baby for all its dreadful defect and slowly loses its poor colour and begins to breathe more easily. And Sister wraps it and puts in in its special cot and says to Fay Buckland, 'Well?'

And Fay Buckland shrugs and shakes her head. 'Sad,' she says briefly. And goes away and Sister stands there and tries to think what they will say to the mother when she comes round from her anaesthetic.

And what will they do about the baby? Because a meningocele, which would have been detected early enough for her to have had a termination if only she'd been having proper care, she tells herself, a meningocele baby has a hell of a life to look forward to.

If we let it look forward, that is.

Seven-thirty p.m.

The annual hospital Christmas show is in progress. The medical students, the third-year nurses, most of the physios and the occupational health students have put it on and it is very funny and very noisy.

There are rude sketches about the senior medical staff, all very insulting, and even more rude sketches about the sisters. There is dancing more energetic than elegant, and there is singing and a lot of noisy stamping from the audience who are watching with a great deal of glee and not a little scorn, especially those who wanted to be in the cast but were turned down by the committee who organised it. They are the ones who shout and jeer the loudest. But the patients who have been brought over to the big lecture room in wheelchairs and allowed to come hobbling over on foot are liking it well enough, because it is, after all, Christmas and these young doctors and nurses, well, they work so hard, don't they? So good and caring and so, well, *good*.

It must be nice, thinks the girl in the third row who has been having treatment for a twisted spine and who is still wearing a big plaster jacket designed to give her back a chance to grow straight, it must be nice to be one of them. All these good-looking young men and the nurses, ever so pretty some of them in their uniforms. Not the fat ones whose uniforms don't fit, or the lanky ones who look so droopy, but the pretty ones, it must be nice to be them. And she imagines being one of them one day, and how nice it will be. Nothing to worry about but helping people be comfortable and everyone thinking you are marvellous.

It would be nice to be a nurse, she decides. And one day I will be. Nothing to worry about, just being nice to people. Lovely.